Information Systems and Healthcare Enterprises

Roy Rada
University of Maryland, Baltimore County, USA

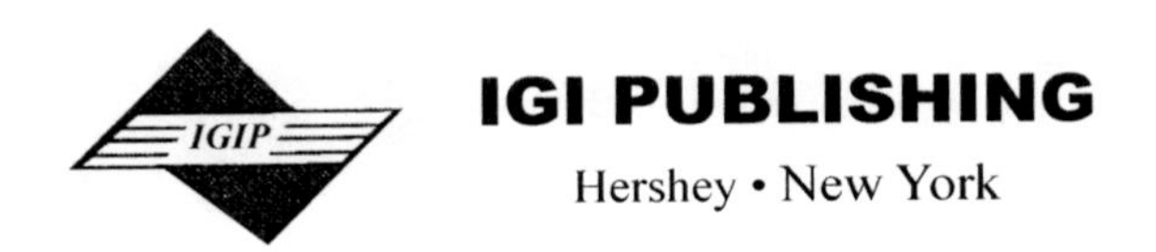

Acquisition Editor:	Kristin Klinger
Senior Managing Editor:	Jennifer Neidig
Managing Editor:	Sara Reed
Development Editor:	Kristin Roth
Copy Editor:	Alana Bubnis
Typesetter:	Elizabeth C. Duke
Cover Design:	Lisa Tosheff
Printed at:	Yurchak Printing Inc.

Published in the United States of America by
IGI Publishing (an imprint of IGI Global)
701 E. Chocolate Avenue
Hershey PA 17033
Tel: 717-533-8845
Fax: 717-533-8661
E-mail: cust@igi-pub.com
Web site: http://www.igi-pub.com

and in the United Kingdom by
IGI Publishing (an imprint of IGI Global)
3 Henrietta Street
Covent Garden
London WC2E 8LU
Tel: 44 20 7240 0856
Fax: 44 20 7379 0609
Web site: http://www.eurospanonline.com

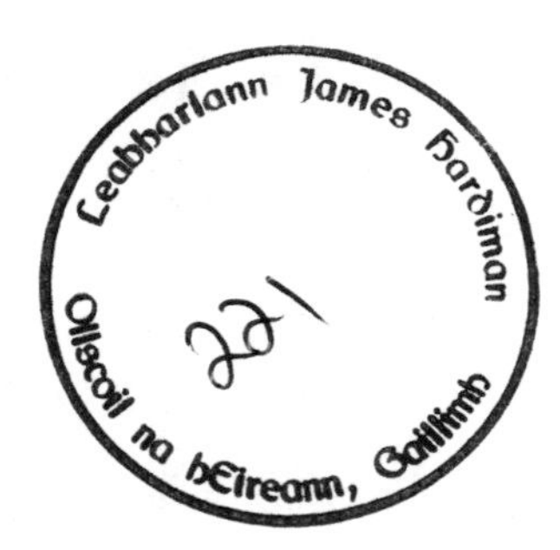

Library of Congress Cataloging-in-Publication Data

Rada, R. (Roy), 1951-
Information systems and healthcare enterprises / Roy Rada.
p. ; cm.
Includes bibliographical references and index.
Summary: "The United States' healthcare industry consumes roughly 20% of the gross national product per year. This huge expenditure not only represents a large portion of the country's collective interests, but also an enormous amount of medical information. This book examines the special issues related to the collection, disbursement, and integration of various data within the healthcare system."--Provided by publisher.
ISBN 978-1-59904-651-8 (hardcover)
1. Medicine--United States--Data processing. 2. Medical care--United States--Data processing. 3. Information storage and retrieval systems--Medicine--United States. I. Title.
[DNLM: 1. Information Systems--United States. 2. Delivery of Health Care--United States. 3. Health Care Sector--United States. 4. Information Storage and Retrieval--United States. W 26.55.I4 R124i 2008]
R858.R33 2008
610.285--dc22

2007007280

British Cataloguing in Publication Data
A Cataloguing in Publication record for this book is available from the British Library.

Information Systems and Healthcare Enterprises

Table of Contents

Foreword

In 2006, healthcare information systems expenditures in the U.S. are estimated to be $31 billion. Hospitals make up the largest portion of these expenditures. Hospital information systems typically represent 2-5% of a hospital's operating budget. Frequently, it is the largest item in the hospital's capital budget. Many claim hospitals and other healthcare organizations are not spending enough on information systems, and that the benefits of past and current expenditures are not fully realized.

I have had the good fortune of observing and participating in much of the history of hospital-centric healthcare information systems. This has been as a student, college professor, consultant, entrepreneur, and company executive.

Most early efforts to automate financial and clinical processes were made in teaching hospital environments and frequently funded by research grants from government and private sources. Early on, computer hardware companies (e.g., IBM, Honeywell) invested in hospital software development hoping to stimulate computer hardware sales in the emerging hospital information systems market. There were also some early innovators funded by venture capital. The first widely accepted healthcare software applications were produced by these commercial efforts. However, in-house software development was widespread.

In the late 1960s, several commercial organizations adopted a business model, called shared services, which involved having the principal hardware required for information processing located at a single location and linking hospitals and other healthcare organizations to this central facility using satellite data transmission (e.g., Shared Medical Systems, now a subsidiary of Siemens). These companies used a standard software offering. Shared services provided an alternative strategy for hospitals and other healthcare organizations to automate their information systems. This alternative grew rapidly and accelerated adoption of information technology in financial and selected clinical areas.

Today, most hospital applications software is supplied by third party vendors. There continue to be a limited number of hospitals that are maintaining their self-developed core applications. Current offerings provide the opportunity for computerization of most hospital departments, support of many clinical processes and computerization of physician offices and other non-hospital healthcare activities. Hospital utilization of these offerings varies from limited to extensive; and operating costs are too high for the benefit gained.

Recently, there has been a renewed interest in hospital IT outsourcing, which involves taking a specific function within the IT department and contracting with a third party to perform that function. Many healthcare organizations have contracted with a third party to perform all functions of their IT department. Offshore outsourcing involves performing one or more functions of the IT department overseas. India, China and the Philippines are among many countries in which offshore companies offer these services. Since healthcare information systems are largely dependent on third party software, many of the cost-benefit advantages of offshore outsourcing are not available to healthcare organizations.

Currently, there is considerable discussion about making a patient's health record available appropriately anywhere in the nation. The federal government's proposed architecture for achieving this national health information network is through creation of regional health information systems that eventually will be linked into a national health information system. At this time, there are a limited number of regional demonstration projects underway. The ultimate cost to achieve a national health information network is very high and the source of funding has not been identified.

In this book, Roy Rada discusses these developments and issues plus many others. He has documented the conceptual foundation of healthcare information systems, its history and current status. This is a definitive work and our industry has needed it for some time.

Ronald L. Gue, PhD
Chairman, Board of Directors
Phoenix Health Systems, Inc.
Gaithersburg, Maryland

Ron Gue was the founder of Phoenix Health Systems. He has a BES and a PhD from the Johns Hopkins University. He began his career as a college professor at the University of Florida and Southern Methodist University. In addition to Phoenix, Gue has been the CEO of two other hospital information technology companies. He also has been a healthcare IT consulting practice leader for a small Chicago firm and for a Big 8 accounting firm. He has been a consultant for numerous private and governmental healthcare organizations in the U.S., Asia, the Middle East and Europe. He is the author of one textbook and many articles published in refereed professional journals.

Preface

The healthcare industry touches everyone, and is information intensive. Information systems have spread slowly from the billing room to the examination room. Successful *information systems applications* must be managed by people knowledgeable in the issues relevant to both healthcare and information systems. This book examines those special issues.

This book is an introduction to healthcare information systems for people with some background in *healthcare* and *information systems*. While no particular knowledge of the reader is expected, the book does not comprehensively define the basic concepts of either healthcare or information systems. Instead, the reader can expect to become immersed quickly into the challenging issues of getting information systems to work in healthcare organizations.

Many books have been written about health information systems, usually with a distinct *audience* for each book. For instance, one can find books for:

- Physicians with practical tips on how to use computers in the private office
- Nursing students on record keeping

This book is for students of information systems and of healthcare administration and for professionals responsible for decisions about information systems in healthcare enterprises. Feedback from information systems students has been encouraging. For instance, one student said: "gave new insight to another industry. The subject matter is important—patients, providers, payers, policies—and sparked an interest in a career path that I had not considered."

The healthcare industry varies across *countries*, as explained in the penultimate chapter of this book. That chapter goes into detail about aspects of healthcare information systems in different countries. Government regulation and financing of healthcare affect the evolution of healthcare information systems in a country. For a reader to get a deep understanding of the practical issues facing practitioners in the healthcare information systems industry, a detailed look at one country's experience is worthwhile. This book thus goes into detail about the finances, government regulations, and major entities that are relevant to healthcare information systems in the United States.

The book has *14 chapters* in a logical sequence. The Introduction defines the field and examines its trends and challenges. The software life cycle is introduced in the second chapter. Providers and payers are two key components within the healthcare industry. How providers and payers work and use information systems is elaborated in Chapters III and IV. The standards and codes that are crucial in the communication among providers and payers are introduced in Chapter V. A provider sends a claim to a payer who examines the claim and makes the appropriate payment, and these transactions are analyzed in Chapter VI. The connection between providers and payers is one part of the network that is crucial to a modern healthcare industry. Healthcare information networks are addressed in Chapter VII. Healthcare is one of the most heavily regulated industries, and the nature of that regulation is addressed in Chapter VIII. Two prominent examples of government regulation of information systems in U.S. healthcare concern the privacy and security rules, and their requirements and how to comply with them are detailed in Chapters IX and X. The people who work in healthcare systems and the vendors that serve them are addressed in Chapters XI and XII. The advances in healthcare information systems are many, but the difficulty of diffusing innovations in healthcare are addressed in Chapter XIII. The final chapter summarizes and concludes.

The reader is asked to address the issues that should lead to the *ability* to do the following as it regards health information systems:

1. Identify needs for development of health information systems
2. Manage a design team
3. Delineate the typical components of a health information system and how they are integrated in new systems spanning diverse organizations
4. Identify the people who create and use information systems
5. Anticipate the factors that determine whether or not a system will be adopted by its users and thus diffuse through the target population

This sequence corresponds broadly with the life cycle of an information system.

The first chapter defines the field of health information systems by comparing and contrasting it with the field of management information systems. The *history* of computerized health information systems is relived through the eyes of those who created the history and demonstrates that many key issues have remained largely the same across time. New technologies of care are in abundance but the ability to cope with them cost-effectively is in short supply. This leads also to problems of data quality and coordination. In other words:

- New technologies demand new skills, but
- If new skills are in short supply, then new technologies may be incorrectly used.

The need for information systems in healthcare is predicated on the trends in the healthcare industry, trends in information systems, and the specific strategies of any given healthcare organization. Those trends are outlined along with the typical expectations that those trends imply for health information systems.

The *Software Life Cycle* chapter looks at the life cycle of information systems and focuses on the requirements and design phases. The importance of involving users in the design of a system is highlighted. Cooperative design requires methods and tools to make it easy for the users to understand the issues faced by the technical designers. To this end, simple diagrams that demonstrate the flow of information among people may help.

While the healthcare providers are much larger in number than the payers and catch more of the public eye, the payers play a crucial role that is underappreciated. The *Providers* and *Payers* chapters emphasize the information systems' aspects of those industries. For providers, the key components are administrative systems, patient management, and clinical support. For payers, the components must support the enrollment of members and the adjudication of claims. The biggest budget in healthcare has been for hospitals, but doctors' offices have unique and important information systems needs too. On the health plan side, case studies are offered of the "Centers for Medicare and Medicaid Services" and of "Blue Cross and Blue Shield" to illustrate the significant differences between the mandatory government plan and the private-sector plan.

The chapter *Data and Knowledge* looks at the range of knowledge representations that are important in healthcare and gives examples of each. It begins with types of data and moves to standardization because communication with information systems depends on standardized languages and protocols. The chapter describes a range of standardized knowledge representations from simple codes to complex rule bases. Decision-making is carefully considered with two detailed examples: one for utility theory and the other for rule-based expert systems. Systems to support research, such as the online library of the National Library of Medicine, are also described.

The interactions between the provider and payer have historically imposed a large overhead cost on the delivery of care. The government has intervened and mandated a standard format in *provider-payer transactions*. Technical details of the format for certain transactions, such as an eligibility inquiry, are presented. Given the intricacy of the transactions and their complex relationships to financial exchange, careful testing of the software implementation of the provider-payer transactions is done. One problem with the human use of the provider-payer transactions is the temptation for providers to submit claims that overstate their case. Fraud occurs when claims are submitted for work that was not done. What kind of fraud occurs and how payers and government combat it with software is also addressed in the chapter on provider-payer transactions.

The connection of components of the healthcare system is a major step in improvement of the healthcare system. Through networking, different entities can better coordinate their efforts. The chapter on *information networks* examines some of the human, organizational aspects of networking and begins with e-commerce networks, goes to supply chain management, and then goes to community and consumer networks. Consumerism is one way that patients can improve the efficacy of the healthcare system by becoming proactive. Many governments are encouraging national health information networks.

The healthcare industry is one of the most heavily regulated industries. The chapter on *regulation* describes the history of government regulation in the U.S. Healthcare regulations cover access to, cost of, and quality of care. The approaches to compliance by healthcare entities are described.

The Administrative Simplification provisions of the *Health Insurance Portability and Accountability Act* require not only standardization of provider-payer transactions but also privacy and security of protected health information. Two chapters in this book examine first privacy and then security in the healthcare industry. While privacy and security are tangential to the core function of the healthcare industry, they are two of the hottest topics for healthcare information systems in the early 21st century. Both chapters provide all the important aspects of what the government regulations require for privacy and security. They also provide case studies of how entities have chosen to comply with the regulations. Through the course of these descriptions the reader is also exposed to some of the tantalizing philosophical, political, and social challenges associated with the very complex issues of privacy and security.

Students of healthcare information systems are particularly concerned about the career options that face them. The chapter entitled *Personnel* looks at the patterns of employment in healthcare and particularly in healthcare information technology jobs. The structure of information technology organizations in healthcare entities is described. Salaries of employees at different ranks and with varying responsibilities are also explored.

Many healthcare entities rely extensively on vendors and consultants to support their information technology needs. The chapter entitled *Vendors* examines life for vendors and consultants in the healthcare industry. That chapter also provides a case study of Cerner Corporation, a major vendor of hospital information systems.

Diffusing a healthcare information system requires overcoming many barriers. The conditions under which a healthcare information system is successfully adopted by its intended target audience are explored in Chapter XIII. Generic strategies for achieving diffusion are balanced with case studies.

Many books on healthcare information systems take the perspective of a particular healthcare professional, such as a nurse or a doctor. This book emphasizes the information systems student *perspective*. Many books for university courses on the topic have a decidedly academic feel with an emphasis on topics related to research, such as artificial intelligence or ethics. However, this book includes a practitioner's view. The book also gives special emphasis to the impact of the regulations deriving from the Administrative Simplification provisions of HIPAA, given the relative novelty of that topic and thus its relative under-representation in existing books. While many books examine the staff involved in healthcare information systems, few consider the role of information technology vendors and consultants, as this book does. While the focus is on provider organizations, particularly hospitals, fair attention is given to health insurance companies.

The book is used in *teaching* university students. Each chapter begins with a list of learning objectives. Every chapter ends with questions that test what a reader has understood or invites readers to do projects (called the "reading" and "doing" questions, respectively). Multiple-choice quiz questions for each chapter are available from the author in plain-text format or with standard XML quiz markup.

Health information systems have been relatively under-developed compared to the information systems in other industries, such as the financial, manufacturing, retail, and publishing industries. The reasons for this under-development are presented along with the steps to change the situation. The investment in health information systems is growing, and the principles and examples given in this book can help the reader take advantage of this growth and *contribute* to it.

Acknowledgment

The author could not have written this book without the support of many people. First, he would like to thank his classes in health care informatics at the University of Maryland, Baltimore County who have been using versions of this book for six years. The book was published by Hypermedia Solutions Limited in three earlier editions, beginning in 2001 as *Information Systems for Health Care Enterprises* and followed in 2003 by the 2nd edition and in 2005 by the 3rd edition. The students have not only provided useful feedback, but the motivation to provide worthwhile material to them has been the reason that this book was written. The author is also very grateful to the support of IGI Global, for working with him for the updates and refinements to create this 4th edition called *Information Systems and Health Care Enterprises*.

The Johns Hopkins Healthcare Informatics seminars and the University of Maryland Baltimore Nursing Informatics seminars have been a source of valuable information. Dr. Scott Finley, Director of Oncology Clinical Information Systems at Hopkins Medical System, helped this author become intimate with the challenges facing a large institution that tries to integrate its oncology information systems needs with the needs of other departments in the institution. Collaboration with the Healthcare Information and Management Systems Society through the author's leadership of its HIPAA Special Interest Group was part of an opportunity to get closer to the diversity of concerns in the practicing healthcare informatics community. Phoenix Health Systems is an outsourcing and consulting company with which the author has had an opportunity to collaborate, particularly through D'Arcy Gue, in developing plans for small group practices to deal with modern regulatory requirements, and the impressive practices of that company have inspired the desire to pay attention to the day-to-day information systems concerns of small health care entities. Working with Mel York of the Department of Public Health in Washington, DC, on regulatory compliance provided a view from the other side.

The Department of Computer Science at Wayne State University gave this author his first opportunity to create and teach an undergraduate, full-semester medical informatics course in 1981. Collaboration with Dr. Laurens Ackerman at Henry Ford Hospital and Dr. George Kaldor at the local Veterans Administration Hospital helped the author provide concrete examples to students of applications of information systems in hospitals.

The author was first introduced to medical informatics by Dr. Alan Levy at Baylor College of Medicine while the author was a medical student. Dr. Levy moved to the University of Illinois and recruited this author to become a National Library of Medicine postdoctoral fellow at the University of Illinois. Subsequently, the author became a senior administrator and researcher at the National Library of Medicine. Reporting to Dr. Donald Lindberg was an opportunity to see one of the fathers of medical informatics in action.

The author is indebted to his family. His loving parents were themselves healthcare professionals and wanted their son to contribute to healthcare. Finally, the author's wife has provided, through her endless goodwill and her support for their children, an environment conducive to writing.

Chapter I

Introduction

Learning Objectives

- Distinguish health information systems from management information systems
- Describe the history of information systems in healthcare
- Identify the diverse books that address healthcare information systems based on audience
- Analyze the challenges facing the healthcare industry as regards rising costs, medical errors, coordination, and professional organizations
- Relate the trends in healthcare to the trends in information technology

Healthcare is one of the greatest single *cost* items for citizens in many developed countries. Information is fundamental to healthcare. Yet information systems to support health are underdeveloped.

What It Is

The discipline of *health information systems* (HIS) involves a synergy of three other disciplines (Tan, 2005), namely, health, organization management, and information management:

- Health is the end-purpose of HIS applications. The ultimate goal in applying HIS solutions is to improve the health status of people.
- Organization management provides the managerial perspective on developing and using HIS applications for health service organizations.
- Information management is how the information is used. To achieve their goals, health managers must rely on health information.

HIS is based partly on the application of *management information systems* (MIS) concepts to health. One difference between HIS and MIS is that HIS objects are more specialized though derived substantially from MIS (see *Table 1.1*). Of course, a healthcare organization has to deal with general problems, like resource management, and in another perspective the discipline of HIS contains the discipline of MIS.

Lindberg (1979) created an analytical framework for comparing HISs. His taxonomy included seven dimensions. For each dimension, values that might identify the position in the dimension of a particular HIS are indicated here:

1. **Patient population:** Healthy patients vs. ill patients; acutely ill vs. chronically ill; general population vs. special population
2. **Organizational setting:** Office vs. institution; individual vs. group practice; public vs. private; screening clinic vs. general clinic; general hospital vs. specialist hospital
3. **Medical service area:** Admissions office; ambulatory care facility; clinical laboratory; dietetics department; intensive care unit; mental health center; operating room; pharmacy; radiology department

Table 1.1. HIS vs. MIS (Adapted from Tan, 2001)

Characteristics	HIS	MIS
object of cognition	clinical and health management decision making	general management decision making
object of systems	health delivery systems, patient populations, health providers, third parties	organizational systems, consumer populations, business professionals, corporations
subspecialties	medical informatics, dental informatics, nursing informatics, pharmacy informatics	management technology, data processing, office automation, tele-communications
reference disciplines	MIS, health sciences, information science	behavioral science, computer science, management science, information economics

4. **Data elements collected:** Patient identification; health provider location; demographic information; past hospitalizations; diagnosis; time qualifiers; billing information; patient complaints; laboratory results; healthcare professional interpretations
5. **Functions performed:** Retrieval of patient records; patient monitoring; fiscal controls; differential diagnosis; therapy recommendations
6. **Uses of output:** Immediate healthcare team; consultant; researcher; administrator
7. **Financial basis:** Patient fee-for-service with individual insurance coverage; patient prepays; insurance carrier; federal government intermediary; state or municipality

One may define a HIS by selecting one or more values from each of the seven dimensions. Along these dimensions one famous HIS, called *HELP*, had these attributes in 1979 at University of Utah, Salt Lake City (Warner, 1979):

1. **Patient population:** Acutely ill
2. **Healthcare setting:** Institution; individual and group practice; private and public; general hospital
3. **Medical service area:** Admissions office; clinical laboratory; surgical recovery room; intensive care unit
4. **Data elements collected:** Patient identification; hospital location; demographic information; past hospitalizations; diagnosis; time qualifiers; billing information; patient complaints; laboratory results; health care professional interpretations
5. **Functions performed:** Retrieval of patient records; patient monitoring; differential diagnosis; therapy recommendations
6. **Uses of the output:** Immediate healthcare team; consultant; researcher
7. **Financial basis:** Patient fee-for-service with individual insurance coverage; federal government intermediary

HELP included an integrated patient record system with input from more than 100 ports in the hospital. The data content included demographic admitting data, diagnoses, screening data such as EKGs, history, test values from other cardiology tests, pathology laboratory results, and more. The system monitored the patient physiological signs when in intensive care and was capable of generating alerts for problem situations.

Technology History

Understanding the healthcare industry in the United States is vital to understanding how information systems serve that industry. The role of technology in healthcare from 1850 till now will be traced.

Pre-1960s

Before *1850*, healthcare in the United States was a loose collection of individual services functioning independently without much relation to each other or to anything else. The history of the American health system can be depicted in four stages (Torrens & Williams, 1993):

- **1850-1900:** First large hospitals established
- **1900-1960:** Science and technology introduced into healthcare, attention to social and organizational structure of healthcare
- **1960-present:** Reorganization of the methods of finance and delivery with use of computers

The healthcare industry initially lagged behind some others in the wide-scale adoption of information systems, but that has now changed.

In the period 1850-1900 only a very *rudimentary technology* was available for the treatment of disease, and the large hospitals, such as Bellevue in New York City, which first appeared in that period, were merely places of shelter for the sick poor who had no home. Indeed, the hospitals were a threat to life, since they were crowded, dirty, and disease-ridden.

After *1900* conditions began to change, stimulated by new discoveries of technologies to help diagnose and treat disease. As more technology developed, it tended to be concentrated in hospitals, with the result that patients and physicians began going to hospitals for the technology to be found there.

Another major change in this period is attributed to the *Great Depression* of the 1930s. The Depression shook the belief in being totally and personally responsible for all aspects of one's life. The government began slowly to assume some responsibility for healthcare.

With the advent of *World War II*, new antibiotics, new surgical techniques, and new approaches to transportation of wounded people were some of the myriad of improvements created by the massive government investment in improved techniques of care. After World War II, new procedures and new equipment flourished to such a degree that technology became the motivating force for hospitals, and most major decisions were based on that technology. This in turn called for waves of new workers, each more specialized and highly skilled than the last. This increasing *specialization* also called for increasing interdependence and a reliance on healthcare systems to integrate the work of many separate groups.

Not only did World War II accustom the country to large-scale healthcare programs, it also encouraged the growth of the *health insurance industry*. During the War, the government froze wages, but did encourage health insurance. This provided the American public with a new form of social organization, the fiscal intermediary or third party. The Blue Cross and Blue Shield plans appeared as nonprofit, community-based healthcare plans that insured against medical costs. With the push also by commercial insurance carriers, the percentage of Americans covered by health insurance rose from less than 20% prior to World War II to 70% by 1960.

Post-1960s

In the 1960s the U.S. government became a major force in the healthcare insurance business by creating Medicare and Medicaid. These programs reimbursed hospitals on the basis of their costs. Hospitals provided *financial cost reports* and received money for services provided to Medicare or Medicaid patients. The amount reimbursed was slightly more than the reported cost. To help produce this kind of billing information, the hospitals turned to information systems.

Initially these billing systems existed primarily in large hospital centers that had the resources to develop and maintain their own billing applications. The applications ran on mainframes. The system was housed in a Data Processing Department whose director reported to the chief financial officer. The *mainframe* supported only a *centralized computing model* in which data was entered by clerks on dumb terminals.

Small hospitals also needed help in creating the financial cost reports. To obtain billing information systems support they turned to *shared systems*. A small hospital would collect its data manually and then send it to a center that would process the data with its computers and send bills to Medicare and Medicaid. Of course, the operators of the shared system charged the small hospital a fee for this service.

The challenge of controlling escalating healthcare costs and the availability of the *minicomputer* in the 1970s supported the appearance of departmental systems in hospitals. For instance, a laboratory could afford to buy a minicomputer and a software system that would help the laboratory perform its functions. Information technology vendors began to provide turnkey systems for the clinical departments. The systems were called turnkey because the clinical department needed only to turn the key on the minicomputer and the system would run. The department could not modify the software but tried to choose a vendor whose system was a close fit to the department's needs. The senior executives of the hospital were involved in funding decisions about these turnkey systems and had to communicate with the clinical departments about them, but were otherwise distant from information system issues.

The 1980s bore witness to three trends in the healthcare environment:

- In 1982, Medicare shifted from a cost-based reimbursement system to a prospective payment system based on diagnosis related groups (DRG). Reimbursement amounts came to depend on the DRG given to the patient and not the actual cost to manage the patient. Whereas prior to this approach to reimbursement a hospital had a financial incentive to provide costly tests and procedures for any given patient, now the hospital was motivated to minimize what it spent on a patient relative to that patient's *DRG reimbursement amount*.
- At the same time as Medicare implemented the DRG approach, the private health insurance industry introduced *managed care*. A managed care plan reimburses a physician based on an estimated annual cost to take care of a patient. That estimated annual cost is also called the capitated rate.
- Healthcare entities began to merge into integrated delivery systems that combined multiple hospitals and clinics that provided various forms of acute, chronic, and rehabilitative care.

These trends coincided on the technical side with the advent of the microcomputer or *personal computer* (PC). The PC would be connected via a local area network to a minicomputer or a mainframe.

Healthcare executives were increasingly motivated to acquire information systems for *departments* that generated substantial profits, such as laboratories, or were crucial in finances, such as the billing department. Each department would tend to acquire from a vendor the "best of breed" system for its department. A system in one department typically did not communicate effectively with a system in another department.

The 1990s witnessed further changes in the reimbursement in physicians. By now, the reader will have appreciated that the method of reimbursement has traditionally driven the evolution of information systems in healthcare. In 1992, Medicare introduced the *resource-based relative value scale (RBRVS)*. RBRVS was intended to shift the emphasis in healthcare from specialty care to primary care and prevention. To this end, primary care providers were given a boost in reimbursement that occurred through RBRVS. Payments are calculated by determining the cost of the resources used and then multiplying that cost by a conversion factor to achieve a relative value. The resource costs themselves are divided into three components: physician work, practice expense, and professional liability insurance.

The emphasis on primary care led to improved methods of handling information in *primary care clinics*. Vendors produced systems that would allow a doctor in a small clinic to develop an electronic medical record, give guidelines semi-automatically to patients, and generally integrate the patient into a disease management scheme.

The end of the 20th century witnessed the birth of the Web and the increasingly widespread use of the *Internet*. The first decade of the 21st century was the decade of the Internet. The U.S. government developed regulations under the HIPAA Law that mandated a standard format to electronic billing across the healthcare industry (often via the Internet). Opportunities for patients to participate in their own healthcare online also increased.

Developments of the past few decades in healthcare financing, planning, policy, and regulation have served to reinforce the increasingly powerful role played by the *federal government* in the direction of information systems for healthcare. The federal government now controls a significant amount of the financial support for healthcare (approximately one-third of the total healthcare expenditures from all sources). By using these massive resources in a unified and centralized manner, the

Figure 1.1. Healthcare Network. Doctors' office, health insurance company, government, employer, hospital, pharmacy, and lab work together

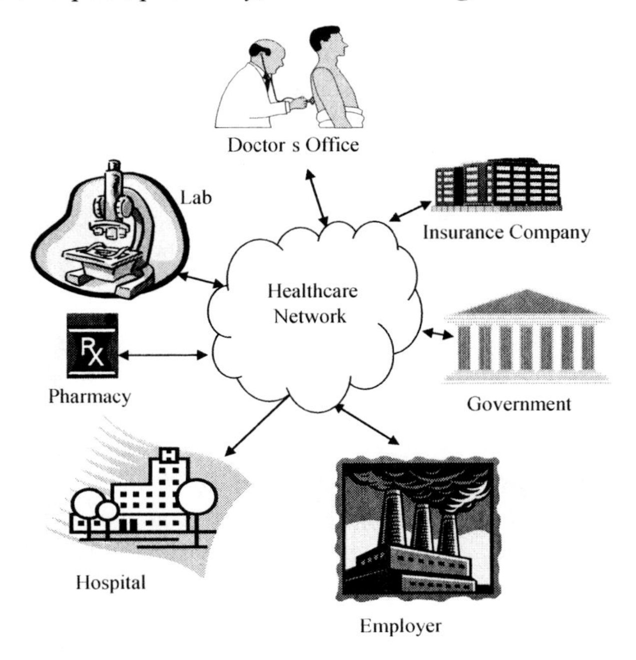

federal government is able to set many of the rules by which healthcare, governmentally funded or not, is provided.

In summary, over the past two centuries the American healthcare system has become enormously interconnected and diverse. Hospitals, doctors' offices, health insurance companies, government, laboratories, patients, and more need to work together (see *Figure 1.1*). Information technology plays a vital role in this *information network*.

Biographical Perspective

The history of computerized health information systems can be relived through the eyes of those who created the *history*. In particular, excerpts from the writing of Donald Lindberg, Kerry Kissinger, and Octo Barnett are provided. From Lindberg is evidenced the "ah-ha" experience that motivated this medical pioneer to enter the field of information systems. Thirty-year-old writings from Barnett about the key factors to success in health information systems remain relevant today.

The Insight

Donald *Lindberg*, MD, in 1960 at University of Missouri was doing research on bacteria and collecting data with a computer. Simultaneously, he was directing clinical chemistry and microbiology at the medical center. The biggest practical problem was getting correct reports from the laboratories to the clinics and wards. From the microbiology lab the pathologists personally signed the report slips, which usually contained a great assortment of spellings of the bacteriological names. Furthermore, the Record Room had, at all times, hundreds of lab reports on which patient names did not match the patient identifier, and these reports were not permitted to be placed in the charts and hence were lost forever. Lindberg (1990) says:

It suddenly occurred to me that the computing system I was using for the antibiotic sensitivity experiments could be used to solve my clinical laboratory problem as well. After all, I reasoned, computer programs always spelled things the same way day after day, and the tabulating printer certainly was faster than the folks running the laboratory typewriters. In addition, I could establish limits, so that at least some of the ridiculous errors could never again be reported out and truly life-threatening findings could be identified for telephone reporting. Once one yielded to this line of thinking, it became immediately obvious that the product of the clinical labs was purely information: hundreds of thousands of items per year. Tables outside the program could contain editing and limit values, pointers to other medical record elements, pricing and quality control data, etc.

Lindberg's experience was unusual in the 1960s. More recently, such insights, as documented for Lindberg, have become more common, and thousands of physicians are now actively advancing the use of computers.

Accounting Systems

Kerry *Kissinger* began work with IBM in the early 1960s installing patient accounting systems. Kissinger's first patient *accounting system* used an IBM 1440 with 16 kilobits of main memory and punched card input. The technological changes since then have been phenomenal, but the basic challenges to the organization remain the same.

The *billing program* had been written by programmers at IBM and was distributed free to hospitals that leased or purchased the IBM 1440. By 1965, 20 hospitals in the U.S. were utilizing this patient billing system. Each decade has spawned a *new generation* of hardware and software capable of doing more things at lower unit cost. The watchword of the 1990s was client server computing and the watchword of the 2000s is Internet-enabled computing.

Despite the many improvements in technology, the human struggles have retained a certain *commonality* and in some ways have become more difficult: each new generation of users struggles with learning how to deploy the technology. Kissinger's team spent 8 months in 1964 working with the hospital to achieve full operation of the billing system. The payback for the hospital was self-evident. The number of technicians and clerks involved in billing operations was reduced by half. Bills were produced sooner and more accurately, and hospital cash flow improved.

Implementation of a healthcare organization patient accounting system in the 1990s took two years to complete and employed a 35-person project team. Everything about the project was more *complex* than earlier projects. The regulatory environment, the number of interfaces to other systems, the network requirements, the testing and data conversion, the procedural changes and training requirements, and coping with multiple, new vendors were all complex and costly in human effort.

The costs and benefits of this 1990s implementation were difficult to measure. The previous system had become too difficult to maintain and had to be replaced. This was a necessary cost of doing business, just as an old building may need to be replaced. The hospital had become locked into a vendor system with little flexibility. The executives did not approve incremental improvements that might have been attempted earlier and that would have avoided massive *one-time costs*. Unfortunately, this scenario is more the norm than the exception in healthcare (Kissinger & Borchardt, 1996).

Evolutionary Development

Octo *Barnett*, MD, was the leader of the Massachusetts General Hospital Computer Laboratory for over 30 years. The Laboratory developed the COSTAR clinical information system and its underlying operating system, called the "*Massachusetts General Hospital Utility Multiprogramming System*" (MUMPS). In reviewing the history of information systems in clinical care, Barnett (1990) had occasion to reflect on how little the basic issues have changed over the decades. Barnett's 1968 article in the *New England Journal of Medicine* contains an analysis that applies equally well today (Barnett, 1968):

Early interest in bringing the revolution in computer technology to bear on medical practice was plagued with over enthusiasm, naiveté, and unrealistic expectations. The use of computers would allow rapid and accurate collection and retrieval of all clinical information, perform automatic diagnosis, collect, monitor and analyze a variety of physiological signals perform and interpret all lab tests immediately and replace the telephone and medical record by fulfilling their function. However attempts to apply computer methods to medicine have had only limited success with numerous failures. ... The initial wave of optimism and enthusiasm, generated by beguiling promises of an immediately available, total hospital computer system, passed. Now, efforts are directed towards the painful, slow, evolutionary process of developing and implementing modules or building blocks for individual functions.

The process of convincing people to build a system, building it, and then successfully using it remains the painful, slow *evolutionary process* that Barnett described in 1968.

In another article of the same vintage, Barnett and Greenes (1969) elaborate three recurring problems for system development as follows:

First the magnitude of the problem is usually grossly underestimated and there is almost always inadequate concern for defining objectives and for planning. Hospital and medical staffs have had little prior experience in innovation in the area of information processing and in many situations the critical decisions are made by individuals in isolated departments who do not process a broad view of the needs of the hospital.

Second, the computer industry has often displayed a considerable lack of understanding and of sophistication. On a number of occasions the sales and promotional aspects of marketing hospital computer systems have been quite misleading and have led to false expectations.

Third, the hospitals have rarely made the depth of commitment of both administrative and professional staff that is required to develop and implement a viable system. The commitment must be in terms of years in order to provide the exposure and experience necessary to cope with the complexity of the problems.

From these problems, the observation is made that an *evolutionary systems development* approach is critical. This issue of developing systems in pieces and integrating them across time versus building whole systems in one swoop has often arisen as contentious in HIS discussions. On the one hand, the systems cannot be completely effective without integrated information, and on the other hand, the amount of change at any one time is typically best kept small.

Challenges

Salient problems facing the healthcare system include rising costs, medical errors, and coordination. Each of these is addressed in the next three subsections.

Rising Costs

New diagnostic *technologies*, such as magnetic resonance imaging devices, lead to increased costs of healthcare. The rapid rise in healthcare costs sets off a series of events. Briefly stated, the rise in costs forces the insurance programs and employers to contain costs. These efforts of the *payers* to contain healthcare expenditures have an impact on the hospitals and physicians. They find their sources of revenue being constrained as a result of the payer's healthcare containment efforts, so they then take actions of their own in reaction to the efforts of the payers. These actions of the healthcare providers, in turn, often affect patients and communities, which must take actions to lessen the impact (Torrens & Williams, 1993).

The result of this chain of events is a circular system that passes along the effects of one particular set of changes to another part of the system, which in turn takes actions of its own to pass the problem along further. This system forces each individual part of the system to determine how to play the game. Each part solves its particular limited problems and very often does so with an elaborate display of talent, energy, and sophistication. Tragically, the need for each individual part to:

- Deal with its limited problems
- Treat other parts as adversaries

prevents the individual parts from coming together to cooperatively solve system-wide problems. The ultimate irony of this *"gaming" system* is that it not only does not solve the initiating problem of rising costs but it works against broad, cooperative efforts to solve the problem.

The *precipitating factors* for these escalating costs are not failures but successes. Despite various problems evident in the quality of care, American healthcare is considered worldwide to offer some of the most sophisticated medical care in the world. The product is highly desired by patients who can afford to pay for it.

Healthcare expenditures grew 6.9% in 2000 and 9.3% in 2002. A survey of employers, healthcare providers, and health plans showed that:

- Employers plan largely to share cost increases with employees through increased employee premiums
- Health plans expect to pass much of their cost on to employers
- Healthcare providers intend to increase preauthorization efforts

The technology of information along with sound human practices is one of the few new technologies that could both improve care and reduce costs. If people agree to standardize data collection, to integrate networks of data, and to semi-automatically monitor practice by criteria both of low cost as well as quality care, then a system could evolve that would work against the negative, gaming situation currently in place. The primary obstacles to such an *information systems solution* are, however, not technological but rather political.

Medical Errors

Some estimates show that about 100,000 people die each year in the United States from *medical errors* that occur in hospitals. That's more than die from motor vehicle accidents, breast cancer, or AIDS. Indeed, more people die annually from medication errors than from workplace injuries. Add the financial cost to the human tragedy, and medical error easily rises to the top ranks of urgent, widespread public problems.

The startling statistics of medical error are at odds with the public perception of the incidence of error. Legitimate liability concerns on the part of healthcare professionals discourage reporting of errors. The Institute of Medicine (Kohn et al., 2000) concluded that the problem is not bad people in healthcare—it is that good people are working in *bad systems* that need to be made safer.

Existing information systems, designed primarily for billing purposes, often fail to record important information about a patient's condition. A comparison of claims and patient records reveals that claims do not accurately reflect over half of the clinically important patient conditions. Even when information system software allows for the entry of additional information, that information often is incorrectly entered. The National Committee for Quality Assurance's audits comparing reported performance data with patient records have uncovered average error rates as high as 20%. These *audits* have uncovered a number of data quality problems, includ-

Figure 1.2. Avoidable Error. The drug administration system can help reduce error. This example is from a practicing nurse.

Avoidable Error

The health care industry is not perfect. The people administering health care are also not perfect. They tire after 12-hour shifts. They at times must make quick decisions with very little support around them. Their handwriting at times is less than ideal, and above all else, they are human. Whether we want to admit it or not, humans make mistakes. Because we in the health care industry are aware of our human characteristics that leave us exposed to the possibility of making mistakes, we do everything possible to prevent those mistakes from occurring in the first place. Information technology can help. Medication errors in hospitals are frequent and may harm patients. Medication errors include incorrect dosing, incorrect drug given, or incorrect timing of drug administration. Medication administration is a primary responsibility of nurses, and error prevention is taught during their training. Still, competent nurses may make mistakes. An example of a device and information system that is in widespread use in hospitals today and that has dramatically decreased the number of medication errors is called Pyxis. Pyxis is a medication-dispensing computer that is maintained by the pharmacy, is located on each unit, and is stocked with medications for each patient on that unit. The patient s medication administration profile is updated in the system by the pharmacy and when medications are due to be given, a nurse, using password entry, signs into the system and obtains the medication. Medications can be obtained only when due and only in the correct dose required. The Pyxis system can be overridden, but the nurse must then take extra steps. This computer-supported dispensing helps to prevent errors by nurses who are rushing and tired and who might otherwise be reading orders written in difficult to read hand-writing. Medication errors can still occur but are less frequent due to the enforced double check (pharmacy and nursing).

ing missing encounter data, homegrown codes, and missing information in patient records (Shaller et al., 1998).

Important to *patient safety* is the ordering, transcribing, and administering of medications (see *Figure 1.2*). A very common iatrogenic injury to the hospitalized patient is the adverse drug event, yet about half of all adverse drug events would be relatively easy to prevent. The most common error is in dosing, which occurs three times more frequently than the next type. The top causes of failure include:

- Prescribing errors due to deficiency in drug knowledge related to incorrect dose, form, frequency, and route
- Order transcription errors due to manual processes
- Allergy errors due to the systems poor notification to healthcare providers
- Poor medication order tracking due to a cumbersome, inefficient system, that is, dose administration is recorded in more than one location
- Poor interpersonal communication, that is, illegible orders

Proper information systems could reduce the incidence of these errors. For instance, computers could help by reducing the number of choices in the *Physician Order Entry* system so that physicians are only shown acceptable drug doses and frequencies.

Coordination

Because of its decentralized nature, the healthcare industry has a very complex business model consisting of a fragmented community of trading partners (i.e., hospitals, providers, group purchasers, pharmacies, clearinghouses, and others). A Presidential Commission reported (*Quality First: Better Health Care for All Americans*, 1998):

Few other industries are decentralized to the same degree. The auto industry, for example, has a tightly coupled set of commerce partners. The mutual fund industry has employers, shareholders, and stock exchanges. In contrast, the health care industry is so fundamentally decentralized and yet so critically needs data-sharing that the use of common or cooperating information systems and databases becomes an operational imperative.

Improvements in information systems also are needed to support the coordination of care. To provide effective care, health professionals and providers need access to a patient's treatment history, test results, and related information. Paper records

Figure 1.3. A Failure to Share. This story about coordination problems is from a family in the U.S. that was from another culture. The hospital and town names have been fictionalized to provide anonymity.

A Failure to Share

My grandmother died because there was no medical history available so that the physician could be aware of her condition and provide appropriate treatment to save her life. She always went to Adventist Hospital for surgery and other procedures. All of her medical histories were at this hospital, and this is where her primary care physician was affiliated. One tragic weekend my grandmother went to see my mom in Adamsville. That morning my grandmother told my mom that she was having stomach pain, and about noon the pain was still there and my grandmother felt tired and short of breath. My mom called the ambulance to take my grandmother to the emergency room. When the ambulance personnel arrived, they took her to St. Mary s Hospital. My mom said no, we want you to take us to Adventist Hospital . The ambulance personnel replied we must take her to the nearest hospital . When my grandmother got to St. Mary s Hospital, the medical staff didn t know what to do. They asked us to give them my grandmother s medical history. Our family gave all the information that we knew to the nurse. After a few hours, my grandmother cried and asked for medication. The nurse responded that the ER physician was trying to contact her primary care provider for further information so that the ER physician could determine the best treatment. Another hour passed, and nothing was done to stop the pain. The ER physician decided to admit my grandmother to the hospital for further evaluation. After they took my grandmother to her room, still nothing had been done for the pain. My grandmother lay in bed and cried. Two hours later my grandmother went into cardiac arrest. Nurses gave her CPR and were able to bring her back, but she was in a coma and connected to numerous machines. For 10 days my grandmother never awoke or responded to the family. Finally, our family had to make the painful decision to remove the machine that was keeping her alive.

The problem was that St. Mary s Hospital did not have any medical records of my grandmother so the ER physician was not able to determine a treatment for her. Her primary care physician wasn t affiliated with the hospital; he didn t have privileges to access the facility. Think of the senseless deaths that are the result of an ER physician being unable to make an accurate decision on which care to give a patient.

are difficult to transfer between organizations. The problems are both technical and administrative (see *Figure 1.3*). Where computer records are kept, the use of incompatible hardware and software configurations makes file sharing difficult.

Improved information systems should generate *population-level data* that can assess the performance of the health system in caring for discrete populations (*Quality First: Better Health Care for All Americans*, 1998). Public health officials would be better able to monitor disease outbreaks or the adverse effects of medications, procedures, or other products. Most existing information systems are not designed for these purposes.

Professional Organizations

An organization's structure is affected by the variety one finds in its environment. Environmental variety in turn depends on both environmental complexity and the pace of change. Mintzberg (1979) identifies four types of *organizational form*, which are associated with four combinations of complexity and change (see *Table 1.2*). Each of the four organizational forms in Mintzberg's scheme depends on fundamentally different mechanisms for coordination.

The *professional bureaucracy* relies for coordination on the standardization of skills. Training and indoctrination first instill those skills in the new professional, and interaction with colleagues through time maintains the standardization (Glouberman & Mintzberg, 2001). The organization hires trained professionals for the operating core, and then gives them considerable control over their work. Control over his own work means that the professional works relatively independently of his colleagues, but closely with the clients he serves. Most necessary coordination between the operating professionals is handled by the standardization of skills and knowledge (see *Table 1.3*).

The *machine bureaucracy* generates its own standards. Its techno-structure designs the work standards for its operators and its line managers enforce them. The standards of the professional bureaucracy originate largely outside its own structure,

Table 1.2. Environmental determinants of organizational structure

Pace of Change	Environmental Complexity	
	Simple	Complex
Stable	Machine Bureaucracy	Professional Organization
Dynamic	Entrepreneurial Startup	Adhocracy

Table 1.3. Form and coordination

Organizational Form	Coordination Mechanism
Machine Bureaucracy	Standardize procedures and outputs
Professional Organization	Standardize professional skills
Entrepreneurial Startup	Direct supervision and control
Adhocracy	Mutual adjustment of ad-hoc teams

in the self-governing association its operators join with their colleagues from other professional bureaucracies. The professional bureaucracy emphasizes authority of a professional nature.

The professional organization is a specific organizational structure with a large operational core, a small middle line, a very small techno-structure for planning and standardizing organizational performance and a considerable support area to relieve the *highly-paid professionals* from as much routine work as possible. The structure is what distinguishes professional bureaucracies from both machine bureaucracies and innovative organizations.

The strategies of the professional bureaucracy are largely ones of the *individual professionals* within the organization, as well as of the professional associations on the outside. The professional bureaucracy's strategies represent the cumulative effect over time of the projects that its members are able to convince it to undertake.

The professional's technical system cannot be highly regulating, certainly *not highly automated.* The professional resists the division of his skills into simply executed steps because that:

- Makes them programmable by the techno-structure
- Destroys his basis of autonomy
- Drives the organizational structure to the machine bureaucratic form

Like the machine bureaucracy, the professional bureaucracy is an *inflexible structure*, well suited to producing its standard outputs but ill-suited to adapting to the production of new ones. Change in the professional bureaucracy does not sweep in from new administrators taking office to announce major reforms. Instead, change seeps in by the slow process of changing the professionals—changing who can enter the profession, what they learn in its professional schools (norms as well as skills and knowledge), and thereafter how willing they are to upgrade their skills.

The dominance of expert work affects the administrative structure in professional organizations. The administration lacks power relative to machine or entrepreneurial organizations and is *decentralized.* It provides professionals with more control over their own work as well as collective control over administrative decisions. The administrators typically spend their time handling disruptions and negotiations. Nevertheless, administrative structures serve a key role in creating the boundary of the organization. Often through this boundary creation, the administration gains power.

A small technical structure and a weak administration lead to a distinctive strategy process. The conventional way, in which central administrators develop detailed, integrated plans, seldom works in the professional organization. Many strategic issues are controlled by individual professionals or require the participation of a variety of members in a complex *collective process*. The resulting fragmentation of activity discourages initiatives. This is one reason for the remarkable degree of stability in professional organizations (Klischewski & Wetzel, 2005).

Trends

Healthcare trends influence an organization's strategy and help drive the relevant information systems trends (see *Figure 1.4*). The organization's strategy along with accessible information technology tools determines what the information systems needs are.

Structurally, the healthcare industry trend is to *integration*. Physicians who once practiced in solo groups are increasingly practicing in large groups. In the past, the boundary between providers and payers was sharp, but that boundary is becoming fuzzy as providers offer health plans and insurers develop provider networks.

In the past, information systems were focused on collecting *billing data* from patient encounters. In the future these systems will pay attention to clinical data that is important in the delivery of care. Financial and clinical data will be collected and maintained.

In the past, decision-support tended to rely on data archives and reflect patterns determined retrospectively. In the future, information systems should monitor data in real-time and provide decision support at the moment of care. Examples of this are *alerts* that are built into a system and let healthcare professionals know immediately upon doing something whether or not the system perceives this action as dangerous somehow.

Figure 1.4. Trends. The national trends influence a particular organization's strategy and its information systems needs.

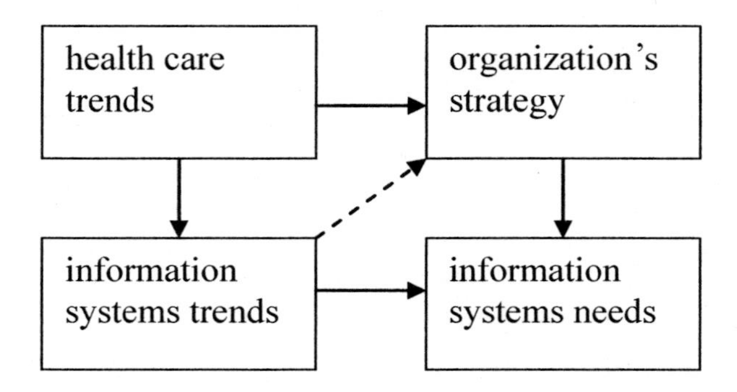

The perspective of workflow has become increasingly important over the last few decades (Rada, 1995). The move towards integrated and managed care, which requires designing healthcare processes around patient needs and incorporating efficiency considerations, has led to an increased interest in process-oriented healthcare information systems based on workflow technology (Poulymenopoulou et al., 2003).

Given an understanding of industry trends and of information system capabilities, an organization needs to have a realistic strategy as to how it will distinguish itself for its customers. One *business strategy* is to emphasize the development of physician networks. For a hospital this can be critical to getting patients referred to the hospital and treated by the doctors in the hospital. Primary care networks serve as important gatekeepers to hospitals.

Ambulatory care is typically less expensive than hospital-based care. Contemporary reimbursement schemes give preference to those who provide such ambulatory care. Thus primary care centers, diagnostic laboratories, outpatient surgical facilities, and other ambulatory care systems might be the strategic goal of a provider to emphasize. Likewise, home healthcare may be targeted.

Having reviewed the trends in healthcare and information systems and having established a strategy for the healthcare organization, the organization can specify its information systems needs. These needs can be viewed as common applications, specific applications, or technical infrastructure.

The common *applications* include things like data repositories that contain patient information. Information about the patient is needed in most other transactions in the healthcare organization. Specific applications would be, for instance, for the diagnostic laboratories, such as pathology and radiology, in an organization. A need for physician office systems is another example of a specific application need.

The *technical infrastructure* needs must be delineated. Does the organization need to have high-speed networks connecting all its components or can it rely on phone modems for connecting some entities? Must large database systems for handling thousands of simultaneous queries be available or is something much less robust adequate? These and other technological infrastructure questions must be answered before the full requirements can be specified.

While the information systems needs of any particular organization are highly context dependent, the general industry and technology trends allow the identification of weaknesses in the current information systems implementations. This extract from Kleinke (2000) highlights the challenge:

Contrary to the claims of its well-financed promoters, the Internet will not solve the administrative redundancies, economic inefficiencies, or quality problems that have plagued the U.S. health care system for decades. These phenomena are the result of economic, organizational, legal, regulatory, and cultural conflicts rooted in a health care system grown from hybrid public and private financing; cultural expectations of unlimited access to unlimited medical resources; and the use of third-party payers rewarded to constrain those expectations. The historic inadequacy of information technology to solve health care's biggest problems is a symptom of these structural realities, not their cause. With its revolution of information access for consumers, the Internet will exacerbate the cost and utilization problems of a health care system in which patients demand more, physicians are legally and economically motivated to supply more, and public and private purchasers are expected to pay the bills.

Improvement in the healthcare industry does not depend on information technology, but a properly oriented use of information technology can make a big difference in the future of healthcare. *Investors* in health information systems should pay close attention to the business situation in medicine.

Other Books

When this author *Rada* taught his first course on medical informatics in 1981, there was no one book appropriate for an entire university course on the subject. The field was still new as an academic discipline. The two books that the author used in 1981 were:

- Lindberg's (1979) *The Growth of Medical Information Systems in the United States*
- Warner's (1979) *Computer Assisted Medical Decision Making*

Warner's book is about his landmark health information system that emphasized decision support. Lindberg's book is an overview of the HIS field conceptually and an analysis of the state-of-the-art in 1979.

There are several kinds of publications in the area of health information systems. One kind is aimed at the *practicing professional*, another kind at students, and another kind at the general public. Within each category certain books may target specific subcategories. For instance, some books are for medical students, some for nursing students, some for students of medical records, and so on. Of course, some books claim to satisfy the information needs of many different audience types.

On the professional side, naturally, there are also further divisions of the audience. For *healthcare executives*, *Information Technology for Integrated Health Systems: Positioning for the Future* edited by Kissinger and Borchardt (1996) has an organization not unlike this book in that it goes from vision to design to implementation. The book assumes a reader knowledgeable in healthcare and information technology and emphasizes the important, broad, practical issues to guide decision-making about information systems acquisitions in healthcare organizations. The book by Wager et al. (2005) emphasizes healthcare data quality and information technology governance in hospitals. Some books targeting the healthcare manager may focus on particular techno-managerial topics. For instance, Worthley's (2000) *Managing Information in Healthcare: Concepts and Cases* focuses on security management.

Some books target the practicing physician. An example is Ruffin's (1999) *Digital Doctors*. Ruffin argues that physicians need to take care of healthcare information systems and presents detailed technical and political information as to why physicians should be Chief Information Officers for healthcare systems.

The United States employs over three million *nurses*—more than triple the number of physicians. Targeting various healthcare information systems professionals and particularly nurses and nursing students is the extensive series *Computers in Health Care*. Books that target nurses, such as Saba and McCormick (2005), take a basic approach to information technology and emphasize the practical interface that the nurse has with the technology or with other healthcare professionals in maintaining the medical record.

Medical records professionals are intimately involved with computerized information systems. An example of a book targeting medical records students is McMiller's (2004) *Being a Medical Records/Health Information Clerk* (3rd ed.). That book gives the students a rather broad introduction to general principles of management along with specifics of how a medical records department works and should be managed.

A book from the management side that teaches HIS assuming that the reader is a *health administration student* is Tan's (2001) *Health Management Information Systems: Methods and Practical Applications* (2nd ed.). This book presents a comprehensive, theoretical view of what management means in the context of healthcare information systems. Much of what is presented is elementary as regards information systems. A book edited by Tan targets the same audience but emphasizes the role of the Internet in healthcare.

Health Management Information Systems: A Handbook for Decision Makers (Smith, 2000) targets students of public health. The book presents background principles from various disciplines and augments them with brief case studies. The case studies come from Britain, Australia, and the United States, and the book attempts indirectly to compare and contrast the healthcare information systems of the three *countries*.

A large collection of books comes from the medical informatics community. People in *medical schools* typically author these books and target students or staff of medical schools. Thus the emphasis tends to be on topics like medical expert systems, patient monitoring systems, and medical library information systems. There have been many conferences of academics that include published proceedings that are a kind of book. The well-known conferences series that produce book-like proceedings are the American-dominated "American Medical Informatics Association" conference series and the European-dominated "MedInfo Conference" series. This portion of the healthcare information systems community tends to use the term "medical informatics" in preference to healthcare information systems or healthcare informatics. A popular book for medical students studying informatics is *Medical Informatics: Computer Applications in Health Care and Biomedicine* (2nd ed.) (Perreault et al., 2002). As a book for students of medical computer science, the book emphasizes concepts, such as medical data, medical reasoning, evaluation of medical systems, and ethics. Another book from the medical informatics community emphasizes evaluation of information systems and ethics (Anderson & Aydin, 2005).

In addition to the books targeting professionals, students, and researchers, there may be other categories. For instance, targeting the *general public* is Karen Duncan's (1994) *Health Information and Health Reform* that provides a layman's rationale for a national health information system and attempts to politically move people to do something about it.

Questions

Reading Questions

1. What are the similarities and differences between health information systems as a discipline and management information systems as a discipline?
2. Summarize the history of technology in American healthcare from 1850 until now.
3. Lindberg and Barnett are physicians working in research environments. Kissinger is an information systems specialist working for a vendor of information systems. Their histories show a greater concern for accounting by Kissinger and on diagnosis and treatment by Lindberg and Barnett. Explain why these different emphases might exist.
4. What views on the critical interfaces for success of HIS were espoused several decades past but remain true today?
5. In what sense are the escalating costs of healthcare the result of a gaming system? Identify the components of this system and how they interact.
6. Provide evidence for this statement: One of the tragedies of medical errors that cause death is that proper use of good information systems might prevent those errors.

7. How does the money invested in information technology by healthcare compare to that in other industries? How is this healthcare investment changing?

Doing Questions

1. This book provides a sub-section called "Other Books" that introduces a simple taxonomy of book types in the subject matter area of the book. This assignment should be submitted with three parts as follows:

First, reproduce the taxonomy and list under each category the author or editor (this exercise may use the term "author" to refer to authors and/or editors) and book title for those entries in that category from the book. Use hierarchical format with indentations to indicate different levels. Do this in Microsoft Word or html. Use black text on white background.

Second go to www.amazon.com and find books that can be retrieved with key words of "healthcare information systems." Select five books (not mentioned in this book's "Related Work" section) that fit each into a distinct category of the taxonomy. You can extend the taxonomy if you find a book that does not fit into the taxonomy from step 1. Provide the taxonomy in indented hierarchical form and list the author and title of each of your five books in the appropriate location in the taxonomy. Mark all you additions in red ink. In other words, the books you enter should be in red and any new terms that you add to the taxonomy should be in red.

Third, provide an explanation for each book as to why it belongs where you put it in the taxonomy. This explanation might relate to the professional position of the author(s), the reviews of the book, the author's preface, or something else that indicates directly or indirectly the intended audience.

2. Relate two incidents where medical errors occurred and where better use of information systems might have reduced the likelihood of the error. Your incidents can come from the literature, your own experience, a personal acquaintance, or some other source, but you should note in the answer also your source. Explain the incident in enough detail that a layperson can understand. Structure your answer as follows:

   - Introduce your answer by providing the overview of the error situation and motivating your approach

- Describe incident ONE in a paragraph or more
- Describe how use of information systems might have reduced the likelihood of incident ONE
- Describe incident TWO in a paragraph or more
- Describe how use of information systems might have reduced the likelihood of incident TWO
- Generalize one of your incidents and describe technical approaches to it

References

Anderson, J.G., & Aydin, C.E. (2005). *Evaluating the organizational impact of health care information systems* (2nd ed.). New York: Springer.

Barnett, G.O. (1968). Computers and patient care. *New England Journal of Medicine, 279*, 1321-1327.

Barnett, G.O. (1990). History of the development of medical information systems at the Laboratory of Computer Science at Massachusetts General Hospital. In B. Blum & K. Duncan (Eds.), *A history of medical informatics* (pp. 141-154). New York: ACM Press.

Barnett, G.O., & Greenes, R. (1969). Interface aspects of a hospital information system. *Annals of New York Academy of Science, 161*, 756-768.

Duncan, K. (1994). *Health information and health reform*. San Francisco: Jossey-Bass.

Glouberman, S., & Mintzberg, H. (2001). Managing the care of health and the cure of disease. Part I: Differentiation. *Health Care Management Review, 26*(1), 56-92.

Kissinger, K., & Borchardt, S. (Eds.). (1996). *Information technology for integrated health systems: Positioning for the future*. New York: John Wiley & Sons.

Kleinke, J.D. (2000). Vaporware.com: The failed promise of the health care Internet. *Health Affairs, 19*(6), 57-71.

Klischewski, R., & Wetzel, I. (2005). Processing by contract: Turning the wheel within heterogeneous workflow networks. *Business Process Management Journal, 11*(3), 237-254.

Kohn, L., Corrigan, J., & Donaldson, M. (Eds.). (2000). *To err is human: Building a safer health system*. Washington: National Academy Press.

Lindberg, D. (1979). *The growth of medical information systems in the United States*. Lexington, MA: Lexington Books.

Lindberg, D. (1990). In praise of computing. In B. Blum & K. Duncan (Eds.), *A history of medical informatics* (pp. 4-12). New York: ACM Press.

McMiller, K. (2004). *Being a medical records/health information clerk* (3rd ed.). Upper Saddle Creek, NJ: Prentice Hall.

Mintzberg, H. (1979). *The structuring of organizations*. Upper Saddle River, NJ: Prentice-Hall.

Perreault, L.E., Shortliffe, E.H., & Wiederhold, G. (2002). *Medical informatics: Computer applications in health care and biomedicine* (2nd ed.). New York: Springer-Verlag Telos.

Poulymenopoulou, M., Malamateniou, F., & Vassilacopoulos, G. (2003). Specifying workflow process requirements for an emergency medical service. *Journal of Medical Systems, 27*(4), 325-335.

Quality first: Better health care for all Americans. (1998). Washington, DC: President's Advisory Commission on Consumer Protection and Quality in the Health Care Industry.

Rada, R. (1995). *Software reuse* (1st ed.). Oxford, UK: Intellect Books.

Ruffin, M.d.G.J. (1999). *Digital doctors*. Tampa, FL: American College of Health Executives.

Saba, V.K., & McCormick, K.A. (2005). *Essentials of nursing informatics* (4th ed.). New York: McGraw-Hill.

Shaller, D., Sharpe, R., & Rubin, R. (1998). A national action plan to meet health care quality information needs in the age of managed care. *Journal of the American Medical Association, 279*, 1254-1258.

Smith, J. (2000). *Health management information systems: A handbook for decision-makers*. Buckingham, UK: Open University Press.

Tan, J. (2001). *Health management information systems: Methods and practical applications* (2nd ed.). Sudbury, MA: Jones & Bartlett Publishers.

Tan, J. (Ed.). (2005). *E-health care information systems: An introduction for students and professionals*. San Francisco: Jossey-Bass.

Torrens, P., & Williams, S. (1993). Understanding the present, planning for the future: The dynamics of health care in the United States in the 1990s. In S. Williams & P. Torrens (Eds.), *Introduction to health services* (pp. 421-429). Albany, NY: Delmar Publishers.

Wager, K., Lee, F., & Glaser, J. (2005). *Managing health care information systems: A practical approach for health care executives*. San Francisco: Jossey-Bass.

Warner, H. (1979). *Computer-assisted medical decision-making*. New York: Academic Press.

Worthley, J. (2000). *Managing information in healthcare: Concepts and cases*. Chicago: Health Administration Press of College of Healthcare Executives.

Chapter II

Software Life Cycle

Learning Objectives

- Construct a preliminary analysis and design for a health information system
- Distinguish between approaches that successfully involve the client and approaches that do not
- Compose a method of collecting requirements from healthcare professionals that visually presents information to them that they readily understand
- Apply different stakeholder matrices to determine the future of a legacy healthcare information system and illustrate the importance of politics

An example of an admissions process for a patient as seen by a nurse depicts a typical use of computers in healthcare (see *Figure 2.1*). While the process is impressive in many ways, it also leaves open the possibility of improvement through re-design of workflow and introduction of further automation. This chapter describes the *software life cycle* for healthcare information systems. The emphasis is on the development of a requirements document and a design document for a system. The emphasis is on working with executives and end-users to understand what will work. Finally, sections on system acquisition and system retirement are presented.

The traditional software life cycle defined in ISO 12207 (Rada & Moore, 1997) begins with requirements capture and ends with retirement. The *system development life cycle* remains largely unchanged over the years, though it calls increasingly for end-user involvement. The system development life cycle is basically the same in healthcare as in numerous other industries. However, what to expect in implementing the life cycle in a health environment is different from what to expect in other environments. The assessment of healthcare information systems requires subjective

Figure 2.1. A Typical Case. These are the observations of an experienced registered nurse (RN) about the use of information systems in her unit.

In the Ambulatory Surgery Unit where I work, the registration process begins with the infamous white card. This card is completed by the physician who requests that the patient be registered for her/his surgical procedure. The white card contains patient demographics, insurance, medical service to which the patient is to be admitted, and procedure.

The Admissions Unit then generates a medical record and a medical record number for the patient by entering this information into a patient management information system. A red card (small plastic addressograph plate that looks like a credit card) is also produced for the patient and includes the patient s identifying information. This red card, a demographics fact sheet, physician orders, previous test results, and old records are sent to our unit the day before surgery. The unit secretary then prepares a paper chart for the patient which includes the necessary paper documentation forms.

On the day of surgery, the patient registers with our unit secretary. The secretary then gets the patient s paper chart. On our unit most documentation is done by paper. The only clinical information system to which we have access is a pathology laboratory system but only to view results and not to make orders. Lab tests and medications are ordered with a paper form. Radiology tests can be ordered by the physician entering the request for the test into a radiology clinical system or via paper.

Converting to an automated system on this unit would involve extreme process reengineering. I would hope that eventually this would happen. In two years, the unit will be in a brand new state of the art building, and I asked my manager if she knew whether we would be using a computer system, and she said that it was discussed, but all of the details were not finalized.

or qualitative methods as well as objective or quantitative methods (Heathfield et al., 1997):

Health care information systems (IS) cannot be treated purely from the objectivist perspective. ... Whilst health care IS have a functional objective, ... the perception of health care IS will always involve an element of aesthetics, politics and sociology. ... The provision of an evaluation framework which takes account of these factors is important in the move towards professionalism in medical informatics.

Assessing a system requires a multi-faceted approach and must rely in part on qualitative methods.

Requirements Phase

Each phase of the software life cycle, such as requirements or design, might itself involve multiple sub-phases. For instance, the requirements phase may have a business requirements sub-phase that is separate from a functional or a technical requirements sub-phase. One approach to the *requirements phase* is described next. An organization might begin by determining its generic functions and specific clinical functions grouped by categories. The interrelationships among application areas and their current level of development should indicate what is not automated, what is moderately supported, and what is currently well supported. A technical strategy provides an overview of the technical environment and technical characteristics of the infrastructure. Integration considerations, particularly for heterogeneous systems, must be addressed. Evaluation criteria should specify the ability to meet functional user requirements under cost constraints. The acquisition strategy gives ground rules for in-house development versus outside sourcing. Selection criteria for outside sourcing include historical vendor performance. Responsibilities of the user, managers, and vendors must be clear.

Following the preceding model of the requirements phase, the U.S. *Department of Defense* (DoD) determined requirements for one of its healthcare information systems. Those requirements are sketched next. The DoD has one of the world's largest healthcare systems and is typically in some stage of a major system upgrade. The deliberations and documents of the DoD process are available to the public to a level of detail not usually available for commercial systems.

The vision and strategic initiatives of the *Military Health Services System* focus on accomplishing goals, which:

- Maintain readiness for joint operations in a global environment
- Improve health
- Right-size the medical work force

The *Clinical Business Area,* which comprises all clinical business processes and functions, supports delivery of health services and supports the vision of a computer-based patient record.

The business process reengineering of the *Department of Defense Vision Information Services* (DVIS) addresses:

- Three functional areas of business process improvements (BPIs), functional system requirements, and product evaluation scenarios
- Three functional areas of Optometry, Ophthalmology, and Optical Fabrication Laboratory

The DVIS workgroup included doctors, laboratory professionals, technical, and health records representatives from the vision, optical, and eye health disciplines.

The *DVIS workgroup* met for two, one-week workshops. The workgroup validated and augmented a previously defined DVIS functional area model-activity (FAM). In addition to discussion and presentations, the DVIS workgroup utilized groupware as a tool to facilitate the workgroup process.

The workgroup identified *process improvements* based on the DVIS FAM. The workgroup identified several hundred improvements to their business processes. Analysts refined them to 80 improvements. These improvements were then separated into eight categories, with each category further divided into system and non-system BPIs. The system BPIs were used in the development of the DVIS Functional System Requirements.

The analysts focused on mapping the vision, optical, and eye (VOE) health providers' *workflow* to the DVIS FAM. After this validation of the FAM, the workgroup separated into four subgroups. The subgroup topics were:

- Group 1. Develop Direction and Manage Resources
- Group 2. Deliver Clinical Services
- Group 3. Manage Optical Fabrication Process
- Group 4. Deliver Preventive Services

The four subgroups then generated BPIs. The entire workgroup then reconvened to share findings. This process allowed the workgroup, as a whole, to propose the necessary BPIs, considering both their particular work and FAM. The group suggested approximately 200 BPIs.

The final *BPI statements* were organized into the following eight categories:

- **VOE-wide processes:** There is a need for broad VOE process improvements, ranging from online information to standardization of policies and procedures throughout DoD and the individual services. Improvements in this BPI category affect all areas of VOE service and its environment.
- **Ensure readiness:** Readiness is the current ability of forces or systems to deploy and perform their planned mission. The current ability of forces to

deploy and perform a planned mission based on their vision, optical, and eye health status is a major BPI area that can be enhanced by the DVIS application. This provides automated query and reports regarding active duty personnel's VOE readiness status. Units and individuals must ensure they have the right information, supplies, and instructions to be VOE ready.

- **Increase productivity and ensure quality care:** The DVIS system supports diverse ways to increase productivity and ensure quality care. These options must be compiled, viewed, evaluated, and implemented. Use of multiple types of studies, analyses, outcome measurements, and benchmarks will determine how best to use resources to ensure efficiency and quality care.
- **Manage and trend patient encounter and patient information:** To increase efficiency and improve service, there is a need to improve the tracking of patients and their orders. There is also a demand for the ability to trend different functions and variance tracking throughout the clinical encounter and healthcare facility.
- **Manage appointments, access, and scheduling:** Automation of scheduling is of utmost importance. This type of support, with its automatic notifications, would allow the clinics to have more flexibility and increase productivity. The automated system would use diagnostic codes to prioritize appointments. There is a need to allow patients to gain access to the automated system to improve care.
- **Manage equipment, facilities, consumables, and fiscal resources:** Proper management of equipment, facilities, consumables, and fiscal resources are vital to quality care.
- **Prevent and record eye injury:** Historically, 10% of war injuries are eye-related. Further studies have shown that in peacetime, and increasingly so in wartime, 90% of eye injuries were preventable. Fact-based effective countermeasures require a central database for eye injuries and diagnoses. This database will track personal and unit eye injury history, and specific eye hazard sites, to enable decision makers to identify effective protection.
- **Promote and organize education and training:** Education regarding vision conservation and VOE readiness is important in order to have a VOE ready force. Plans, training programs and manuals must be developed to facilitate patient education using various training methodologies (automated patient instruction sheets, handouts, interactive software, and videos).

The eight categories identify *overall improvements* needed *in the* VOE system. Each category focuses on one main topic that affects the workflow of VOE professionals.

The delineation of requirements for a vision system in the military indicates at the top level the kinds of requirements that one can expect for a major component of a healthcare information system. Other *components* of the military health system might have similar requirements.

Design Phase

Designing or redesigning processes in order to better meet customer needs is vital to business adaptability. Over 60% of all U.S. hospitals are involved in reengineering activities and billions of dollars are being spent in the name of reengineering (Walston & Kimberly, 1997). The professional character of healthcare providers has profound implications for how a systems analyst must proceed to analyze and design a system to support the organization. Whoever is involved in information systems (IS) development in healthcare has to nurture *collective participation* (Wetzel, 2001). Decisions cannot be made:

- Solely by a centralized administration, nor
- Based upon detailed in-house knowledge provided by a large techno-structure

Neither the administration nor the techno-structure possesses the required power, work resources, or available knowledge of organizational processes.

The low motivation among professionals to participate in collective efforts may also aggravate the situation. IS improvements are often perceived not to be in the interest of the professional. In some cases the benefits that IS implementation may bring the entire organization may reduce resources to certain individual units that will then resist the implementation. IS development projects may need to permanently sell the project to different units in the organization. The recognition of subtle *power plays* and existing alliances between various hospital units assumes a greater role in healthcare systems design and implementation than in organizations where well-defined teams have strong authority over IS development.

IS development has to set *priorities* concerning which part or aspect of the organization should receive primary support and how this decision effects or influences other types of activities. Simple issues concerning how computers could be employed without disturbing sensitive conversations or how teams will share computers deserve careful consideration and are part of the design effort.

Interdepartmental cooperation is critical in hospitals. The cooperation is highly regulated and at the same time unique to each hospital. The systems analyst must appreciate this complexity.

A Failed Design Case

The management of a local hospital in a rural community in the United States initiated the acquisition of a hospital-wide *order processing system* (Huynh & Angihothri, 2000). This system is to communicate and process orders primarily from doctors. These orders are patient related and include tests, x-rays, and medications. At present, a paper-based order processing system is used, as in many hospitals. To start the project, the hospital organized a committee with the president, chief information officer, the manager of nursing, a resident, a laboratory system coordinator, and a radiology coordinator. The wide range of needs from various departments, the diversity of orders, and the different order handling procedures all needed to be addressed.

Given time and resource constraints, the *preliminary study* was limited to the West Wing of the hospital. The West Wing was the largest and most active of the wings of the hospital, and its requirements were perceived to be in common with those of the rest of the hospital. First the processes existing were carefully documented. The West Wing specializes in heart patients, and has 40 nurses and 35 beds. The floor manager, nurses, and unit clerks were interviewed about the order processing system, and work at the reception center was observed. Two other departments that would receive orders and return values were also studied. Those departments had various needs as regards online notification and message content. Surveys of staff were circulated.

Next, a flowchart was developed to indicate the flow of information and what happened to the information. Data was collected and manually run through the *flowchart* to confirm its validity. The hospital processed an average of 95,000 orders per month and 25% of these came from the West Wing. Interviews were again done with staff with the flowcharts in hand to register their feedback.

According to the original plan, the next step was to be a second phase of data collection and revisions to the design. At this stage, however, a *restructuring* in management took its toll on the project. Top management became involved in other projects and did not give adequate support to this effort. Senior management did not convey the re-engineering message to the staff in a continuing way.

The intended users of the proposed system had not bought into the plans. Many of the hospital staff were not familiar with the plan to automate order entry and were not necessarily supportive of changes. The actual intended users of the system, principally physicians and nurses, were little involved in the requirements and design generation process. There was *poor response rate* from doctors to the surveys that were circulated. In fact, only one doctor replied to the survey. The radiology department noted that it did not intend to surrender any of its control over its current radiology system that would, however, be otherwise expected to interface with a new ordering system.

In reflecting on the needs of the hospital, the intention of redoing order processing in one sweep throughout the hospital was naïve. The logic of ordering is complex in the working hospital and connected to numerous existing systems, which cannot be readily removed. The cost/benefit analyses need to be carefully considered in advance, and the management and staff need to share a *vision* of where they want the hospital to go.

Successful Design

A *successful approach* to system design is illustrated next. The approach is for the acquisition of a hospital information system for a small acute care hospital with 230 beds and 560 employees. The project was embedded in the organizational development of the hospital and had participation from all departments: internal medicine, surgery, anesthesiology, nursing, administration, and technical. The new system was successfully acquired and then worked in several parts of the hospital beginning with patient administration.

Three generic needs of the design team can be sketched as follows (Krabbel et al., 1996):

- Designers need to understand the relationships and interdependencies among activities. Each activity concerns the individual accomplishing a task and the organization assuring that the performance of the task meets diverse organizational requirements. For instance, a patient may want to stay in the hospital another night, and the healthcare provider may feel this is justified based on the patient's personal situation. However, the organization may want to consider whether the insurance will cover another night. These dual concerns of the individual and the organization require the designer to continually interact with users in providing first one (the individual) view and then another (the organization) view.
- The heterogeneity of user groups requires consideration of competing interests. The designers have to fight against narrowed perspectives and, at the same time, endlessly attempt to motivate an integrated solution against possible

disadvantages for the individual units—this requires an ongoing negotiation process.

- Since healthcare organizations often have little professional focus on organizational development, designers may have to initiate infrastructure developments.

The three factors relate to current and future work practices. These practices need to be understood by the design team and communicated with the staff of the hospital.

The patient puts high demands on the information processing requirements and design of hospital information systems:

- A patient requires different specialists and their coordination
- His condition changes and necessitates changes in planned actions
- He moves from place to place, but staff need the ability to locate him
- The patient may need attention any moment of the night or day

This patient situation requires fluidity in the behavior of the staff. Again, an emphasis on current and future *workflow* is vital to successful design.

Cooperation Pictures

The starting point for the analysis of current work practices is the use of qualitative interviews at workplaces. Interview partners are chosen following the concept of a functional role. The choice of actual person to be interviewed in each role should be made by the hospital. The interviews are performed in serial by small developer teams. The main focus lies on the learning and communication processes and not in the complete registering of each activity. The interviews must be held at the actual workplace to get an impression of the environment. *Scenarios* are used to represent the results of the interview. The beginning of a scenario is illustrated as follows:

- At least one nurse accompanies the physician during the daily ward round.
- The ward round takes place every morning. Each patient is visited. The nurse is responsible for carrying the patient record files.
- The physician gives orders for examinations, for changing the medicine, and the treatment and writes them down on the ward round form.
- After the ward round, the nurse transfers the examination orders to order forms, changes in medicine to the chart...

Through these scenarios analysts quickly gain an understanding of the context and task performance in the workplaces.

Pictures promote the understanding, illustration, and feedback of the current work practices of joint ventures. The transfer of information and objects of work may be visualized. *Pictures* may represent:

- Places between which information and objects are exchanged
- The kind of exchange in the shape of annotated arrows
- Errands to be performed by staff and how patients make their way to different units

In a picture for the admissions process there are:

- Six entities making phone calls to the admissions office
- Computer records sent to administration
- Paper records sent to the nursing unit
- The patient sent to the nursing unit
- Paper records sent to medical records and retrieved from medical records

The picture (see *Figure 2.2*) also shows other entities and activities.

The *Cooperation picture* distinguishes between places outside and inside the hospital and certain roles, like a chief physician. Annotated arrows represent cooperation. In the hospital context the delivery of documents by the hospital staff, phone calls, data exchange via computer, and the patient making his way to the different units of the hospital are distinguished (see *Figure 2.3*). The arrows are annotated by pictograms indicating these different kinds of cooperation. A more detailed picture could focus on the process of an X-ray examination, where numbers are added to the arrows to indicate work sequences for a typical case. The focus in this analysis lies on the purpose of cooperation, since this is the more stable factor compared to the how of cooperation, which might change.

The cooperation pictures illustrate which errands have to be made by the hospital staff and how the patient makes his or her way to the different units of the hospital. They *objectify the cooperation* through "places" and annotated arrows. This contrasts with the popular means of representing information systems in which merely abstract information passing is described.

In many workshop sessions, Wetzel (2001) found that cooperation pictures were very useful in initiating *active participation* of the heterogeneous groups in elaborating, discussing and sharing their activities. Cooperation pictures supply an ap-

Figure 2.2. Cooperation Picture: After admission of a patient in the hospital domain. The flow of information between the nursing unit and x-ray and laboratory is depicted by the arrows. The boxes represent units within the hospital. Adapted from Krabbel, Wetzel, and Ratuski (1996).

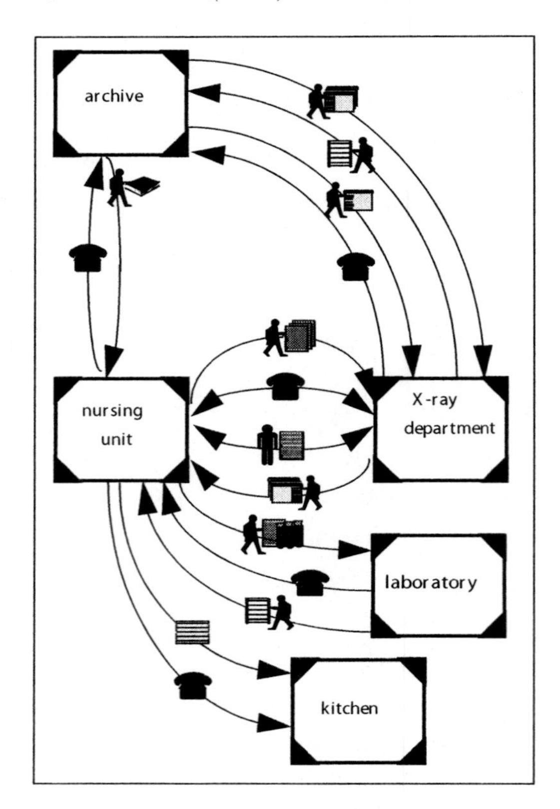

Figure 2.3. Symbols. Selected symbols and icons for Cooperation Pictures are indicated here. Patients and staff are differentiated in combination with different objects like the patient record and the X-ray bag. Adapted from Krabbel, Wetzel, and Ratuski (1996).

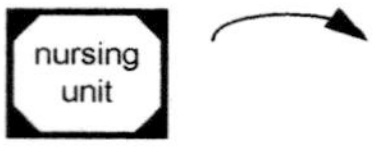 nursing unit	Symbols for organizational units and information transmission
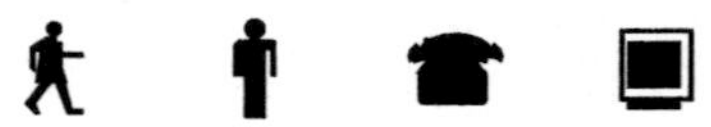	Icons for employee, patient, phone, computer
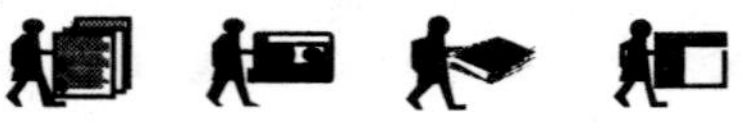	Icons for employee with documents, tape, patient record, X-ray bag

propriate subject of discussion, which put users directly into the position to reflect together about their own organization. Users were able to elaborate on the picture and provide reasons for particular tasks. All workshop participants were surprised that within a regular admission of one patient, seventeen phone calls are made. Immediately, a discussion ensued about how to improve the process. For many users, the picture manifested for the first time that their work does not consist in caring for a patient only but that a significant portion includes tasks for cooperation and documentation purposes.

Tables supplement pictures by providing more detailed information at selected areas. They add information by naming the objects at the arrows in the picture and by describing the purpose or implications of individual activities (see *Table 2.1*).

The Kernel

Systems in the market sometimes neglect the cooperative parts of the task and only note the requirement, such as "registration of the x-ray order." Those systems may presume the physician performs the order entirely. Thus, the physician writes a note to himself about what patients should have x-rays, goes to the computer, and makes the required entries. The information for the nurse and others would thus be missing, and the physician would be doing more work than normal. The computer system must respect not only the accomplishment of the basic task of ordering the test but also of *coordinating* the work among the members of the health care team.

Parallel to the analysis of current work practices, a *task-oriented design* of functions needs to be ongoing. The complexity of the HIS necessitates agreement about the subdivision of tasks. For reducing complexity and supporting negotiation, a document called the Kernel System and another called Systems Stages, are introduced.

For a HIS the content of the *kernel* is debatable. From the organizational point of view, the kernel should support tasks of key units that show a high cooperation profile. It must satisfy urgent needs of the organization and supply a basic and uniform infrastructure. For the case study here, the kernel included patient administration and billing, admission/discharge/transfer, procedure codes, and communication.

Table 2.1. Purpose table

Single Activities	Purpose
Nurse carries the order to the radiology department.	Radiology department can schedule the test.
Radiology technician phones ward to confirm date for patient to be brought to radiology.	The patient schedule is coordinated between the ward and radiology.

These were connected to non-kernel systems, including surgery, radiology, laboratory, medical records, dietetics, and administration.

Each user group has its own profession and perspective. These groups compete and are able to varying degrees to exert their will on other groups. Each group wants an optimal solution for its own work, whereas aspects of integration are less important. Additionally, each group may want to be autonomous and to be served immediately. If not enough players advocate an integrated solution, then the project will fail. The agreement on the kernel system is a key step in *integration*. A pictorial representation of workflow and of the kernel can help understanding.

The kernel will typically be too large and complex to be readily understood without further explanation and analysis. Accordingly, *system stages* are introduced in which the workflow through the kernel is divided into steps. In the case under study, the stages began with these three steps:

1. Patient administration
2. Admission, transfer, and discharge
3. Nursing workload

These do not need to be done in that sequence but making steps for people to understand the exercising of the kernel facilitates understanding. As systems will be assessed for their suitability, the existence of this step-by-step walk through the kernel can make it easier for staff to test the systems and determine their suitability to the hospital.

Prototype

Two further steps are appropriate in this preparation of the hospital to procure a HIS:

- System visions need to be elaborated
- Prototypes for selected functions built

The *system vision* would give users expectations of what to see in the system. Examples of systems visions for this case study are:

The ward group workplace shows an information area and a working area. The information area provides general guidance without logging into the system. The working area is accessible only after logging into the system and then provides the user with tasks.

Prototypes are operational models of selected aspects of the future system. Prototypes are developed with regard to single tasks, the arrangement of group workplaces, or the design of cooperation tools. The prototypes make concrete the system visions. They allow users to interact with a computer screen and get a realistic sense of how the system might behave for them, although the prototype is not connected to real data or the rest of the hospital activity. The prototypes would show actual screens with dummy patient names and staff names with tasks to do, proper color-coding or whatever else had been deemed important in the scenarios and visions.

Another Success Case

Another *case study* is used to illustrate the complexity of the design process for a HIS. Calgary General Hospital in Calgary, Canada designed a modularized HIS that depended heavily on a kernel containing masterfiles (Ross et al., 1991). A masterfile is an index for large amounts of information on a particular subject. The Calgary masterfile is hierarchical and includes:

- The hospital masterfiles contain information general to the hospital, such as valid financial classes
- The department masterfiles contain information specific to a department, such as telephone number
- The procedure masterfiles contain the most specific information and cover each procedure, test, or diet that patients may receive

At *Calgary General Hospital* there are 800 diagnostic imaging procedures alone. Masterfiles indicate all required entries related to a specific test or procedure. For instance, an entry may specify that "height, weight, and blood pressure are required for the test."

Individuals from different departments in Calgary view the same function performed within the hospital differently. Upper management has the global view. Within departments, staff may have a clear understanding of how their area performs but may be unfamiliar with how those functions support other departments. Since all departments access the masterfiles, all departments should have input into the design of the masterfiles. Calgary also found appropriate the establishment of a *masterfile analyst role* that was filled by a nurse with broad experience of different departments. The work of this role is not finished when the system is implemented but is a permanent position, as the masterfile needs to be maintained across time.

The preparation for acquisition of a system from the marketplace is an enormous task. The hospital should not simply buy a system. The hospital should carefully analyze its own *workflow* and understand what it wants to achieve. Such self-study will be crucial to the use of any purchased system. Even if multiple systems exist that could equally well satisfy the needs of the hospital, the ability to successfully use a system requires careful forethought, training, and planning, all of which are best initiated before the system is purchased rather than afterward.

System Acquisition

System acquisition is the process that occurs from the time the need for a new system is acknowledged until the time a contract for a new system has been signed. The steps of *system acquisition* are essentially the same in healthcare as in any other industry. Those steps are explored in the chapter about vendors. Here, a few healthcare specific features are mentioned.

The first step is to establish a *Project Steering Committee*. In a small physician practice, this committee would include one of the physicians and the office manager. In a large organization, the CIO might chair the steering committee, and the committee should include representatives from those groups most to be effected by the intended system.

The steering committee defines the project objectives and the system objectives. For instance, *project objectives* in acquisition of a billing system might be to become familiar with what the market has to offer and to identify five vendors that seem promising. *System objectives* might be to be able to transmit electronic bills to all health plans semi-automatically upon the completion of each patient visit. The steering committee should prepare a schedule for meeting these project objectives and detail the system requirements. Both steps may benefit from consultation with system acquisition experts or with colleagues who have been through a similar experience.

The next step is to identify vendors that seem reputable and expert in the domain for which a system is sought. To get information about the vendor field, the steering committee might turn to an *outside research source*, such as KLAS. KLAS (www.healthcomputing.com) measures and reports on vendor performance and is devoted exclusively to healthcare information technology vendors. Alternately, someone from the steering committee might attend a Health Information and Management Systems Society Annual Conference at which approximately 1,000 vendors exhibit their strengths.

At the next step, the entity may either send a:

- *Request for information (RFI)* or
- *Request for proposals (RFP)*

to the vendors. The RFI is designed to obtain basic information on the vendor's products, services, and cost guidelines. The RFP by contrast provides the vendor with a comprehensive list of system requirements and asks the vendor the cost it would charge to meet all the requirements. If an entity does first a RFI, it might subsequently prepare and send a RFP to those vendors whose responses to the RFI were best. If the system is small and the response to the RFI somehow convincing, the entity might chose to skip the RFP phase.

After receiving replies to an RFP, the entity will evaluate each proposal against a set of criteria. Site visits and reference checks may also be in order. A *cost-benefit analysis* will be done to consider not only the upfront costs but also the maintenance costs and to quantify the expected lifetime benefits. The entity will then enter negotiations with the vendor providing the RFP with the lowest cost-to-benefit ratio.

Implement

Implementing a system means different things to a software house than to a small hospital. On the one hand, for a software engineering firm to implement a design means to write the code to follow the design. On the other hand, for a healthcare entity, implementation typically means to deploy software from a software vendor. *Implementation* is addressed here in the sense of deployment. For the deployment of a healthcare information system to succeed typically requires standardizing workflow and data (with sensitivity to variability among settings), long-term training, and managing expectations (DeVault, 2004). After an explanation of these phases, a case study is given.

Standardization

An enterprise system will have many parameters that have to be set at deployment time, and these often relate to the *standardization* of workflow and data. While one might imagine that these issues of workflow and data would have been completely covered in the design or acquisition phase of the project, in fact, much remains to be done at the time of deployment.

To standardize *workflow* means that, for similar roles in different parts of the entity, that similar tasks in a similar sequence with similar tools are used. This will make it easier to tailor the system to the entity because the amount of variability in the same role will be limited. Additionally, such workflow standardization may help the organization work towards best practices in its role specifications.

Data representation determines how data is stored and how it can be subsequently retrieved and compared. For instance, if a laboratory urine analysis is stored in one way by one hospital laboratory but in a different way by another laboratory in the same hospital, then the hospital will face some extra effort not only in deploying the system but also in maintaining and effectively using the system. Comparing data across the two laboratory urinalysis values will be complicated. Standard vocabularies are available for some data elements, such as the International Classification of Diseases for disease categories, but at the time of deployment substantial data standardization effort may be required.

While standardization offers numerous advantages, some *variability* is also critical. The difference between doctors' private practices and their hospital activity is a case in point. A physician office visit typically follows a linear workflow in which the patient arrives, registers, sees the nurse, sees the doctor, a treatment is provided, notes are made, and the patient leaves. In the hospital setting, this workflow will involve many more people involved in parallel activities: the hospital patient may see several doctors; a doctor may see the hospital patient but not engage in a treatment action; and so on.

While respecting this diversity, the system implementers want to find occasions to bring commonality into the implementation both for the expedience of the software tuning efforts but more importantly for the smoothness of adoption of the system by users. An example of how *commonality* can be found involves the notion of making rounds. Making rounds is defined in the dictionary as going from place to place, as on business or for entertainment. Examples from a dictionary are a delivery truck making the rounds or students going the rounds in the entertainment district. For a doctor to *make rounds*, the doctor takes care of each and every one of his or her patients who has current needs. This rounding exercise is different in the hospital than in the private office. A doctor in the hospital may at times be able to do rounds in which information about a patient is collected for the doctor, the doctor visits the patient, the doctor makes an assessment and plan, and then proceeds to the next patient to repeat those steps. The information system that supports rounding has provided for the doctor in the hospital situation something like what the doctor experiences in the private practice situation. While the doctor in the hospital might be doing rounds, the information system might provide an interface and functionality that simulated the doing of rounds, and thus create a commonality for the application across the settings of the private practice and the hospital.

Training

Training is vital to successful deployment. If the users are not made comfortable with how to use the newly deployed system, the system will not be used. Training costs may be substantial, and the training program must be multifaceted.

The private practice setting is more predictable than the hospital setting. Thus, the training in the private practice setting is less difficult. For the *hospital setting*, a sophisticated program may be needed to assure that the multiple shifts of professionals are trained in a way that allows the system to be adequately used. For an enterprise-wide system in a hospital, one approach is to train clinical users in the first week on the basics of using the system for patient care, such as navigating the system, entering basic information about the patient (charting), and reviewing results from the laboratory tests. In the second week, those users might be taught how to place orders and enter diagnoses, and in the third week, advanced functionality would be taught.

The *scope* of the training must be narrowed to the basics at the beginning. Standardization in workflow or data should reduce the complexity of the training problem. The mode of delivery of training would include classroom, online, and one-on-one.

Managing Expectations

What will (and will not) be accomplished in the initial phases of system implementation should be clearly delineated and communicated. This definition sets the *expectations* of the users. If the expectations are too low, then users will doubt the value of the effort. If the expectations are too high, then users will become frustrated after they realize that the reality differs from the expectation.

The *shortcomings* of the system must be honestly shared with the users, as well as the strengths. For instance, computerized physician order entry (CPOE) will typically take more time of physicians in entering orders then the physicians needed to spend previously in their paper-based approach. However, CPOE has many benefits for the patients and the rest of the healthcare system, and the physician users should be told these pros and cons of CPOE.

Managing expectations and scope go hand-in-hand. The initial expectations should be modest, and the initial scope of implementation should be modest. As the implementation proceeds, the *expectations and scope* can broaden.

Case Study

While the broad, enterprise issues have been delineated in the preceding subsections and appropriately emphasized standardization, training, and expectations, implementations also have down-to-earth technical challenges. The following case study illustrates such challenges along with the importance of training. The implementation of Cerner's *Pharmnet System* in Metro Health Systems of Cleveland, Ohio is the subject of this case (Unfricht & Enderle, 2000).

The Pharmnet application supports the *Pharmacy* and is a three-tiered architecture with a graphical user interface, Cerner middleware, and an Oracle database backend. Through the interface, pharmacy and information system staff can display patient and medication information and enter medication orders. Servers were installed in the pharmacy to run both the backend and the middleware.

A *Cerner engineer* delivered a three-day course to hospital analysts on how Pharmnet works. The Cerner engineer also installed the system. The complexity of the system necessitated that the hospital employ a systems analyst, an Oracle database administrator, an operating system administrator, and a network administrator. Without these in-house specialists, the hospital would have needed a contract with someone else (such as Cerner) to provide such services. The Cerner-supplied engineer did work with the hospital database administrator to try to ensure that no tables or data files would overflow. In particular, the database must be able to accommodate information from the hospital about admits and discharges of patients, as well as medication orders.

When the system went live, the *database* was quickly overwhelmed. This was secondary to a larger than expected drug ordering volume. Also, the admission and discharge data from the hospital contained more unnecessary information than was anticipated. Before the implementation could proceed, the engineers need to develop various methods to filter the admission and discharge data so that the Pharmnet application would not crash. The database administrator proved less prepared and available than had been expected and other staff members needed to contribute in order to make the implementation succeed. Additionally, the hospital needed to buy additional disks for the pharmacy computers to accommodate the size of the database.

After one month with the Cerner engineer full-time on site at Metro Health Systems, the implementation was stable enough for the Cerner engineer to leave and for Metro Health Systems to maintain the Pharmnet system by itself. The users had become comfortable with the system. *Metro Health Systems* continued a contract with Cerner to provide long-distance support.

Legacy Phase

The hospital information systems that were designed to solve accounting problems are often still operating. They are now *obsolete*. As various departments added their own systems for admissions, radiology, laboratory, emergency room and pharmacy services, they created an electronic Tower of Babel, with none of the systems capable of speaking to one another. The solutions range from starting from scratch with a single supplier to upgrading the legacy software.

A survey of hospitals revealed that most hospital IT staff thought of the system's development life cycle without a legacy phase (Gassert & McDowell, 1995; Wong et al., 1995). The truth is that (Lemaitre et al., 1995): "Legacy systems are crucial for organizations...But they become obsolete with aging...Managing the software life cycle from the requirement phase through the *legacy phase* is a key issue in software engineering."

Each phase of the software life cycle is substantially impacted by a large variety of factors (Beath & Orlikowski, 1994), and as the software process moves into the retirement phase, the complexity of factors that impinge on the process is great and the process tends to leave the domain of the engineer. The cost of the legacy phase needs to be considered from the beginning, and the notion of *whole life costing* is important (Bradley & Dawson, 1999):

Whole life costing refers to the cost of ownership of a product from initial concept until eventual retirement with all cost categories taken into consideration. ... In recent years, the falling cost of computers has lead to increasing use of whole life cost in the marketing and advertising of IT products though there is very little published case study data available.

Retiring a system is difficult and little is known about how to do it.

A search on MEDLINE in 2004 with the phrase "legacy information systems" retrieved over one hundred articles. Some are about designing new systems that integrate fragmented legacy systems (Garde et al., 2003). Others are about *tools* for integrating across legacy applications (Akiyama, 2001), such as separating the back-end of the legacy system from its front-end (O'Kane, 2001) or using standards-based solutions (Hartel & de Coronado, 2002). While new systems or tools may be crucial, understanding how an organization evolves with its information systems is more crucial but is less studied. The following case study emphasizes the experiences of a hospital with an aging system.

Case Study

A legacy, oncology information system for patient care, called the *Oncology Clinical Information System* (OCIS) will be examined. The administrators for OCIS worry that OCIS is outdated and do not know to what extent to invest in software revisions to OCIS or in replacements for OCIS. They are uncertain as to how to assess the utility of a legacy system, and since the workflow of the cancer center is intimately connected to OCIS, the administrators are worried about disruption to workflow.

OCIS was developed in the *1970s* at a major cancer center (hereafter called simply the Cancer Center), and for a quarter century was the dominant information system in the Cancer Center (Enterline et al., 1989). The Cancer Center is itself part of a major hospital, which, in turn, is part of an integrated delivery network. In OCIS's early years, computer systems for comprehensive support of clinical care were novel, and OCIS was a major success. However, maintaining a "home-grown" system is expensive, and in healthcare the trend is towards acquiring commercial systems rather than tailoring in-house systems (Kuhn et al., 2003). The Cancer Center faces pressure to replace OCIS with commercial systems. Issues relevant to the aging of OCIS include:

- Workflow
- Software life cycle
- Legacy systems

and these issues are addressed next.

OCIS was developed to support doctors in *decision-making* by storing and displaying data trends. The initial assessment of OCIS was positive and included:

- People were not required to use OCIS. Yet, the information from the system was widely used, and this voluntary usage attested to the value of OCIS.
- The financial costs and benefits of OCIS compared favorably with other hospital information systems.

Given the technical constraints of the 1980s, output to users was only on paper and professional data coordinators did all data entry.

The *data coordinators* worked with the healthcare providers to ensure that important data was captured and new reports were developed to display that data in the best format. The data coordinator:

- Had a comprehensive knowledge of the capabilities and limitations of the OCIS applications
- Was knowledgeable and experienced in medicine and healthcare delivery

Furthermore, the data coordinators attended daily rounds and were active participants in the care giving team. With this background, the data coordinator was well situated to:

- Enter clinically meaningful data about the patient into OCIS
- Provide reports for the clinicians that took advantage of the best retrieval and formatting capabilities of OCIS
- If OCIS was not currently supporting the type of data retrieval or report that the clinician should have, then the data coordinator worked with the OCIS programming staff to add this functionality

By assuming these responsibilities, the data coordinator eliminated the need for any other member of the clinical team to enter data into OCIS. The physicians and nurses typically operated in a read-only mode.

In successful organizational systems, a "socio-technical" facilitator role is considered vital (Deakin et al., 1994). The *socio-technical facilitator* is knowledgeable in both the human and computer aspects of the organization and works with people to help them take advantage of the computer. The socio-technical facilitator role for OCIS was played by the data coordinator.

The functionality of OCIS did not much change. However, positive comments about the utility and cost-effectiveness of OCIS that were apparent in the old days are missing in the modern days. What has changed markedly is the role of the data coordinator. The data coordinator no longer does rounds with the physicians and is not expected to have any medical training. A data coordinator with the outpatient unit spends most of her day typing laboratory values from outside laboratories into OCIS. The data coordinators are no longer socio-technical facilitators. The role of the data coordinator became that of a *data entry clerk*.

The diminished socio-technical facilitator role is a problem for OCIS. However, the data coordinator role change was seen by staff as an *irreversible change*. Funding is not available for a new socio-technical facilitator role. Other problems, such as the interface, were seen to be currently more critical.

Interviews with the leaders of the hospital, the Cancer Center, and OCIS revealed that *politics* would determine the future of OCIS. The term "politics" is used here in the sense of (*American Heritage Dictionary of the English Language* (4th ed.), 2000):

- Maneuvering within an organization
- The often conflicting relationships among people

Politics is known to influence decisions about technical issues in many healthcare environments (Keselman et al., 2003).

Stakeholder Matrices

A technologist asked to take the next step with OCIS might:

1. Collect user functional requirements and compare them to the functionality of OCIS
2. Recommend the least expensive system that meets the desired functionality

However, the technologist may be poorly equipped to deal with the subjective nature of the administrative factors that influence the fate of an old, legacy system. A *stakeholder matrix* is needed to help an analyst collect non-technical information about the likely future of an information system.

A stakeholder matrix might be established with two dimensions corresponding to (1) stakeholders and (2) topics. A typical stakeholder matrix (Cavan et al., 1998) might have these:

- **Stakeholders:** Physicians, nurses, ancillary staff, administrators, and system developer
- **Topics:** Direct effects on patient care, impact on the healthcare process, usability, integration (does the system integrate well with other existing systems that must be used around the same time), and cost effectiveness

The preceding stakeholder matrix is traditional and fails to capture some *administrative realities*.

A few studies in requirements engineering reveal the importance of political activities in software development (Bergman et al., 2002):

Large-scale system requirements is constructed through a political decision process, whereby requirements emerge as a set of mappings between consecutive solution spaces justified by a problem space of concern to a set of principals. These solution spaces are complex socio-technical ensembles that often exhibit non-linear behavior in expansion due to domain complexity and political ambiguity. Stabilization of solutions into agreed on specifications occurs only through the exercise of organizational power.

For the National Aeronautics and Space Administration's *Jet Propulsion Laboratory (JPL),* the development of successful requirements for a large software system required repeated "sense-making" among technical, project, and organizational individuals (Bergman & Mark, 2003). The challenges to successful software requirements development apply also to the retirement phase of the software life cycle. In other words, political concerns and *power struggles* in the organization will be critical for a large, legacy system.

JPL has special characteristics not necessarily present at a health center. In particular, at JPL promotion from the technical to the project level or from the project level to the organizational level requires expertise at the preceding level. In other words, everyone at the project or organizational level was previously a *technical expert.* Such omnipresent technical expertise puts negotiation at a certain common level. However, the project and organizational individuals with influence over the retirement of OCIS are not necessarily technically expert. The absence of a common technical base would put increased reliance on political factors for determining the fate of a software system.

Those who analyze the aging of a legacy information system might benefit from extended stakeholder matrices. Two such matrices are:

- One for non-supervisory staff is designed to collect functional requirements
- One for leaders is designed to support organization-wide decisions about the system

The leader's matrix asks about history, vision, resources, and politics. For roles that perform largely routine tasks or have little or no supervisory responsibility, such as a receptionist, the people filling the roles may tend to have a narrow view of the issues. Questions to them would be largely restricted to topics regarding their own performance of tasks on the system, and the analyst would more or less be soliciting functional requirements (see *Table 2.2*). For *leaders* the questions would be more far reaching and would address for the system (see *Table 2.3*):

Table 2.2. This stakeholder matrix is for collecting functional requirements for a clinical information system. Roles are on the left and questions across the top. The cells of the matrix are completed with the responses of the people in the role.

Roles	Questions		
	What functions do you find helpful?	What functions would you like modified?	What functions would you like added?
Physician			
Nurse			
Ancillary staff			

Table 2.3. This stakeholder matrix has questions for leaders regarding a legacy, clinical information system. Roles are on the left and questions across the top. The cells of the matrix are completed with the responses of the people in the role.

Leaders in	Questions				
	How has the system changed?	What is your vision for the system?	What resources are needed?	What political forces are relevant?	What should be done next?
medicine					
nursing					
health system admin					
ancillary services					
information systems					

- History
- Vision
- Resources
- Administration (or politics)
- Next steps

Historians say that history is subjective (Ragsdale, 2003):

No truth is solid and everything depends on the imagination if not the whim of the observer. History is "constructed," not discovered. At best this means a skeptical relativism, at worst a free hand to subordinate history to political agendas.

Accordingly, the analyst should consider historical interpretations from various stakeholders.

Ways to assess an aging system and to decide what should or should not be done with it are little understood. A state-of-the-art system might *evolve* through software modifications to an existing, legacy system or through the death of a legacy system and the acquisition of new systems. Vision and politics play an important role in shaping decisions about whether to modify or replace a legacy system.

Questions

Reading Questions

1. Compare and contrast the design approaches in the sections "A Failed Design Case" and "Successful Design."
2. How were pictures and purpose tables used in the success case and why did they help?

Doing Questions

1. Try to identify someone or find information somewhere that provides further information about an analysis and design case for a healthcare information system. Describe how that case was done and compare and contrast to the cases described in this chapter.
2. Consider that you are to design a Web-enabled information system to connect you and your primary doctor's practice. This is not the design of an interface for the patient but also an information system that works with the doctor's office. Consider in your design what the people in the office need to do to maintain their side of the deal.

Enlightened by the analysis and design method of Krabbel, Wetzel, and Ratuski (1996) you must demonstrate a

1. Scenario
2. Cooperation picture
3. Purpose table

for your system. For the cooperation picture obtain your own symbols and provide a table explaining what symbols mean what. You can do this by choosing from clip art widely available. A handful of icons or symbols is enough for the symbol table. The cooperation picture does not need to depict the entire scenario but rather to indicate your understanding of the significance of a cooperation picture. A few icons and labeled arrows is enough. The purpose table needs only to describe what you put in the cooperation picture.

References

Akiyama, M. (2001). Migration of the Japanese healthcare enterprise from a financial to integrated management: Strategy and architecture. *Medinfo, 10*(1), 715-718.

American Heritage Dictionary of the English Language (4th ed.). (2000). Boston: Houghton Mifflin Company.

Beath, C., & Orlikowski, W. (1994). The contradictory structure of systems development methodologies: Deconstructing the IS-user relationship in information engineering. *Information Systems Research, 5*(4), 350-377.

Bergman, M., King, J., & Lyytinen, K. (2002). Large scale requirements analysis revisited: The need for understanding the political ecology of requirements engineering. *Requirements Engineering Journal, 7*, 152-171.

Bergman, M., & Mark, G. (2003). In situ requirements analysis: A deeper examination of the relationship between requirements formation and project selection. In *11th IEEE International Conference on Requirements Engineering* (pp. 1-12). Monterey Bay, CA: IEEE.

Bradley, M., & Dawson, R. (1999). Whole life cost: The future trend in software development. *Software Quality Journal, 8*(2), 121-131.

Cavan, D., et al. (1998). Preliminary experience of the DIAS computer model in providing insulin dose advice to patients with insulin dependent diabetes. *Computer Methods Programs Biomedicine, 56*(2), 157-164.

Deakin, A., Gouma, P.-I., & Rada, R. (1994). The plan-facilitator and the plan-document: A new aspect of computer supported management. *Journal of Intelligent Systems, 4*(1-2), 83-111.

DeVault, P. (2004). Adopting an enterprise health care automation and information system: The initial implementation. *The Permanente Journal, 8*(4), 39-42.

Enterline, J., Lenhard, R., & Blum, B. (Eds.). (1989). *A clinical information system for oncology*. New York: Springer-Verlag.

Garde, S., Knaup, P., & Herold, R. (2003). Qumquad: A UML-based approach for remodeling of legacy systems in health care. *International Journal of Medical Informatics, 70*(2-3), 183-194.

Gassert, C., & McDowell, D. (1995). Evaluating graduate and undergraduate nursing students' computer skills to determine the need to continue teaching computer literacy. In R. Greenes, H. Peterson, & D. Protti (Eds.), *8th World Congress on Medical Informatics. MEDINFO 95* (pp. 1370). Vancouver: North Holland.

Hartel, F., & de Coronado, S. (2002). Information standards within the National Cancer Institute. In J. Silva, M. Ball, C. Chute, J. Douglas, C. Langlotz, J. Niland, & W. Sherlis (Eds.), *Cancer informatics: Essential technologies for clinical trials* (pp. 135-156). New York: Springer.

Heathfield, H., et al. (1997). Evaluating large scale health information systems: From practice towards theory. *AMIA Annual Fall Symposium* (pp. 116-120).

Huynh, M., & Angihothri, S. (2000). Healthcare process redesign: A case study. In A. Armoni (Ed.), *Healthcare information systems: Challenges of the new millennium* (pp. 27-49). Hershey, PA: Idea Group Publishing.

Keselman, A., Patel, V.L., Johnson, T.R., & Zhang, J. (2003). Institutional decision-making to select patient care devices: Identifying venues to promote patient safety. *Journal of Biomedical Informatics, 36*, 31-44.

Krabbel, A., Wetzel, I., & Ratuski, S. (1996). Participation of heterogeneous user groups: Providing an integrated hospital information system. In J. Blomberg, F. Kensing, & E. Dykstra-Erickson (Eds.), *PDC'96: The Fourth Biennial Conference on Participatory Design* (pp. 241-249). Cambridge, MA.

Kuhn, K., Giuse, D., & Haux, R. (2003). IMIA Working Conference on Health Information Systems 2002 in Heidelberg--practical HIS experiences. *Methods of Information in Medicine, 42*(1), vi-viii.

Lemaitre, D., Sauquet, D., Fofol, I., Tanguy, L., Jean, F., & Degoulet, P. (1995). Legacy systems: Managing evolution through integration in a distributed and object-oriented computing environment. In *Annual Symposium Computer Applications Medical Care* (pp. 132-136).

O'Kane, K. (2001). Migration of legacy mumps applications to relational database servers. *Methods of Information in Medicine, 40*(3), 225-228.

Rada, R., & Moore, J. (1997). Sharing standards: Software reuse. *Communications of the ACM, 40*(3), 19-23.

Ragsdale, H. (2003). Comparative historiography of the social history of revolutions: English, French, and Russian. *Journal of the Historical Society, 3*(3-4), 323-372.

Ross, S., Gore, M., Radulski, W., Warnock-Matheron, A., & Hanna, K. (1991). Nursing's role in defining systems. In M. Ball (Ed.), *Healthcare information management systems* (pp. 114-124). New York: Springer Verlag.

Unfricht, D., & Enderle, J. (2000). Automating the pharmacy: Implementing Cerner's Millennium PharmnetSystem. In *IEEE 26th Annual Northeast Bioengineering Conference* (pp. 59-60) Storrs, CT: IEEE.

Walston, S.L., & Kimberly, J.R. (1997). Reengineering hospitals: Evidence from the field. *Hospitals and Health Services Administration, 42*(2), 143-163.

Wetzel, I. (2001). Information systems development with anticipation of change focusing on professional bureaucracies. In *Hawai'i International Conference on System Sciences, HICCS-34* (pp. 10). Maui, HI: IEEE.

Wong, B., Sellaro, C., & Monaco, J. (1995). Information systems analysis approach in hospitals: A national survey. *Health Care Supervisor, 13*(3), 58-64.

Chapter III

Providers

Learning Objectives

- Distinguish the types of healthcare systems serving middle-class families, poor families, and military personnel
- Diagram the major components of a hospital information system and indicate at least two subcomponents of each
- Describe the flow of information in patient management
- Demonstrate how characteristics of patient information peculiar to a clinical unit, such as radiology, lead to unique characteristics of the information system underlying that system
- Compare a typical suite of offerings from a major healthcare information systems vendor to the functionalities that a healthcare provider needs
- Distinguish the software needs of a small group practice from those of a large hospital

The official definition of a *healthcare provider* is broad. It encompasses institutional providers such as hospitals, nursing facilities, home health agencies, outpatient facilities, clinical laboratories, various licensed healthcare practitioners, and durable medical equipment suppliers. Any individual or organization that is paid to provide healthcare services is a healthcare provider.

Populations

Understanding the healthcare industry in the United States is vital to understanding how information systems serve that industry. In particular, healthcare for middle-income families, poor families, members of the military, and veterans is provided by very different healthcare systems, which, in turn, will have different information systems needs. There is not any single "*American healthcare system*." There are many separate subsystems serving different populations in different ways. Sometimes they overlap; sometimes they are entirely separate from one another.

Four subsystems of healthcare in the U.S. address four different subpopulations. These subpopulations are (Torrens & Williams, 1993):

- Regularly employed, middle-income families with continuous programs of healthcare insurance
- Poor, unemployed or underemployed families without continuous health insurance coverage
- Active-duty military personnel and their dependents
- Veterans of U.S. military service

An endless set of variations is possible from different combinations of these four. Additionally, the diverse types of healthcare systems in the United States relative to the populations that they serve will be outlined.

Middle-Income Families

The most striking feature of the *employed, middle-income system* of care is the absence of any formal system. Each family puts together an informal set of services and facilities to meet its need. The service aspects of the system focus on physicians in private practice. The system is financed by nongovernmental funds.

For public health needs the family benefits from the services of *public health departments* for services like sewage disposal. Those public health services that target the individual, such as vaccinations, have to be arranged by the family through the family physician.

Ambulatory patient services are also obtained from *private physicians*. When laboratory tests are ordered or medications prescribed, private for-profit laboratories or pharmacies are used. Typically the patient pays some of the cost of these services out-of-pocket.

Inpatient hospital services are usually provided by a local *community hospital* that is usually voluntary and nonprofit. The specific hospital to be used is determined by the physician. Long-term care is most likely obtained at home through the assistance of a visiting nurse. If institutional long-term care is needed, it is probably obtained in a for-profit nursing home.

When emotional problems are confronted, first private services via the physician are utilized. If hospitalization is required, it might first be in the psychiatric section of the local hospital. In those cases in which very extended institutional care is required and the patient's financial resources are relatively limited, the family may request hospitalization in the *state mental hospital* (the U.S. has about 300 state mental hospitals). This event usually represents the first use of government health programs by the middle-income family and frequently shocks the family for the style of care provided.

The patient has considerable latitude in this system. On the other hand, the system of care is poorly linked. The system can be very *wasteful of resources* and usually has no central control or monitor to determine whether it is accomplishing what it should. One approach to providing further system coordination has been through health maintenance organizations (HMOs) that contract to provide an organized package of health services in an integrated and intentionally coordinated program.

Poor Families

If it was important to study the system of healthcare for middle-income families because it represents the "best" of American medicine, then to study the system of healthcare for underemployed or *poor families* is important, for it represents the "worst" of American medicine. Again, there is no formal system per se and the family must put together what services it can. However, the poor do not have the resources to choose where and how they obtain their health services. The great majority of services are provided by local government agencies, such as the county hospital. The patients have no continuity of service as the middle class family has from its family doctor.

When a poor family's newborn baby needs its vaccination, the family goes to the district health center of the health department, not to a private physician. To obtain ambulatory services, the poor family frequently turns to the *emergency room* of the county hospital. The county hospital is the analogue to the "family physician" for the poor. The emergency room serves as the port of entry to the rest of the health system. To gain admission to the county hospital clinics, the poor typically first go to the emergency room and then get referred to the clinic.

When the poor need inpatient hospital services, they again turn first to the emergency room of the *county hospital,* which refers them. The teaching hospitals associated with medical schools also often have wards that are free for the poor, and the poor may go to the emergency rooms of these facilities to get referred to these wards.

The long-term care of the poor begins usually with extended stays in the county hospital. This is not by design but because the hospital is reluctant to discharge them when no responsible other care seems available. For nursing home type care, the major difference between the middle income and poor families is that some government program, such as Medicaid, usually covers the long-term care of the poor.

Military

Military personnel enjoy a well-organized system of healthcare at no cost. The military health system goes where active-duty military personnel go, and assumes responsibility for total care that is unique among American healthcare systems. No initiative is required by the individual to start the system. For instance, vaccinations on induction into the service are mandatory. The system emphasizes keeping people well. Great stress is placed on preventive measures, such as vaccinations, regular physical examinations, and education. Unlike any other healthcare system in the U.S., the military health system provides healthcare and not just sickness care.

Routine ambulatory care is usually provided by *medical corpsmen* in a dispensary, sickbay, first aid station, or similar unit that is very close to the military personnel's actual place of work. These same medical corpsmen are responsible for the preventive and education aspects of the care and physicians or nurses typically supervise them. For hospital services the person is referred to a small base hospital, but if the problem requires more specialized attention, then the patient is referred to a military regional hospital. These regional hospitals offer extensive, state-of-the-art services. For long-term psychiatric problems, the patient is probably given a medical discharge.

In general, the military medical system is closely organized and highly integrated. A single patient record is used, and the complete record moves from one healthcare service to another with the patient. When the need for care is identified, the system arranges for the patient to receive the care and provides any necessary transportation. The system is *centrally planned*, uses non-medical and non-nursing personnel to the utmost, and is entirely self-contained. Generally, the patient has little choice regarding the manner in which services will be delivered, but this drawback is counterbalanced by the assurance that high-quality services will be available when needed.

Dependents and families of active-duty military personnel have access to the regular military healthcare system services when such services are not fully utilized by the active duty personnel. In addition, the military provides health insurance to the dependents through its *Civilian Health and Medical Program of the Uniformed*

Services (CHAMPUS). CHAMPUS is provided, financed, and supervised by the military, but dependents access care in the same way that other middle-class families would access it from private facilities.

Veterans Administration

Parallel to the system of care for active duty military is another system, the *Veterans Administration Health Care System*, operated within the continental U.S. for retired, disabled, or otherwise deserving veterans of previous military service. This VA system focuses on hospital care, mental health services, and long-term care. It operates close to 200 hospitals and more than 200 outpatient clinics.

Patients typically also have a variety of other social services and benefits outside those provided by the VA Health Care System. A further feature of the system is its unique relationship with organized consumer groups in the form of local and national veterans' clubs and associations. In no other healthcare system in this country does organized consumer interest play such a constant, important, and influential role.

Admission to the *VA hospitals* can be gained through its ambulatory patient care services or via referral from physicians in private practice. Salaried, full-time medical and nursing personnel provide the services in VA hospitals. The VA system is the largest single provider of healthcare services in the U.S.

Without an understanding of the interaction among these four major components (the middle-income, poor, military, and VA) of the American healthcare system, one cannot design appropriate information systems to serve an integrated healthcare system. Additionally, the competition among the four subsystems of healthcare creates unfortunate patterns of usage. Although the four systems are separate from one another, they all *compete* for the same resources since they are all dependent on the same economy and the same supplies of health personnel. This competition tends to mean that the services for the underemployed get the smallest share of the resource pie. The competition for resources also creates some waste. For example, in the same region, a county hospital, a teaching hospital, a military hospital, and a VA hospital may all be operating exactly the same kind of expensive service, although only one facility might be needed. Because each institution is part of a separate system, serves a different population, and approaches the resource pool through a different channel, no purposeful planning or controlled allocation of resources is possible.

Components

The major structural components in a typical large healthcare information system, such as hospital information systems, are:

- Administrative systems
- Clinical support systems
- Patient management systems

Administrative systems include accounting, finance, and strategic systems. Clinical support systems include pathology laboratory, pharmacy, and radiology. Patient management includes admission/registration, medical records, and order entry.

Functional analysis helps to define what the information system is to do. Structures, on the other hand, are prerequisites for effective function. Functional analysis shows that the patient is first examined, then procedures are ordered or treatments initiated, followed by reporting on these efforts. Care management includes accounting

Figure 3.1. Functions of Patient Management. The waterfall of actions from patient care management to communications with external parties is matched by a feedback loop (Adapted from Smith, 2000).

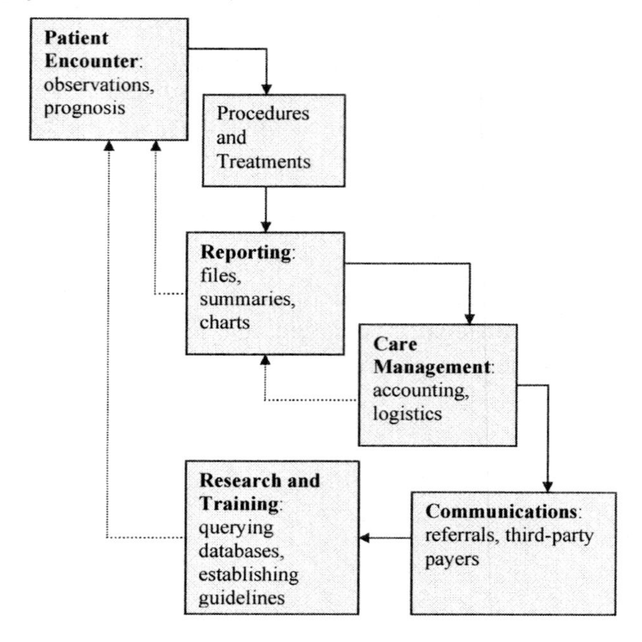

and other administrative functions. Research and training may occur relative to the collected information and feed into the next round of patient management (see *Figure 3.1*).

The migration of patients from inpatient to outpatient settings necessitates new functions in the outpatient section. *Outpatient systems* assist with appointment scheduling, registration, medical records, insurance eligibility, service pricing, and billing and collections. These features are reflected in the core functions of the systems in larger provider organizations. The outpatient management system may also directly connect with a hospital information system so that access to records of a patient and various resources is most direct. Physician offices may have a miniature version of all these systems and also may be connected to hospital systems.

Administrative Systems

The *administrative systems* include patient accounting, scheduling, financial management, and strategic information systems.

Patient Accounting

Patient accounting systems are one of the most popular HIS applications. By the mid-1980s many different accounting systems were in use. The patient and payer accounting application performs the following major tasks (DeLuca & Enmark, 2002):

- Patient service pricing
- Patient billing and insurance claims
- Electronic data interchange
- Receivables management
- Payer logs

Patient service pricing determines the price of a service or checks the price of a service when proposed by another module in the healthcare information system. This pricing determination is a complex function. A wide range of services may be provided for patients in various categories, such as inpatient, outpatient, and emergency room, and the pricing varies with all these factors. Furthermore, diagnostic related groups may be assigned by another module and for some payers will determine the price that can be attached to services for a patient. Additionally, various exclusions and limitations may be required for contracts with various service contractors, and this further complicates the pricing function.

The charges for services must be converted into bills. Different payers have historically expected different formats for the *claims*. Historically, insurance companies, Medicare, Medicaid, intermediaries, employers, guarantors, and patients may each have expected a different format for a bill. The diversity of claims formats has changed with the implementation of the Health Insurance Portability and Accountability Act.

For a given patient, whether inpatient or outpatient, multiple bills may need to be generated to accommodate a range of payers for those services for a single patient. Increasingly claims are submitted electronically and payments also sent electronically. The accounting system would handle this *electronic data interchange*.

Receivables management keeps track of the bills that have been generated and what has not been paid is flagged for a further collection effort. Thus, if a patient is late in paying or has underpaid, then the receivables management subsystem might automatically generate a reminder bill. If a reminder bill is unsuccessful, then the receivables management subsystem may next notify the collectors of the need to pursue the patient.

Payer logs are generated, usually on an annual basis, by the accounting system to facilitate negotiations with payers. If a provider treats many patients of one payer, then the payer may give that provider particularly favorable business conditions.

Scheduling

Enterprise scheduling helps bring disparate organizations together and optimizes resources (Kissinger & Borchardt, 1996). A scheduling system controls the use of services or limited-access resources, such as magnetic resonance imaging (MRI) equipment. Scheduling systems may automate various administrative tasks, such as searching for available slots, maintaining a waiting list, generating medical record pull chart instructions, scheduling recurring appointments, and scheduling multiple resources, such as room, equipment, and staff. A surgery center, for example, may require the ability to block and schedule rooms, equipment, and staff based on predefined requirements. As a first step, a surgery center may allocate rooms based on specialty (see *Figure 3.2*). In this case, specialists from different groups know when they may schedule their patients for procedures in the surgery center. If they do not confirm the room at least 24 hours in advance, the room may be released for rescheduling.

Scheduling systems were developed to serve *niche markets*. Systems developed originally for inpatient facilities may be strong in their ability to support resource

Figure 3.2. Allocate Rooms. Surgery rooms allocated by specialty across weekdays. OR means operating room.

	OR #1	OR #2	OR #3	OR #4
Monday	General Surgery	Orthopedics	Cardiac Surgery	Pediatric Surgery
Tuesday	General Surgery	Orthopedics	Vascular Surgery	Gynecology
Wednesday	General Surgery	Plastic Surgery	Neurosurgery	Urology

scheduling, like an MRI, but may be weak in their ability to schedule services, like a doctor examination. Conversely, scheduling for outpatients may be strong in their ability to support services scheduling but weak in resource scheduling.

To realize the potential of scheduling to help an organization requires either connecting existing systems or replacing them with an enterprise-wide system. Several vendors now offer *enterprise-wide scheduling systems* that they created by expanding on the niche products.

A number of control and operation issues challenge the organization trying to implement a system-wide enterprise scheduling solution. First, most departments are reluctant to allow staff from other facilities to schedule appointments in their facility. This *control problem* must be resolved administratively. Second, the new system will have to offer all the functionality of the previous niche systems, otherwise the niche units will object to the new system. Third, the new system will have to link to both legacy systems and the hospital information system in order that adequate information is available to semi-automatically exploit enterprise-wide scheduling.

An example of the challenge of linking a scheduling system to the *legacy system* follows. St. Agnes Hospital in Fresno, California uses vendor X's hospital information system. St. Agnes has linked X to vendor Y's scheduling application. Requests for appointments are called into a centralized scheduling site where operators schedule the procedures on the Y system. Demographic information is then automatically retrieved from system X. Scheduling results are then routed from Y to X. Scheduling information is maintained on X to provide access to hospital-based users. Furthermore, St. Agnes uses Y's materials management module that links into Y's enterprise-wide scheduling system. With this link, materials are automatically ordered based on the scheduled procedures.

Many *linkages* are possible. Scheduling systems may be linked to transportation systems. Additionally, many tests that must be ordered when certain procedures are scheduled can be automatically put into the order-entry system by the procedure scheduling system. Further integration is possible as staff allocation systems calculate staffing based on procedure schedules. The possibilities are endless.

To facilitate the development of enterprise-wide scheduling, a standards development organization has developed messaging standards for scheduling. The basic structure involves placer, filler, and querying applications. A placer application requests the booking, modification, or cancellation of a schedule; a filler application owns a schedule for services or resources, and a querying application gathers information about a particular schedule. The filler application connects the placer and query applications. Standardizing the format of messages among these applications helps health information systems integrate scheduling.

Financial Management

A *financial management system* includes general accounting and resource management:

- **General accounting** includes payroll and accounts payable that feed into general ledger, which in turn supports budgeting (see *Figure 3.3*). The payroll module tracks hours worked, computes vacation days and tax withholdings, and so on. The module produces the paychecks. The accounts payable module converts a purchase order into a financial obligation and eventually a check to a supplier or vendor.
- **Resource management** includes human resources, maintenance management, and fixed assets management. The human resources module maintains employment history and might be used to link quality control and incident reporting to the individual employee record. The fixed-assets module lists each piece of capital equipment, its physical location, depreciation schedule, current book value, and insured value.

Figure 3.3. General Accounting. This diagram shows the payroll and accounts payable feeding into general ledger and then budgeting.

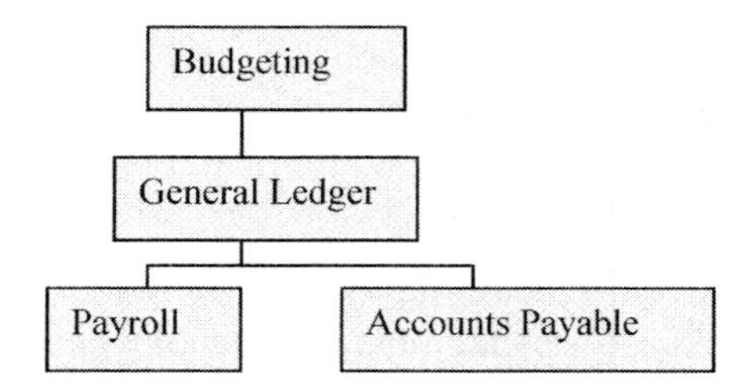

When integrated with the resource management system, the accounts payable system becomes more complex but can provide further services, such as allowing the receiving unit to automatically match the arrival of a purchased item with the purchase order and confirm that what has arrived is indeed what was ordered.

Strategic Information Systems

An organization needs a strategy for achieving its vision. Information systems can provide support in refining and implementing this strategy. Such information systems may be called *strategic information management systems*.

Strategic information management systems may have multiple sub-systems:

- A cost accounting sub-system will collect a large amount of cost data and produce a cost per procedure. From this can be computed such things as cost per case and then per case profitability.
- Case-mix analysis modules analyze the diagnosis distribution of outpatients and inpatients. Reports on utilization aid in analyzing patient trends and physician order patterns. Case-mix systems may typically be part of a patient accounting system.
- Financial modeling systems perform simulations of revenue and expense patterns based on differing assumptions. For example, changes in case mix can be the basis for different revenues and, based on the results of financial modeling, the organization may decide to encourage a shift of patients from inpatient to outpatient.

At the opposite end from strategic information systems are the bread-and-butter tools that staff use, such as *office automation tools*. Office automation provides for centralized calendaring, telephone messaging, and electronic mail. Office automation can help in many routine ways and provide a substantial productivity boost at relatively low risk. Some of the features, such as calendaring, that are supported with office automation might be incorporated in more advanced systems such as workflow management systems. The ability to compose, share, and track messages is important for many communications that occur in the management of the organization but are not directly linked to patient care.

Patient Management

Managing the patient and his record is a complex process. The patient has to be admitted or registered and associated with a unique identifier. Diagnoses should be coded into some standard nomenclature. Orders that are entered should be connected to a billing system and to the medical record system.

Admission

Patient admission is for admitting a patient to a hospital. Admission includes the following functions to:

- Collect enough demographic, clinical, and financial information to supply the patient care, clinical, patient accounting, and medical records applications with data.
- Produce forms that patients must sign, to include admitting forms, consent forms, and insurance benefit assignments.
- Notify housekeeping, security, volunteers, and other departments as room transfers and discharges occur. The midnight census is balanced through this application, and daily room and bed charges are generated.

Registration is similar to admissions but is for registering an outpatient rather than admitting an inpatient.

An admission and registration information system might be a freestanding system. Alternately, the admission and registration functionality might be provided in another package, such as a patient care system or an accounting system. These other systems need the information provided by admission and registration and need to know the structure of that information. If a healthcare organization gets different systems from different vendors, the healthcare organization then needs to decide which admission and registration system to use. Whatever the choice, the healthcare organization then faces the difficult task of *integrating* the systems that may make contrary assumptions about the admitting and registration data.

A vignette of a registration system is presented for a remote laboratory system. The patient goes to the laboratory to have testing done.

The patient first provides either a paper order or a pointer to an electronic order. The order from the physician details the patient demographics, insurance information, tests to be performed, and diagnosis. The nurse or phlebotomist inputs the order or retrieves the electronic data, if the physician placed the order electronically. After the patient name is entered into the registration system, the information is passed to the medical records management system. The medical records management system determines if the patient has a record on file. If so, it compares the data on file to previous records and asks the nurse/phlebotomist to verify anything that may have changed. If this is a new encounter, a medical record number is assigned to the patient and the data is passed back to the registration program. If the patient was found to have previous records, the registration system then passes the patient medical record to the patient account system which verifies that there are no outstanding balances due to rejected claims. If there are outstanding claims, the nurse/phlebotomist is asked to verify the patient's insurance information. At the same time, the patient account system also checks the patient's insurance guidelines to verify that all required information to submit a claim has been provided and to determine if the insurance may deny the claim due to limited coverage or limited frequency. (An insurance company may deny a claim because the diagnosis provided by the ordering physician, according to the insurance company, does not warrant the test or procedure. An insurance company may also deny a claim because the test or procedure may only be performed once over a certain period. For example, Medicare will only pay for a PAP smear once every three years). After resolving any patient account issues, the registration system generates a requisition with accompanying forms, if needed. Finally, the data collected through registration passes to the laboratory system. Regardless of how the order was placed, some state laws require a paper requisition be submitted. (So much for the paperless office!)

The admission or registration process is one of the most crucial in patient management because the identity of the patient is first determined here.

Medical Record

The *medical record* may be seen as a set of attribute-value pairs for a given patient at a given time. For example, an attribute might be heart rate and the value might be 60. The basic medical datum has four elements:

- The patient identifier
- An attribute (for example, heart beat)
- A value of the attribute (for example, 60 beats per minute)
- The time the value of the attribute was collected

Depending on the attribute, the value could be narrative (for example, history of illness), numerical (for example, heart rate), signals (for example, electrocardiogram), or images (for example, chest x-ray). Before the era of instrumented tests, a record did not necessarily contain many test results, but now the record typically includes numerous test values.

The earliest medical records were *time-oriented*. Hippocrates said the medical record should accurately reflect the course of the disease. A record would thus be a list of attribute-value pairs sorted according to when the value was recorded—in other words, chronologically sorted.

Lawrence Weed proposed in the 1960s an alternate structuring of the medical record that focuses on identifying the problems of the patient and the plans to resolve the problems. This is called the *problem-oriented medical record* structure. In the problem-oriented medical record, the notes are recorded for each problem assigned to the patient. Each problem is described according to the patient's complaints, physician's findings, interpretations, and plan. The modern day American medical record is a mixture of the problem-oriented medical record and the time-oriented medical record.

Originally, medical records were *physician-centered* in that a physician knew only the records that he or she maintained. The Mayo Clinic in 1907 began the movement to patient-centered records, in which different Mayo Clinic doctors taking care of the same patient would share the medical record. Generally, in the United States the hospital or clinic that cares for a patient retains the record. The physician tends to consider him or herself to be the owner of the record because he or she created it and only allows the patient to see it under special circumstances. The HIPAA Privacy Rule basically requires healthcare providers to give a patient a copy of his or her medical record anytime the patient requests it.

Electronic medical records offer numerous benefits. Multiple users from remote sites can simultaneously access the same medical record. Different views of a given record can be dynamically generated. For instance, the physician may want to see all the blood glucose values from a half-year period sorted chronologically or might want to see all the laboratory values of a particular day. Decision-support tools can be readily integrated into an electronic medical record. Summary data across patient records can be readily generated.

Historically, managing patient information (collecting information accurately, storing it, retrieving it, and properly sharing it) has been handled poorly. A quote (Nightingale, 1863) from *Florence Nightingale* published in 1863 sounds like it could be said today (see *Figure 3.4*). Collecting accurate data consistently is a problem of the doctors and nurses. Managing the medical record in a hospital is in part the responsibility of the medical records department.

The medical record is a guide to, and continuous record of, treatment while the patient is in the hospital. After discharge it becomes an archival record available for

Figure 3.4. Nightengale. This quote from Florence Nightengale (1863), the mother of nursing, reflects the disorder of patient records in the 19th century but might be said today as well.

> *an urgent appeal for adopting ... some uniform system for ... records of hospitals. There is a growing conviction that in all hospitals, even in those which are best conducted, there is a great and unnecessary waste of life ... In attempting to arrive at the truth, I have applied everywhere for information, but in scarcely an instance have I been able to obtain hospital records fit for any purposes of comparison.*

retrieval if the patient is re-admitted or requires further treatment as an outpatient. Medical records also support medical audits. Finally, they support research. To accomplish this myriad of functions, sound *records management* is needed.

Medical records management assigns a medical record number to a patient who is being seen for the first time by this provider. When the patient is admitted or registered, the communication between the admitting/registration system and the medical records management system must determine whether a patient has already a record in the system or is a first-time patient. To facilitate these determinations the medical record management unit maintains a *master patient index* that contains enough of a record for each patient to allow accurate determination of whether an arriving person already has a record in the system or not. Unfortunately, this Master Patient Index combined with the information that some patients bring to the provider prove inadequate too often, as a patient is either matched with the record of someone else or is given a new, empty record when in fact the patient already has a record in the system.

The medical records department is responsible for *transcription processing*. Doctors may orally dictate reports that need to be rendered into textual form or they may hand-write information on one form that needs to be transcribed into another form. In addition to transcription, the medical records department is responsible for tracking the location of charts and for assuring that charts are complete. If, for instance, some document needs a signature but has been put in the chart without a signature, then the medical records department should detect this omission and obtain the correct signature for the document.

To avoid some transcription costs and to facilitate access to records stored digitally rather than in paper, a popular approach in medical records departments has been to scan and digitize medical records and store them as images. The high-capacity physical media for storage of digital information, the increasing computer power for processing of images, and the advances in imaging and workflow technology have underpinned the growth of *document imaging systems*. When the Jewish Hospital Healthcare Services adopted a document imaging system, delays in getting old charts were reduced and records became available to more than one person at a time (Odorisio, 1999).

Since all medically oriented systems contain some portion of the patient's medical record, the point at which a system qualifies as a *record system* requires clarification. An admission system, though it contains demographic data, is not a patient record. A radiology system that contains an x-ray is not a patient record. The key factor in the design of the computerized record system is that it should be a physically distributed system with logical central control of the entire record. The central system should provide integrated and coordinated use of the data (Smith, 2000).

In the future within either patient care systems or medical records systems, certification modules may be included. A *certification module* will help providers assess whether a patient's symptoms meet the criteria for treatment and whether this intervention should have in-patient or outpatient status. This kind of assessment is particularly important where the provider is accepting capitated payments.

Order Entry

The most basic capability of patient care management is *order entry*. A physician might write an order onto a patient chart, and then a nurse or unit secretary enters that order into the nursing station terminal. Alternately, the physician might enter the order directly into the computer. Such direct order by the physician facilitates pre-emptive quality control feedback by allowing the doctor to receive a warning about potential drug-drug interactions incurred by a new drug prescription or other such warning.

The order entry data will also be connected with the *service pricing system*. Thus orders that generate charges are automatically and immediately added to the patient's bill. This electronic capture of charges is one of the immediate, financial incentives for order entry within the healthcare organization.

The patient care management system should not only send the orders from the originating department to the department that might fulfill the order but should also permit the flow of information in the other direction. Thus an order of a x-ray to the radiology department might go directly to the radiology department from the ward, lead to the scheduling of the patient for the x-ray, and be followed by an electronically submitted radiologist's report being associated with the patient record online as soon as the *radiologist's report* is completed. The same flow of information and service would apply to pathology laboratory orders.

The concept of *computerized order entry* is commonplace in enterprise-wide information systems. If someone in a factory needs to order more screws, then placing that order via the computer makes sense. In healthcare the concept has been slow to be accepted in practice, but new forces may accelerate the adoption of computerized order entry. In particular, the interest is in *computerized physician order entry (CPOE)* that includes decision support and is specific to prescriptions. In this context, CPOE refers to computer-based systems of ordering medications, which semi-automate the medication ordering process and include computerized decision support systems of varying sophistication.

CPOE ensures standardized, legible, complete orders by only accepting typed orders in a certain format (Kaushal & Bates, 2001). Basic *clinical decision support* may include suggestions or default values for drug doses, routes, and frequencies. More sophisticated decision-support systems can perform drug allergy checks, drug-laboratory value checks, and drug-drug interaction checks, and offer reminders about corollary orders (such as prompting the user to order glucose checks after ordering insulin) or drug guidelines to the physician at the time of drug ordering.

Adverse drug events (ADEs) are injuries that result from the use of drugs. An example of a preventable ADE is the development of rash after the administration of ampicillin to a known penicillin-allergic patient. *Medication errors* refer to errors in the processes of ordering, transcribing, dispensing, administering, or monitoring medications, irrespective of the health of the patient. One example is an order written for amoxicillin without a route of administration. Studies show that CPOE can substantially decrease medication errors. One study demonstrated that CPOE reduced medication error rates by 55%—from 10.7 to 4.9 per 1,000 patient days (Bates et al., 1999). Another study demonstrated a 70% reduction in ADEs after implementation of a CPOE system (Evans et al., 1998).

The cost of purchasing and implementing large commercial CPOE systems varies substantially, but may be on the order of tens of millions of dollars. Healthcare systems must garner both financial and organizational support before introducing CPOE. CPOE requires a large *up-front investment*. In addition, CPOE impacts clinicians and workflow substantially. Its complexity requires close integration with multiple systems, such as the laboratory and pharmacy systems.

The *Leapfrog Group* is a consortium of more than 100 large companies that provide health benefits to over 30 million Americans (www.leapfroggroup.org). The Leapfrog Group's mission is to:

- Make the American public aware of a small number of highly compelling and easily understood advances in patient safety
- Specify a simple set of purchasing principles designed to promote these safety advances

Leapfrog Group member companies agree to adhere to a common set of purchasing principles in buying healthcare for their enrollees (their employees), including:

- Rating and comparing major healthcare providers' safety efforts
- Holding health plans accountable for implementing the Leapfrog purchasing principles

The Leapfrog Group has developed a CPOE standard. In order to meet Leapfrog's CPOE standard, hospitals must:

- Require physicians to enter medication orders via computer linked to prescribing error prevention software
- Demonstrate that their CPOE system intercepted at least 50% of common serious prescribing errors
- Require documented acknowledgment that the physician read the directives to any override

The CPOE system will warn the physician when a particular prescription from the physician goes against some rule(s) in the CPOE system; and the physician must explicitly override the warning before the CPOE system will proceed with the prescription. The Leapfrog Group will invite hospitals with CPOE systems to warrant that their systems meet these three CPOE standards.

Other entities *support* CPOE. A Medicare Payment Advisory Commission suggested instituting financial incentives for CPOE implementation. California enacted legislation stipulating that acute care hospitals implement information technology, such as CPOE, to reduce medication-related errors. Healthcare providers face both "carrot" (financial reward) and "stick" (laws) pressures to implement CPOE.

Military Health System

An example of an integrated system on a large scale is the Department of Defense Military Health System (MHS). The *Composite Health Care System* (CHCS) integrates data from multiple sources and displays the data at the point of care in the form of a life-long computer-based patient record (CPR). This CPR is available for viewing whenever and wherever needed to support medical readiness and quality healthcare. The CHCS provides a seamless, merged, enterprise-wide repository of health data that will facilitate the worldwide delivery of healthcare, assist clinicians in making healthcare decisions, and support leaders in making operational and resource allocation decisions (DoD, 2006). The CHCS is a compendium of commercial and government-developed software using an open system architecture.

The CPR will capture, maintain, and provide patient-focused information for health service delivery at any time and at any location over the beneficiary's period of eligibility. CHCS connects *medical treatment facilities* (MTFs) within a given geographic region. It consolidates individual MTFs into regions using the capabilities of a health data dictionary, master patient index, and clinical data repository. The health data dictionary enables communication among unlike information sources and the clinical data repository provides a virtual infrastructure for interoperability.

CHCS provides real-time availability to eligible medical and dental patient records, access to critical patient-based medical and dental information, and access to population data for automated queries. CHCS supports *clinical practice guidelines* and enhances the information workflow of MHS health care providers. All data is documented electronically, from the patient check-in to the completion of the healthcare encounter. An electronically accessible medical and dental record is generated and maintained by CHCS, allowing for quality measurement and utilization management within a facility and regionally. The system generates custom reports allowing for patient and provider-specific inquiries, as well as population health studies. As a by-product of the encounter, coding is accomplished.

The CHCS operational *architecture* consists of a common presentation layer (at the user workstation), a database layer, and an applications layer comprised of a variety of healthcare software packages. System elements are interconnected via interface devices, local area networks (LANs), and wide area networks (WANs) that support heterogeneous distributed hardware platforms and operating systems.

The Tri-Service Infrastructure Management Program Office is responsible for providing a common *communications infrastructure* to support CHCS. This communications infrastructure includes, but is not limited to, a LAN of sufficient size to accommodate all CHCS users, including medical and dental clinics outside the main MTF, and a WAN sized to facilitate data exchange from internal and external sources.

The *CHCS database* resides on a regional server suite located at the Defense Information System Agency computer support facilities. The CHCS Project Office requires six regional server sites to support CHCS worldwide. Each regional server site supports numerous, geographically dispersed CHCS host sites. The CHCS host sites are assigned to regional server sites based on availability and quality of communications links, and other technical and programmatic factors.

CHCS allows users to customize how they interact with the system. The *user interface* includes prompts and context-sensitive, online help. Functional capabilities support results retrieval, consult tracking, order entry, problem list, patient encounter, summary of care, alerts, and procedural coding.

The CHCS *enterprise security solution* is designed to provide each site flexibility in configuration while also enforcing standard role-based access across MTFs. The security product is installed at each MTF with a standard set of roles, which have

Figure 3.5. Account Administrator. This schematic screen from the U.S. Department of Defense Composite Health Care System shows how the roles of individuals fit into the Role column.

Schematic of screen for Account Administration			
Applicant Name	Primary MTF	Role	Account Name
Kori Kindred	Tripler	Nurse_RN	KKindred
LCDR Bob Lawry	Tripler	Pharmacy_supervisor	BLawry1
Joe Under, MD	Tripler	Provider_attending	UnderJ

been constructed by the CHCS Functional User Workgroup. Each role has been granted access to CHCS functions based on the work that the role performs. These functions can be altered at each MTF to suit the nuances between sites.

The set of *roles* is large, allowing a very granular set of functions to be assigned. This is intended to limit the amount of user-level granting that must be done. Granting specific functions on a user basis is labor intensive. The CHCS security solution utilizes a Web-based interface to allow CHCS account administrators to perform the basic functions needed for granting access to the CHCS system (see *Figure 3.5*).

Clinical Support

Various departments support patient care in specialist ways. These departments have such *specialized needs* that they typically have special information systems. The clinical departments in this support category include operating rooms, pathology, pharmacy, and radiology.

Overview

Historically, the information systems for specialist departments were provided by vendors distinct from those who provide the core functions, such as admissions and patient records. Thus problems of *integration* have been notorious. However, more recently, individual vendors provide both the core modules and the support modules, and the integration issues are addressed through standardization of messages.

Pathology, pharmacy, and radiology are particularly likely to be extensively *computerized*. They often obtain or generate data in digital form. For instance, the test machines employed by pathology and radiology often have computers in them and generate digital output. These departments also do not tend to directly treat patients, and thus have greater flexibility in determining how specimens, information, or patients will reach the department. For instance, tubes with blood are collected from patients and conveyed to the pathology laboratory where they are assembled into long queues and fed into the blood analyzer. The pathology and radiology departments may be responsible for providing interpretations of test values, and this task is readily supported by computerization.

Operating room systems and intensive care systems emphasize the *scheduling* of various healthcare professionals in interaction with the patient. The schedule may go room-by-room and identify the various professionals that are needed in each room at each moment. For example, in surgery the anesthesiologist's schedule along with the surgeon's schedule needs to be precisely known for a given patient's procedure in a given operating room.

Every unit of the healthcare system that provides clinical support can benefit from computerization. Consider for instance the *food service*. The following functions can be performed with information systems: food inventory control, institutional menu standardization and planning, nutrient analysis, patient selective menu operation, and menu item forecasting.

Pathology

The *pathology laboratory* includes hematology, chemistry, anatomic pathology, microbiology, and blood bank. Particularly for hematology and chemistry the machines in the laboratory may be directly connected to the patient care management system so that results are automatically sent from the laboratory to the patient record without human intervention. The order for these tests may typically require the scheduling of work by a technician to collect the necessary specimen, such as a blood sample, the affixing of an appropriately generated label to the container of the specimen, and the feeding of this specimen into the machine that analyzes the specimen.

By storing values of many tests across time for a given patient, the laboratory system can provide for the physician interactively various summaries of the data across time. Rules in the system can flag abnormalities and give *guidance* to the physician as to what the values might mean diagnostically.

Pharmacy

Medication orders are entered into the *pharmacy system*. The pharmacist may then use various computer-generated documents to guide the delivery of the medications to the patients. Some contemporary hospital systems have special pharmacy machines on the wards that operate somewhat like robots and supply various drugs to the caregiver from the robot based on the drug orders the robot received from the caregiver.

Some pharmacy tasks can be readily automated, such as analysis of appropriateness of drug dosage with respect to patient age and usual dosage level. More generally, the pharmacy system may develop a drug profile of a patient and a prescription history of the doctors and from these two sources support various *decisions*.

Radiology

Radiology systems typically deal with images that are very large in terms of bits stored. Special image processing and transmission systems have been devised to support *radiology departments* and the circulation of radiological images in the healthcare network. The radiology system will support the scheduling of patients for radiological exams and the managing of the patient through the radiology department. Since the radiologist's report is typically a natural language report, radiology systems might capture the radiologist's report orally and immediately convert it into textual form.

Traditionally radiology images were stored on film that was cumbersome. Of course, only one copy of the image typically existed. Thus when one caregiver had the image, no other caregiver could have it at the same time. Finding and transporting images was a major task. *Digital radiology systems* permit the images to be stored, transmitted, viewed, and annotated digitally.

All radiological images can be captured digitally. X-rays can be captured by *non-film detectors*. All other modalities already involve electronic data capture, including ultrasound, nuclear medicine, computerized tomography scanning, and magnetic resonance imaging. Systems dedicated to digital radiological image management are called *picture archiving and communications systems* (PACS). However, PACS are expensive and require:

- High-resolution acquisition
- High-capacity storage
- High-bandwidth network
- High-resolution displays

Some radiology centers still store images on film. Conventional x-rays are taken on celluloid film. Digital studies (computerized tomograms, magnetic resonance images, ultrasounds, and nuclear medicine images) may also be stored on film.

Physicians in clinics could make diagnostic and therapeutic decisions more quickly if the radiologist's interpretation of the image was quickly available *online*. However, most radiology departments do not interpret images in real time but rather on an elective basis in which a radiologist schedules some fixed time to view images collected at an earlier time. Thus, the benefit of digital speed of image transmission is reduced.

Image processing experts working with radiologists have not been able to develop robust systems that automatically interpret all radiological images. *Intelligent systems* to assist the radiologist in interpreting images do exist, and these require the image to be in digital form.

Sample System

One way to explore what healthcare providers need as regards enterprise information systems is to examine one of the most successful products on the market. The following description is based on Cerner Corporation's "Millennium" enterprise information system. *Millennium* includes administrative systems, patient management systems, and clinical support systems for a hospital and other components of a healthcare network (Cerner, 2000).

Administrative Systems

Millenium's *administrative systems* cover the administrative needs of a healthcare provider, including finance and accounting, customer relationship management, executive decision support, and supply chain management. A central data repository stores activity-related information for management of a healthcare organization. This repository includes the electronic medical record and information to help the organization link with information from other organizations, such as indexes to third-party dictation systems.

The *financial and operational management system* supports revenue accounting, billing and accounts receivables. It includes a structured repository for the storage and viewing of health plan information, records, contracts, eligibility and coverage data. The agreement management system automates the managed care processes around membership, eligibility tracking, claims processing and contract management.

The *demand management system* supports the operations of a call center, including protocol-based triage, referral management, and person information. The call center management system enables call centers to automate the telecare function for providers or health plans. These and other functions constitute the customer (or patient) relationship management aspect of Millennium.

A *comparative data warehouse* is available for benchmarking information. Data is provided from client's information systems, as well as national and regional data sets. The warehouse is hosted at Cerner's World Headquarters and accessed via the Web. The executive decision support modules access this warehouse to help an organization complete its strategic plans, including clinical metrics, case profiling, and performance profiling of individuals and organizations. A materials management system module automates the business operations around supply chain management.

Patient Management

The *patient management system* includes a clinician's desktop that supports viewing and modifying the electronic medical record. Physicians can gain access to the electronic medical record to view results and documentation from any Internet-based terminal.

An *acute care management system* collects, organizes, and evaluates clinical and management data. With it, the care team can manage individual activities and plans, as well as measure outcomes. The system has two major parts:

- One automates documentation related to acute care delivery, such as nursing order entry
- The other supports acute care planning, including pathways used to audit care and nursing care plans

Other systems exist for surgery, emergency medicine, and intensive care.

The *surgery information system* addresses the needs of the surgical department, including anesthesia management and operating room management. Case cart management and peri-operative documentation are supported. The emergency medicine information system provides emergency department functionality, including tracking and triage, as well as a graphical reference to patient location and order status.

Clinical Support

The Millennium system provides support for laboratories, radiology, pharmacy, surgery, and other areas of a large hospital that support the provision of care by physicians.

A *laboratory information system* addresses the information management needs of general laboratory, microbiology, blood bank services, and anatomic pathology. It automates the ordering and reporting of procedures, the production of timely reports, and the maintenance of accessible records.

The *radiology information system* allows a diagnostic radiology department to replace its manual, paper-based system of record keeping with a computer-based system. Interfaces to pictorial archive retrieval systems (PACS) are also offered to integrate the radiology information system to the PACS.

The *pharmacy information system* supports the clinical pharmacy. It enables the pharmacist or technician to enter pharmaceutical orders on a screen. Interfaces to automated dispensing devices are supported. Medication fill lists, intravenous fill lists, and medication administration records can be produced automatically.

Other Entities

Beyond the core components for a large hospital, the Millennium system has components to work for other entities. Descriptions follow for the physician office system, the home care management system, and the Internet-based home system.

A private practice module connects physicians in private practice to health systems for referrals, authorizations, claims, eligibility, and reporting. This *physician office management system* supports the clinical and business activities that occur within a physician office and ties the office together with others in the community. It supports patient tracking, clinical records access, eligibility checking, order and referral processing, and reference library access.

The *home care management system* supports the clinical and business processes of home health organizations, such as visiting nurse associations and hospices whether they are Medicare-certified or not. It facilitates the documentation of care activities in the home.

Internet-based home system extends medical care to the consumer's home. It provides a way for the consumer to interact on a regular basis with a healthcare provider, and it supports health appraisals and personalized health plans. Relevant health information can be shared among providers and the patient, under control of the patient.

Millennium is a large suite of complex software tailored to the healthcare provider market. Several other companies have similar products.

Physician Group

The description in this chapter of the information systems of providers has focused on the activities of hospitals. The *small group physician practice* is, however, also very important and very different from the hospital in its information systems needs.

The major professions, medicine, law, and the church, emerged in the *19th century* from the trades and crafts. In those early days, patronage and a liberal education were all that were required. By 1860 the elements of professional standing were tolerably clear (Reader, 1966):

You needed a professional association to focus opinion, work up a body of knowledge, and insist upon a decent standard of conduct. If possible, and as soon as possible, it should have a Royal Charter as a mark of recognition. The final step, if you could manage it—it was very difficult—was to persuade Parliament to pass an Act conferring something like monopoly powers on duly qualified practitioners, which meant practitioners who had followed a recognized course of training and passed recognized examinations.

The professional assumed authority in the specific sphere of his expertise.

Traditionally physicians were solo practitioners charging a fee for service. The *solo practitioner* was the norm till the 1960s. Physicians now typically formally band together in partnerships or groups. The bureaucratic nature of group practice may be expected to impose certain rules and regulations. For example, a group practice will have more detailed protocols to follow than a solo practice.

Another organizational attribute of physician practices concerns the extent to which the practice is for primary care or specialist care (see *Figure 3.6*). The primary or general practice is dependent on patients. The *specialist* is dependent on referrals from general practitioners (or other specialists). The specialist becomes subject to some peer review by the general practitioner, who will get the results of the specialist's work. However, the specialist will also be in an indirect position to do some quality review of the work of the general practitioner.

The typical physician group practice is supported by three medical assistants per physician. *Medical assistant* refers to a broad category to include receptionist, transcriptionist, appointment schedulers, billing clerks, and examination assistants. The workflow for a medical assistant might look as follows:

- When doctor arrives ask about hospital visits and emergency room calls in order to post charges for those services
- When patient arrives, set-up chart for assistant, and write name on day sheet

Figure 3.6. Referral System. GP is general practitioner. SP is specialist. Dashed line is primary care patient flow. Solid line is referred patient flow.

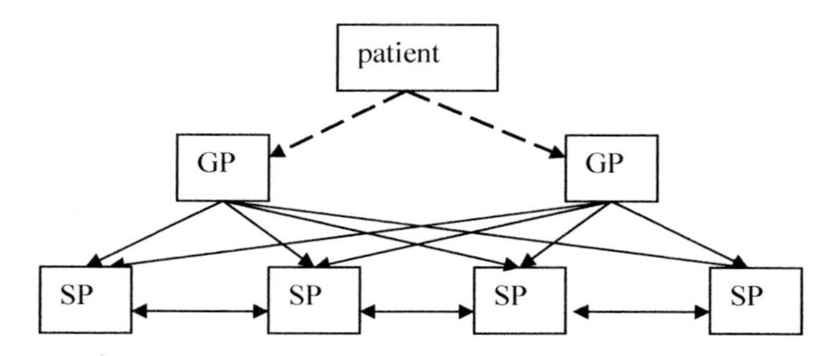

- New patients fill-out registration form
- After patient seen, post charges, ask for payment, make next appointment
- Post check to patient account
- Attach lab reports to front of patient's record and place on doctor's desk
- File lab and other reports in chart
- Make phone calls for forms and payments
- Copy charts for forwarding to new doctors and insurance companies
- Distribute materials brought from doctor's hospital box
- Check office supplies

Most of the work of the group practice is done on *paper*. In particular, the medical record is typically in paper form. Most offices keep records in manila folders. Each patient will have a folder. Sometimes doctors dictate their patient notes, and their secretary transcribes the material into typewritten form for the record. The medical record in the group or solo practice is expected to have these features (Reschke, 1980):

- Patient name on all pages
- All pages secured with fasteners
- Forms organized with tabs for easy access
- Organized chronologically
- Missed appointments documented
- Telephone message documented
- Dictation proofread and initialed
- Allergies documented

- Diagnostic reports initialed prior to filing
- Reason for visit documented
- Clinical findings documented
- Treatment plan documented
- Patient instructions documented
- Patient education documented
- Prescriptions list
- Allergies list
- Informed consent on chart
- Referral letters on chart
- Consultation reports on chart
- Problem list kept current

The part of the group practice that is most often automated is *billing*. This quote from a 1980s textbook remains largely applicable (Lindsey, 1980):

Since the advent of medical and hospitalization insurance, the medical assistant has found a great deal of his or her time now spent billing various insurance companies so that the doctor's fees can be collected.

However, in the past 20 years what has changed is the introduction of software to support the billing. An example of one such product to support billing follows, called Business1 (www.per-se.com). *Business1* is a patient financial management system that supports traditional patient accounting, contract management, and professional billing. Business1:

- Gives users access to various aspects of the patient demographic, insurance and other information
- Uses a rules engine to help ensure that all required information is collected for efficient closure of the revenue cycle

Each provider can mark certain fields as required fields to comply with provider admission policies and payer requirements. With color-coded alerts, users can identify and locate pages that are incomplete. These up-front edits ensure that the payer's billing requirements are met.

Figure 3.7. Accounting Viewer. This schematic of a screen from the Per-Se Business1 software shows the 'accounting viewer'. In this screen two products have been identified and billed.

Guarantors	Invoice ID	Provider	Payer Name	Total Charges	Amount Received
John Smith	HH0089	SEMB	Mut. Ohio	14,823.00	7,588.13
			Line Items		
	Item	Rev. Code	Description	Units	Charge
	1	128	Room-Board	5	2,138.80
	2	210	Coronary Care	5	4,170.00

The Business1 accounting viewer provides a summary of receivables for the patient and guarantor. The *accounting viewer* contains information about both the receivables and the episode from which the receivables were generated (see *Figure 3.7*). As payer contract provisions become increasingly more complex, the billing clerk must have an understanding of how provider cases are consolidated or split into the products from which invoices are generated.

Future

The *progress* with digital information in healthcare has been slower than some wanted or predicted. However, many developments are in process. Pressure from employers for computerized physician order entry systems will increase the use of computers in healthcare. New hospitals are being built with extensive electronic infrastructure, as the following two examples illustrate.

HealthSouth (www.healthsouth.com) spent $100 million to build the *HealthSouth Medical Center*. The project was a partnership among HealthSouth, medical equipment manufacturers, healthcare specialty firms, and Oracle Corporation. HealthSouth's goal was to improve patient care by bringing together technological advances in healthcare that, due to incompatible computer systems, lack of integration among equipment manufacturers and other obstacles, had had limited impact.

The *Indiana Heart Hospital* eliminates paper and film-based medical records. The hospital functions with fully electronic patient records that clinicians can view from inside or outside the hospital. The design eliminates medical record storage rooms, paper charting areas, and central nursing stations. It focuses on providing information that helps doctors and nurses deliver higher-quality care at the patient bedside ("Two all-digital hospitals in the works," 2002).

Questions

Reading Questions

1. What are the interactions among the four top-level components (administrative systems, clinical support systems, medical applications, and patient management) of a health information system?
2. What is the relationship between patient accounting and financial management?
3. What are the responsibilities of the medical records department?
4. What are functions of a pharmacy information system?

Doing Questions

1. Visit a hospital or clinic and observe the admission or registration process. Document the extent to which information systems are utilized.
2. Describe how a master patient index might be developed and maintained and what problems might be encountered during routine use in terms of entering the same person with two different identities in the system.
3. A clinical documentation system is the portion of a computerized patient record that allows patient data entry at the point of service. Compare and contrast the clinical documentation system available from three vendors. Note the prominent connections of each vendor product to other components of the health information system as described in the chapter. Predict what you would see and hear in terms of the healthcare professionals (all levels) in their use of the clinical documentation system in a hospital.

References

Bates, D., et al. (1999). The impact of computerized physician order entry on medication error prevention. *American Medical Informatics Association, 6,* 313-321.

Cerner. (2000). *1999 Annual Report*. Retrieved October 1, 2006, from www.cerner.com

DeLuca, J., & Enmark, R. (2002). *The CEO's guide to health care information systems* (2nd ed.). Chicago: American Hospital Association Press.

Department of Defense. (2006). *Clinical Information Technology Program Office*. Retrieved May 5, 2006, from http://citpo.ha.osd.mil/

Evans, R.S., et al. (1998). A computer-assisted management program for antibiotics and other anti-infective agents. *New England Journal of Medicine, 338*(4), 232-238.

Kissinger, K., & Borchardt, S. (Eds.). (1996). *Information technology for integrated health systems: Positioning for the future*. New York: John Wiley & Sons.

Lindsey, B. (1980). *The administrative medical assistant*. Bowie, MD: Robert Brady Company.

Nightingale, F. (1863). *Notes on hospitals* (3rd ed.). London: Longman, Green, & Company.

Reader, W. (1966). *Professional men*. New York: Basic Books.

Reschke, E. (1980). *The medical office:Organization and management*. New York: Harper & Row.

Smith, J. (2000). *Health management information systems:A handbook for decision-makers*. Buckingham, UK: Open University Press.

Torrens, P., & Williams, S. (1993). Understanding the present, planning for the future: The dynamics of health care in the United States in the 1990s. In S. Williams & P. Torrens (Eds.), *Introduction to health services* (pp. 421-429). Albany, NY: Delmar Publishers.

Two all-digital hospitals in the works. (2002, May 27). *Healthcare IT Weekly, 1*.

Chapter IV

Payers

Learning Objectives

- Diagram the basic operations of a health plan
- Identify salient characteristics of information systems applications in health plans based on case studies
- Compare and contrast the main government health plan with the main commercial health plan
- Explain why clearinghouses and contract managers have a role
- Identify the stakeholders and accountability criteria for health plans

Most of what has been discussed in this book focuses on the provider and its relation to the patient as regards information systems. However, in the American health care system the connection between the provider and payer is critical to the smooth functioning of the system (Starr, 1997). This chapter focuses on the *payer* (or health plan). In many other countries, the operation would be different, but some way is always used to track the expenditure of resources and to pay health care workers.

Context

In its most straightforward, capitalist form, the financial arrangement for health care service requires a patient to pay the doctor directly. However, the American healthcare system, while it started that way, has evolved into one dependent on *insurance*. The history of insurance is next presented and then followed by some definitions.

History

In the 19th century, doctors took care of patients who paid for their services directly. Later some employers hired doctors to work at the factory to assure that workers who became ill could as quickly as possible return to work. Workers in the early part of the twentieth century opposed employers' picking their doctors for them. These arguments were refined over time to support prohibitions against *employers* hiring *doctors* to whom employees were expected to go in the case of medical need. The employees preferred the employer to provide indemnity insurance whereby the employee can go to any healthcare provider and have the insurance pay for expenses engendered. The states supported this opposition to employer-selected healthcare by stifling or prohibiting it. Pre-paid group practices to which an employee is expected to go were not allowed by the states.

In the twentieth century, the federal government passed several major pieces of legislation with implications for health care insurance. A U.S. Supreme Court decision first applied federal scrutiny to insurance markets in 1944. An *antitrust* dispute led the court to rule that insurance transactions were indeed interstate commerce and thus subject to federal antitrust laws. Largely at the behest of insurers who feared federal oversight, the next year (1945) Congress passed the McCarran-Ferguson Act. The McCarran-Ferguson Act exempted health insurance markets from federal antitrust prosecution as long as those markets were regulated by the states.

The *HMO Act of 1973* was the first major federal effort to promote alternatives to indemnity insurance. The act fostered the development of qualifying HMOs by overriding state *statutory* and *common law prohibitions* on the operation of prepaid group practices and the corporate practice of medicine. The HMO Act required employers with more than twenty-five employees that offered at least one health insurance plan to also offer an HMO, if requested by a local HMO.

Definitions

The American healthcare system shows complex relationships among

- Patients
- Employers who typically subsidize their employees' health insurance

- Health insurance companies that collect premiums from enrollees (patients) and pay providers for care delivered to patients
- Providers who care for patients but are paid by insurance companies

An example of the variety of players in the health system is provided by the *Wisconsin Health Information Network* that links 16 hospitals, eight clinics, three nursing homes, 1,300 physicians, seven health plans, and four clearinghouses. Definitions of health plan and clearinghouse are provided next.

A *health plan* is an individual or group health plan that provides, or pays the cost of, medical care. On the other hand, plans, such as property and casualty insurance plans and workers compensation plans, which may pay healthcare costs in the course of administering non-healthcare benefits, are not considered health plans.

Health plans often perform their business functions through *agents*, such as plan administrators (including third party administrators), entities that are under 'administrative services only' contracts, claims processors, and fiscal agents. These agents may or may not be health plans in their own right; for example, a health plan may act as another health plan's agent as another line of business. The three most prominent kinds of health plans in the United States are indemnity, health maintenance, and government plans (Altman et al., 2003).

Traditional *indemnity plans* offer the widest range of choice to consumers. Blue Cross & Blue Shield organizations offer well known indemnity plans. The consumer obtains medical services from the physician or hospital of his choice. He submits his bill to the insurance company and the insurance company makes whatever payments it has pre-agreed it would make for such services. The *consumer* typically pays a percentage of the bill till some threshold is reached.

For the indemnity (indemnity means security against damage, loss, or injury) plans, the patient typically pays 20% and insurance pays 80%. However, this is 80% of what insurance deems is 'usual and customary reimbursement' (UCR). Often this UCR is less than the physician charges so the patient pays more than 20% of the charge. Say the physician charges $1,000 for repair of inguinal hernia, but the insurance company says the UCR is $800. Insurance then pays 80% of $800. The patient is then responsible to pay $360 and not $200.

Health Maintenance Organizations (HMOs) are designed to provide medical care at a pre-arranged monthly fee. Instead of paying a 'premium' to an insurance company, the consumer pays a *membership fee* to an HMO. In return, the consumer receives all medical care from the HMO. Instead of treating patients and then trying to collect money from either the patient or the insurance company for the cost of the treatment, HMOs bypass the insurance company completely and make their 'deal' with the consumer. Managed care is often reimbursed on a capitation scheme. The physician agrees to provide a specified list of services to each patient assigned to him or her for a set dollar amount each month. The insurer pays the specified amount regardless of what this patient does. Typically, this fee is between $3 per patient per month to $15 per patient per month. Obviously these risk-sharing agreements can lead to very different results for the physician depending on circumstances. If the physician has 100 patients in the plan and the capitated fee is $15 per member per month, then if the physician sees 20 of these patients at a cost to the physician of $1,800, then the physician has lost $300. If the physician sees only 5 of the 100 patients and their total services are $200, then the physician has a gross profit of $1,300.

The *government* is involved in one form or another in various health plans to include:

- Medicare and Medicaid programs
- Healthcare program for active military personnel
- Veterans healthcare programs

Other government programs exist, such as the Indian Health Service program.

The health insurance market may also be viewed as consisting of three distinct segments: *large group*, *small group*, and *individual*. These are not simply points on a continuum; they constitute entirely different product lines, often sold by different sales forces and serviced by different insurers or corporate divisions (Hall, 2000).

The large group market accounts for two-thirds of private health insurance. The large group market consists of employer-based insurance for groups of more than fifty workers. Regulation of these groups is determined by whether they are self-insured (the employer bears the financial risk for most claims) or not. More than half of groups of more than 500 workers are self-insured. For these groups, the *Employee Retirement Income Security Act (ERISA)* preempts the core of state-law insurance regulation. *Preemption* includes regulation of solvency and other financial matters, consumer protection regulation, and regulation of the content of health insurance. For large groups that are not self-insured, these matters are subject to state regulation.

Because the employer selects and pays for employees' insurance, there is little tendency for insurance to be selected with the health condition of particular subscribers in mind (adverse selection). This allows the market to function well with little or no medical underwriting (that is, screening and evaluation of individual health risks), since underwriting is focused on group averages. Another advantage to *employer-based insurance* is the subsidy it confers to subscribers, because the employer pays a large portion of the premium and because this premium contribution is not taxed as income to the employee. Finally, larger groups typically offer employees a choice of plans.

At the other extreme, the *individual market* consists of insurance purchased outside the workplace, such as by self-employed or unemployed people, or people with jobs that do not provide health insurance. The individual market segment accounts for less than 10% of private health insurance. Its regulation is almost entirely the province of the states. States typically regulate solvency and other financial matters, the content and wording of policies, and managed care activities.

Because the purchase of individual insurance is determined entirely by purchasers' *health needs*, adverse-selection concerns are great. Thus, medical underwriting is very prominent, in the form of premium variations, coverage limitations or exclusions, and outright denials of coverage. On the positive side, purchasers in the individual market can choose from the full array of product types and variations in coverage.

Basic Operations

What are the basic operations of a typical health plan? First it *enrolls* members. Either members or their sponsor pay premiums to the health plan. What is the main service provided by a health plan? It pays providers for health care delivered to enrollees. The plan agrees with certain providers to *reimburse* them for certain expenses that they incur in treating enrollees of the plan. The plan might also directly reimburse the member for expenses the member paid directly to the provider, though this is increasingly uncommon.

A typical provider function relative to a payer begins with the first encounter between the provider and patient. The provider wants to confirm that the patient is eligible for health care services from the provider and checks this *eligibility* with the health plan. If eligibility holds and care is delivered, then the next major communication between the provider and the payer is the submission of a claim for reimbursement from the provider to the plan.

In 1958, the Health Insurance Association of America and the American Medical Association (AMA) attempted to standardize the insurance claim form. However, payers did not universally accept this form, and as the types of coverage became more variable, new claims forms, requiring more information, were developed. In 1975, the AMA approved a Universal Claim Form called Health Insurance Claim Form or HCFA-1500. It could be used for both group and individual claims. *HCFA-1500* answered the needs of many health insurers who were processing claims manually. Prior to HIPAA, all services for Medicare patients from physicians and suppliers (except for ambulance services) had to be billed on the HCFA-1500 form.

The HCFA-1500 form (see *Table 4.1*) contains *fields* for values about the patient and the physician. The diagnostic codes applicable to the patient are associated

Table 4.1. Stylized Rendering of Part of HCFA-1500. The HCFA-1500 was the claims form widely used in the 1990s. The shaded section shows the procedure (or service or supply) for which the patient is being billed along with the date of the procedure, the diagnostic code of the patient disease which justifies the procedure, and the charge for the procedure.

Patient Name	Patient Address		
Insured's Name	Insured's Address		
Procedure, Services, or Supplies (CPT Code)	Date	Diagnosis Code	Charge
1			
2			
3			
4			
Physician's Signature	Federal Tax ID		Total Charge

with each procedure, service, or supply for the patient. The charge is given, and the physician signs the claim.

Having received a claim, the health plan needs to *adjudicate* the claim. This requires determining whether the services were appropriately rendered and whether the costs are justified. If the health plan feels that inadequate information has been provided to judge the fairness of the claim, the plan will ask the provider to send additional information to the plan. Sometimes the plan will ask the provider to send a copy of the entire medical record of the patient to the plan. Eventually, the health plan must issue a response that includes its payment and an explanation of the relationship between its payment and the claim.

These operations can be elaborated in many ways. The health plan employs many roles for helping assure its smooth operation. In addition to the obvious roles of soliciting enrollees and paying claims, the plan has a layer of operations that includes underwriters and profilers. *Underwriters* are involved in the determination of what health care costs a potential enrollee is likely to incur and what premiums would be required to cover the risks of insuring this enrollee. Profilers analyze providers and recommend providers that are likely to reduce the costs to the plan.

The health plans also work with outside entities other than providers, employers, and enrollees. Clearinghouses are one prominent example, but equally important to the viability of a plan are *brokers*. Brokers and agents give advice to people about available health plans and get paid a commission by a health plan for each enrollee that the broker or agent brings into the plan.

For a payer to perform its functions efficiently, information systems are vital. Time and personnel resources to perform these functions manually are too high. Consider the following examples of how *manual processes* might work for enrollment, claims adjudication, and claims payment.

For *enrollment*, the payer would receive an application for enrollment of a beneficiary and would:

- Visually inspect the form for missing fields or invalid information.
- Look-up the rules for enrolling that beneficiary in a printed reference to determine eligibility. The printed references might vary by employer, or in the case of individual plans, by characteristic of the beneficiary. For example, the printed reference might state that employees of a particular company must be employed for at least 90 days before being eligible for insurance. The payer would then need to check the enrollment application to see that this condition had been met. This process of manual verification of enrollment eligibility would be time consuming and error-prone.
- If the application is valid, then the payer adds the beneficiary to the list of individuals currently enrolled in the plan.

For *claims adjudication*, suppose a pharmacy is filling a prescription for a patient and wants to determine the patient's co-payment, the pharmacy would phone the payer, who then might need to do the following:

1. Verify whether the patient was enrolled in the prescription drug program by looking up the patient's name in a printed enrollment log.
2. Check the printed benefits history for that patient to ensure the patient had not exceeded the maximum annual prescription benefit already.
3. Find the pharmacy in a printed provider log.
4. Find the medication name in the printed formulary, since there is a higher co-payment for medications not on the formulary.
5. Report the co-payment back to the pharmacy.

Now suppose the pharmacy filled the prescription and submitted a paper claim to the insurance company. The payer might then need to do the following:

- Go through steps 1 through 4 above again.
- Check to see if the pharmacy's charges were usual and customary (UCR) and determine the payment amount based on this and the co-payment. If the payer

determined the charges exceeded the UCR, the payer would need to indicate by how much the charge exceeded the UCR on the claim payment statement.

- Issue a check and a statement to the pharmacy.

The above manual processes are time-consuming and inefficient. Currently, for many payers and pharmacies, filling the prescription is tied to electronically submitting the claim—the two occur at the same time. Claims adjudication and payment may occur in a matter of seconds.

CMS

The *Centers for Medicare & Medicaid Services* (CMS) is a federal agency within the U.S. Department of Health and Human Services. CMS was known prior to 2001 as the Health Care Financing Administration. CMS runs the Medicare and Medicaid programs—two national health care programs that benefit about 75 million Americans. CMS also runs the State Children's Health Insurance Program (SCHIP), a program that is expected to cover many of the approximately 10 million uninsured children in the United States. CMS also regulates all laboratory testing (except research) performed on humans in the United States. CMS spent over $360 billion in 2000 buying health care services for beneficiaries of Medicare, Medicaid and SCHIP (www.cms.hhs.gov).

The *Information Technology Objectives* of CMS include:

- Meaningful information is readily accessible to CMS's beneficiaries, partners, and stakeholders
- IT is effectively applied to support program integrity

The functional view of CMS divides the organization into eleven *Functional Areas* as follows:

1. CMS management
2. Program development
3. Program operations management
4. Medicare financial management
5. Program integrity organization
6. Medicaid and child health insurance program administration

7. External communication
8. Administrative services
9. Outreach and education
10. Health industry standards
11. Program quality organization

The information systems that support this host of functions and organizational areas at CMS are:

- Beneficiary data management system
- Provider data management system
- Insurer data management system
- Health care plan data management system
- Utilization data management system
- Survey data management system
- General ledger data management system
- Business management information system
- Health care finance information system
- Health care stakeholder information system
- Health care assessment information system
- Health care services information system
- Geographic locations information system
- Document information system
- Human resources

The information systems are, in turn, decomposed into numerous *subsystems* of which a listing of those whose acronyms begin with the letter 'A' or 'B' indicates the complexity:

- AAPCC Adjusted Average Per Capita Cost System
- APPSGHP Automated Plan Payment System
- ARKA Arkansas Part A System
- ASPEN Automated Survey Processing Environment
- ATARS Audits Tracking and Reporting System

- BAAADS Budget's Apportions Allotments Allowances Database System
- BESS Part B Medicare Extract and Summary System
- BEST Carrier Beneficiary Alpha/State System
- BUCS Budget Under Control System

Each of these systems is complex enough to contain multiple other subsystems.

BCBS

The *Blue Cross and Blue Shield System*:

- Consists of approximately 45 member plans that are independent, locally operated companies under the coordination of the Blue Cross and Blue Shield Association
- Provides health care coverage for approximately 80 million people in the U.S.
- Contracts with 80% of hospitals and 90% of physicians in the U.S.
- Employs 150,000 people

Administrative costs average 12% of health care payments and gross revenue was approximately $1 trillion for the year 2000.

Operations

A large *Blue Cross & Blue Shield Plan* is a complex of entities and not purely a health insurance company. In one example, the 'plan' includes a health maintenance organization, a disease management group, and a plan services group in addition to the traditional BCBS Plan (Paramore, 2001). Information is exchanged among these components. For instance, the Plan Services Group sends health information covering

- Eligibility information
- Membership lists
- Claims information

to the Disease Management Group.

In its *connection* to *providers* and *members*, the BCBS Plans show another complex of relations (see *Figure 4.1*). In the provider direction, the Plan is connected to clearinghouses, pharmacies, and other providers. Other providers include hospitals, individual physicians, clinics, long-term care facilities, and skilled nursing facilities. In the members' direction, the BCBS Plan is linked to groups, enrollees, and brokers. From the BCBS Plan to the hospitals and physicians the following information goes:

- Eligibility rosters
- Capitation reports
- Membership lists
- Pre-authorizations and certification communications
- Claims information
- Daily error reports
- Paid claims information

Figure 4.1. Plan, Members, and Providers. The BCBS Plan is connected to provider organizations on the one side and to enrollees or insured groups on the other. On the enrollee side, brokers match enrollees to plans, while on the provider side, clearinghouses match transactions among providers and plans.

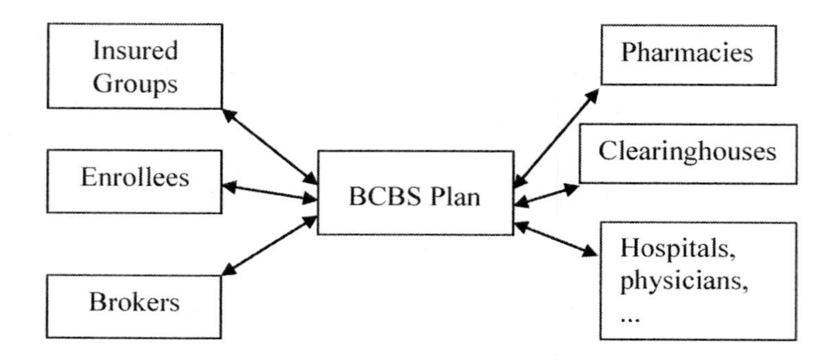

- Case management negotiations
- Utilization data

From a BCBS Plan to the Groups goes some of the preceding plus 'High Dollar or Stop Loss' information.

A BCBS Plan has natural connections to *other plans* and to vendors, regulatory agencies, and financial institutions (see *Figure 4.2*). To the BCBS Association the Plan sends:

- Appeals and complaints
- Transplant network information
- Fraud and abuse case information

To other BCBS Plans, a BCBS Plan sends:

Figure 4.2. BCBS and Others. The Plan connects to other Plans in the upper half of the diagram. In the lower half, the Plan connects to a variety of organizations that regulate, support, and review activity.

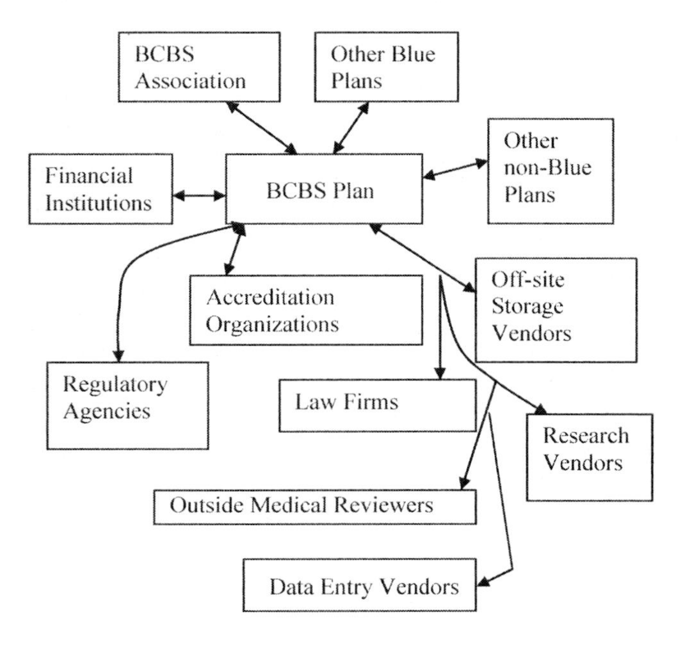

- Secondary cross-over information
- Eligibilities
- Claims information for fraud investigation

To non-Blue Plans, the Blue Plan may send:

- Subrojation information
- Coordination of benefits information
- Claims information for fraud investigation

In the other direction, the Blue Plan will send to financial institutions "verification of benefits" data. To regulatory and accreditation organizations the Plan will send auditable and accreditation information and medical information to support medical audits. To off-site storage vendors, the Plan sends paper applications and underwriting and claims information.

These *complex relationships* of the BCBS Plan are not unique to BCBS Plans but are typical of the health plan situation in the U.S. The health plan is not only collecting enrollee premiums and paying providers but is engaged in a complex set of financial, quality control, and medical activities with numerous other entities.

One Case

One of the regional Blue Cross and Blue Shield Plans is *Blue Cross and Blue Shield of North Carolina* (BCBSNC). BCBSNC has about 1.8 million members and performs 14 million transactions annually. To improve its connectivity with its various stakeholders, BCBSNC extended its legacy systems to make them more accessible to external stakeholders. BCBSNC implemented an Internet-based solution that offers its employer groups and healthcare providers easy access and control over routine but important business functions (Hulme, 2003).

BCBSNC converted the current legacy application, running over an SNA network, to a *Web-based application* communicating over a TCP/IP Intranet. This Internet-based solution streamlines millions of *transactions* between BCBSNC and its healthcare providers and employer groups. The new system gives more than 9,000 hospitals, doctors, other healthcare providers, and employers access to membership, eligibility, benefits, and claim status information. The new system also lets providers and employer groups submit health care claims, request pre-authorizations, and submit enrollments.

CMS vs. BCBS

The most salient difference between CMS and BCBS is that BCBS has more control over who is enrolled and who can provide services. This *control* allows them to be more accountable to their stakeholders in terms of ensuring an acceptable quality of care at a reasonable cost.

BCBS has a high degree of control over who can *enroll* in individual plans. Based on the applicant's age, sex, and health status, BCBS can gauge the amount of services the individual is likely to require. If it determines that the individual is likely to be a high cost, frequent user, it can:

- Refuse to cover the applicant
- Cover the applicant, except for his/her pre-existing conditions
- Cover the applicant but charge a very high premium

A BCBS Plan will typically have less direct control initially over who is enrolled in its small and large *group plans*. It may or may not enforce pre-existing condition limitations on beneficiaries of these plans. Still, it can mitigate excessive costs and exert indirect control by raising premiums. If a particular group uses a large amount of resources, BCBS could raise premiums the next year to an amount that the employer might no longer be able to afford. Increasing premiums would benefit BCBS by either mitigating the financial risk of providing coverage for a high cost group (if that group decided to pay the premiums) or forcing an undesirable, high cost/liability group to drop the coverage.

On the provider side, a BCBS Plan exerts control by deciding which providers can participate in the plan. It carefully *monitors* claims in order to track provider's utilization and habits. A provider who orders many expensive treatments or medications, or who often refers patients to specialists could be dropped from the plan. The BCBS Plan may also exert control over existing providers by giving them feedback on their performance. It may send them 'report cards' of their performance as compared with their peers, particularly with regard to utilization (e.g., number of tests ordered, referrals to specialists, and number of times they have ordered non-formulary medications).

Without sophisticated *information systems* (IS), a BCBS Plan would be unable to exert this kind of control over enrollment and providers. IS are essential for BCBS to be able to determine patient and provider utilization rates, and to determine how much it costs to insure a particular demographic group, patients with various medical conditions, and specific employer groups. Without detailed cost and utilization data, BCBS might take on excessive risk by not charging sufficient premiums to cover the costs of high-utilization individuals and employer groups. Or, it might undertake excessive risk by allowing a high-utilization/high-cost provider to continue to participate in the plan. Finally, using IS to track utilization data would enable BCBS to provide performance information to its stakeholders.

About 90% of a BCBS Plan's business is typically derived from *insured groups*. Insurance brokers advise the insured groups to enroll in a BCBS Plan. The obvious implication is that a BCBS Plan should make its IS as helpful to brokers and groups as possible. A BCBS Plan's web site will help groups and brokers easily and quickly find premium quotes and enroll new employees or groups. Since CMS does not address groups or brokers, CMS has little need for these functions.

CMS has little control over who is enrolled in Medicare, Medicaid, or SCHIP. Eligibility is not based on health status but on age, disability criteria, and/or income. CMS has no way to mitigate the cost of insuring patients who frequently use significant amounts of health care resources. Also, CMS is not able to exert control over high-cost, high-utilization providers unless these providers also happen to commit some gross act of misconduct or fraud. CMS has several approaches to handle *skyrocketing costs*:

- Reduce benefits to existing beneficiaries
- Change eligibility requirements so fewer people will be eligible
- Increase government financial support
- Reduce payment to providers
- Reduce costs by improving the efficiency of existing programs/services

The first four options are politically unattractive and most would require an act of Congress to implement. The fifth option is attractive because the majority of CMS's stakeholders (beneficiaries, providers, taxpayers, and government) want that option, and CMS can implement that option with the help of IS. CMS has undertaken initiatives using IS to attempt to improve efficiency and effectiveness.

Intermediaries

To support the complex relationships between providers and payers, a variety of entities play an intermediary role. Clearinghouses are the prototypical *intermediary*. Contract management services play another kind of intermediary function.

Clearinghouses

The network of connections among American health care entities for the purposes of *money transfer* reflects a complex diversification of specializations. Between the provider and payer lies another network of entities that might be generically called clearinghouses. A *healthcare clearinghouse* is a public or private entity that processes or facilitates the processing of nonstandard data elements of health information into standard data elements. Such an entity is one that currently receives healthcare transactions from healthcare providers and other entities, translates the data from a given format into one acceptable to the intended recipient, and forwards the processed transaction to appropriate health plans and other healthcare clearinghouses, as necessary, for further action.

The clearinghouse provides more than simple connectivity (see Figure *4.3*). Additional *functions* include:

- Reformatting transactions into standard data formats
- Error checking
- Editing, aggregating, distributing and routing transactions
- Producing management and analysis reports

To perform these functions, the clearinghouses 'open the transaction envelope' for routing and switching purposes yet ensure security and integrity of the data through administrative procedures, technical tools, and contractual agreements.

A prominent form of intermediary organization (or clearinghouse) is called a *third-party billing agent*. Third-party billing agents help providers generate claims.

Figure 4.3. Clearinghouse. The functions of the clearinghouse are indicated in the internal cells. The arrows indicate the flow of information to and from the clearinghouse.

		CLEARINGHOUSE FUNCTIONS					
PROVIDER	⇒	receive payer transactions	sort by destination	format to payer specifications	transmit to payer	⇒	PAYER
	⇐	report to provider	sort by provider	verify transaction receipt	pick up responses	⇐	

These third-party billing agents or the providers directly contact with health plans or other "clearinghouses." Hospital information system vendors, telecommunication companies, consortia of provider organizations, and others may support other intermediary activities.

One large electronic clearinghouse for commercial, health care claims supports eligibility and referral inquiries, rosters, and encounter information. For the physician office, the company takes a batch claim file, and its computers sort the information and electronically submit it to the appropriate payers. It automatically checks for clerical errors and omissions, then 'clean' claims are routed to the individual payer the same day. Electronic verification and confirmation is sent back to the physician for each claim. The clearinghouse has access to more than 600 commercial, dental, Medicare, Medicaid and Blue Cross/Blue Shield payers. *Electronic claim submission* to these payers allows for quicker payment to providers through increased administrative efficiency and accuracy.

Contract Management

Managed care organizations control costs by defining, in advance, how a facility will be reimbursed for specific services. They attempt to build into the reimbursement methodology incentives for reducing utilization without compromising quality. The result is complex procedural and reimbursement guidelines that are difficult to map to a stream of claims generated by the provider. *Hospital billing systems* cannot accommodate these complex reimbursement arrangements. The solution may be a contract management system that calculates expected reimbursement based on the contract rules. The contract management system may be run by a claims processing vendor for the provider or may be installed on the site of the provider.

Contract management systems support a variety of reimbursement arrangements, including fee-for-service, diagnosis-related groups, per diem rates, and capitation. Contract management systems also support combinations of these arrangements. For example, a contract may support a fixed reimbursement for a procedure plus a diminishing per diem for each day after the third day in a hospital.

Contract management maximizes *revenues* for a provider, while ensuring that services are reimbursed according to contractual terms. If a provider has several contractual relationships with managed care organizations, paying for contract management is a sound investment. Numerous anecdotes attest to recovering additional revenues in the millions of dollars in the first few months after use of a contract management system.

Accountability

Some take a jaundiced view of the impact of the American system on the ability of the patient to influence change, as witnessed in this excerpt (Fogoros, 2001):

Very few patients go out and buy their own health insurance. Most receive their health insurance through their employers, the government, or not at all. Thus, patients don't really have the power to shop around and choose among health plans (except within very strict limits), nor do they have any true power to walk away from the health plans presented to them. Their lack of the ability to choose a plan, and the ability to exit a plan, essentially destroys any claim they may have to the title "customer." Indeed, their economic position in the health care system is more akin to that of "commodity." (They are, in fact, called by the industry "covered lives," and are traded back and forth like pork bellies.) Thus, health plans see relatively little reason to afford patients the same respect that businesses traditionally afford their customers.

What are the balances among the stakeholders that lead to *accountability*?

Organizations are accountable to their stakeholders, and health care organizations typically have more stakeholders than other businesses (Salain, 2006). "Accountability" is "the process by which one party is required to justify its actions and policies to another party." In the case of a health plan, the *stakeholders* include:

- Individual patients
- Purchasers (private and public)
- Health care providers (physicians and non-physicians)
- Government entities (federal and state)
- Other health plans
- Investors (for publicly-held organizations)

In many cases, health plans are involved in reciprocally accountable relationships with their stakeholders. For example, while a health plan has extensive obligations to its health care providers (e.g., prompt payment of clean claims, due process in disciplinary proceedings), the providers have a responsibility to the health plan (e.g., a duty to maintain licensure and privileges, a duty to not discriminate against health plan members).

Accountabilities to particular stakeholders may vary with *circumstances*. For instance, a health plan has obligations to each enrollee to provide accurate information about accessing benefits. Those obligations change when an enrollee becomes a patient. The health plan must then ensure that claims are paid on a timely basis and that medically needed care is available. Behaviors for which health plans are accountable include:

- Financial reliability and performance
- The provision of reasonable access to qualified health care providers
- The provision of information to promote member health
- Legal and ethical conduct
- Continuous improvement of the quality of health care provided through the health plan
- Competent administration

Within a particular *behavioral domain*, a health plan often has several sets of standards against which its performance is measured. For example, a multi-state health plan may have its performance in a single behavioral domain—continuous quality improvement, for example—measured against *standards* imposed by:

- Multiple state insurance regulators
- Multiple state health regulators
- U.S. Department of Health and Human Services
- American Accreditation HealthCare Commission
- Large employer benefit administrators

The web of accountabilities in which each health plan is embedded imposes complex administrative and operational responsibilities on the health plan.

Technology supports the exchange of information between employers and health plans. This includes enrollment information from *employers* and outcomes information from the health plan. Some employers and payers exchange enrollment information online.

The *Health Plan and Employer Data Information Set* (HEDIS) is a set of performance measures designed to standardize the way health plans report data to employers. (Another perspective on HEDIS is presented in the next chapter under the topic of data standards.) HEDIS focuses on four major performance areas:

- Quality
- Access and patient satisfaction
- Membership and utilization
- Finance

Quality indicators include childhood immunization rates and mammography rates. Patient satisfaction measures reflect the members' satisfaction within their plans. Membership and utilization data includes enrollment and dis-enrollment statistics by age and sex. Finance includes per-member revenues and rate trends. HEDIS is increasingly important for health plans as buyers of health care pay more attention to HEDIS data in deciding what plans to use. Technology is required for accurate and timely extraction of HEDIS data from the various transactions to which payers have access (Kissinger & Borchardt, 1996).

Questions

Reading Questions

1. What is the definition of a health plan?
2. What are the basic operations of a health plan?
3. What characteristics do the Blue Cross and Blue Shield case and the Medicare case have in common?
4. What is the role of a clearinghouse?

Doing Questions

1. What are three functions performed by payers and not by providers? Describe in a few sentences how an information system supports each of these functions in a way that manual processing would not practically permit.
2. Consider the CMS functional operations including Program Integrity Organization and Health Industry Standards. They are decomposed into parts that include for Program Integrity Organization:
   - Utilization monitoring
   - Fraud, waste, and abuse
   - For health industry standards

- Unique identifiers development
- Standard forms development

How might Health Industry Standards facilitate the performance of Program Integrity Organization? Give an example of a case (a fictional one is acceptable) where Standards helps Integrity.

References

Altman, D., Cutler, D., & Zeckhauser, R. (2003). Enrollee mix, treatment intensity, and cost in competing indemnity and HMO plans. *J. Health Econ, 22*(1), 23-45.

Fogoros, R. (2001). *Managing your health plan* Retrieved May 5, 2006, from http://heartdisease.about.com/library/blhcs03.htm

Hall, M. A. (2000). The Geography of Health Insurance Regulation: A guide to identifying, exploiting, and policing market boundaries. *Health Affairs, 19*(2), 173-184.

Hulme, G. V. (2003, November 26). Integration key to competition. *Insurance & Technology,* 1-2. Retrieved May 2006 from www.insurancetech.com

Kissinger, K., & Borchardt, S. (Eds.). (1996). *Information technology for integrated health systems: Positioning for the future*. New York: John Wiley & Sons.

Paramore, M. (2001). Permitted disclosures under HIPAA and Gramm-Leach-Bliley. *Third National HIPAA Summit* from http://www.hipaasummit.com/past3/agenda/day2.html Washington, DC: Health Care Conference Administrators, LLC.

Salain, R. (2006). Forging local level partnerships to make health programs possible. *North Carolina Medical Journal, 67*(1), 58-62.

Starr, P. (1997). Smart technology, stunted policy: Developing health information networks. *Health Affairs, 16*(3), 95-105.

Chapter V

Data and Knowledge

Learning Objectives

- Identify key standards in the health care information systems arena and indicate how they support interoperability
- Identify the coding systems used in health care and their conceptual frameworks
- Contrast aggregated clinical data with aggregated administrative data
- Delineate the pros and cons of various representation and reasoning schemes for medical knowledge—flow charts, databases, decision theory, and rule-based expert systems
- Develop a utility analysis for a medical decision
- Develop a rule-based expert system for a medical decision
- Construct a situation under which a decision-support system is likely to succeed in practice
- Differentiate vision and robotic systems from medical diagnosis systems
- Use effectively a medical literature retrieval system

In the 1960s and early 1970s, the emphasis in hospital information systems was on operational control—active monitoring of routine task performance, with emphasis on doing highly structured tasks better, faster, and cheaper. This *operational control* has been extensively achieved with systems such as patient accounting and medical records. The next era of application, which followed in the late 1970s and early 1980s, shifted attention toward functional effectiveness in the form of management control (Tan, 2001). In practice, this is often accomplished by data aggregation, analysis, interpretation, and presentation (Bali, 2005). Since the 1980s, a major trend has been the development of knowledge-based systems to support clinical care.

Data

The Joint Commission on Accreditation of Healthcare Organizations (JCAHO) emphasizes the distinction between *aggregated* and *comparative* data. To aggregate in this context means to combine standardized data and information. Comparative data is data about the internal operations of an entities and data about other comparable entities; an entity then compares its performance with those of others by analyzing the internal and external data.

Aggregated Clinical Data

Prior to computerization, a hospital might have maintained a *card catalogue* that documented the number of surgeries of each type performed in the hospital. These and numerous other procedure and disease patterns were coded with nationally or internationally standardized codes. With the increasing prevalence of electronic medical records and other databases, card catalogues are no longer needed. Instead, a query can be generated against the patient medical record database to answer questions, such as how many surgeries of a certain type were performed in the hospital. With the computer, the range of queries that can be quickly answered is much greater than was the case when card catalogues were the source of information. Whether with card catalogues or electronic medical records, the coded data constitutes aggregated clinic data.

Another source of aggregated data is a *registry*. Registries are lists that generally contain the names and other identifying information of patients seen in a particular area of a health care provider. For instance, a register might show the people seen in the Emergency Room. Research also benefits from registries. The mission, design, size, methodology, and use of technology vary with each kind of registry. Examples of some of the most widely used registries include cancer, AIDS, birth defects, diabetes, organ transplants, and trauma. Cancer registries are the most common and are elaborated here. Physicians and epidemiologists concerned with assessing cancer incidence, treatment, and results have long accepted the collection, retrieval, and analysis of cancer data as essential. The types of cancer registries are defined as either hospital-based or population-based (Smith, 2000).

The primary goal of *hospital-based cancer registries* is to improve patient care. The data are used:

- To make certain the optimal care is provided
- To compare the institution's morbidity and survival rates with regional statistics
- To determine the need for education programs
- To allocate resources

Data items routinely collected include patient identification and demographic information, cancer diagnosis, treatment given, prognosis factors, and outcomes. Hospitals generally have no legal requirement to keep cancer registries.

The three types of *population-based cancer registry* are:

- Incidence only
- Cancer control
- Research

Most *incidence only registries* are operated by a government health agency and are designed to calculate cancer rates, usually required by law. *Cancer control registries* often combine incidence, patient care, and end results reporting with various other cancer control activities, such as cancer screening and quit smoking programs. Many *research-oriented registries* are maintained by medical schools to conduct epidemiological research focused on etiology. Information is shared with public servants and health care providers, and often published in medical journals. The legislative mandate or funding sources normally determine the focus—incidence monitoring, cancer control, or research.

Aggregated Administrative Data

Aggregate administrative data is important for management of an entity. For example, *Medicare cost reports* are filed annually by hospitals, home health agencies, and nursing facilities that accept Medicare payments. These reports must meet various regulatory requirements and are subject to compliance audits. The report contains utilization data, charges by cost center for Medicare and in total, Medicare settlement data, and other financial data. Medicare uses these reports to determine an entity's reimbursements and to determine Medicare policies generally. Of course, an entity's management wants its Medicare cost reports to put the entity in a position to earn the highest reimbursements from Medicare.

Census statistics and discharge statistics are two further examples of aggregate administrative data. *Census statistics* show how many patients were in a facility at any given time and include such data information as the bed occupancy rates. From *discharge statistics* the entity determines the average length of stay at the entity, death rates, autopsy rates, and infection rates. Census and discharge statistics help an entity plan and monitor patient services.

Aggregate data may combine both clinical and administrative data. Cost per case or average reimbursement per diagnostic group are examples of clinical data combined with administrative data. Administrators may use cost per case or average reimbursement per diagnostic group to help manage finances. Patient satisfaction may be inferred from *clinical-plus-administrative aggregate data*, such as the time it takes to get an appointment at a clinic.

Comparative Data

Comparative data is, of course, for comparisons but particularly refers to data for comparisons between attributes of an entity and attributes of other entities. Comparisons may be made to an entity's competitors, to the industry, or to best-in-class entities. A common attribute to consider is outcomes.

Outcomes measures can be applied to individuals or groups to measure the results of clinical or administrative processes. For example, the percentage of Medicare claims that are denied is an *outcomes measure*. Outcomes measures for one entity can be compared to those of other entities or to some standard. Comparing to a standard is called benchmarking. When multiple outcomes measures are used in an assessment, the approach is sometimes called the 'balanced scorecard'. Entities may select from many external health care data sets to compare their performance against the performance of others.

The National Committee for Quality Assurance (NCQA) engages in accreditation and performance measurement of managed health care. To this end, NCQA developed the *Health Plan Employer Data and Information Set (HEDIS)*. HEDIS data can be used to establish benchmarks or for accreditation of individual entities. Employers may use the NCQA assessments that were based on HEDIS data in determining the health plans into which they want to enroll their employees. (Further details about HEDIS are in the preceding chapter about payers.)

The *Joint Commission on Accreditation of Healthcare Organizations (JCAHO)* is an accrediting body. The mission of the Joint Commission is to improve the quality of care through the provision of health care accreditation that support performance improvement in health care entities. Since 1997, JCAHO has integrated performance measurement data into the accreditation process through the implementation of the ORYX initiative. This initiative permits rigorous comparison of the results of care across hospitals.

Through its *ORYX* initiative, JCAHO provides measure sets in a variety of core areas, such as management of heart failure. The entity to be accredited must provide its data relative to these JCAHO measures. For example, one of the performance measures for heart failure management addresses the extent to which patients were given adequate discharge instructions. The measure in particular specifies:

- **Name:** Discharge instructions
- **Description:** Heart failure patients discharged home with written instructions addressing activity level, diet, discharge medications, follow-up appointment, and weight monitoring
- **Numerator:** Number of patients given these instructions
- **Denominator:** Heart failure patients discharged
- **Data Reported as:** Aggregate data generated from count data as proportion

Other important sources of benchmarking data include the Centers for Medicare and Medicaid Services (CMS) for clinical indicators, the Gallup Organization for patient satisfaction data, and the Centers for Disease Control for public health data.

In 2004, the JCAHO and CMS began working together to align measures common to both organizations. These standardized common measures are referred to as *Hospital Quality Measures*. Measure alignment benefits hospitals by making it easier and less costly to collect and report data because the same data set can be used to satisfy both CMS and JCAHO requirements. The Hospital Quality Measure sets currently utilized by JCAHO and CMS cover acute myocardial infarction, heart failure, pneumonia, and surgical infection prevention.

Standards

Coordination is the top event in a hierarchy that proceeds from data that is communicated in a common language and goes through decision-making before coordination is possible. The sequence is:

1. Data
2. Common language

3. Communication
4. Decision-making
5. Coordination

Before a project can progress, it must choose a common language. For person-to-person conversation, the language might be English. For messages between computers, the choice is less obvious. Common languages for computer-computer communication derive from standardization efforts.

Definition

A standard is defined as something established by authority, custom, or general consent as a model or example. *Standards* arise either from official standards activity or arise by the force of practice. An official standard is a de jure standard, while those that arise by practice are de facto standards. For instance, the Open Systems Interconnection (OSI) standards of the International Organization of Standards are de jure standards, while Microsoft Office is a de facto standard (Rada et al., 1994).

Practically speaking a standard is simply what people use. Microsoft Office is a *de facto standard* because many people use it and not because it was created by a formal standards development organization. The most important aim of standardization is to produce standards that are wanted and used.

A *de jure standard* should be impartial in the sense that it should not give exclusive advantage to the product or service of any individual supplier. A standard is cost-effective when the effort to make and gain compliance with the standard costs less than the benefit. In areas of rapid development, the balance must be struck between inhibiting innovation by standardizing too soon and proliferating wasteful or mutually incompatible solutions by leaving standardization until too late. De jure messaging or data exchange standards (see Figure 5-1) exist for exchanging clinical data (Health Level Seven), images (DICOM), clinical observations (ASTM), bedside instrument data (IEEE), prescription data, and administrative data associated with claims (X12).

Interoperability refers to the ability of one computer system to exchange data with another computer system. Three levels of interoperability are (Benson, 2002):

- *Basic interoperability* allows a message from one computer to be received by another but does not expect the information to be interpreted.
- *Functional interoperability* is an intermediate level that defines the syntax of messages. This ensures that messages can be interpreted at the level of data fields. For example, when one computer has a field for 'Ear Exam', that

Figure 5.1. Messages. Medical record in center connected to other activities via messaging. The square boxes are the activities. The arrows indicate the flow of messages. The italicized term refers to the standard organization that has a standard relevant to that message or transaction.

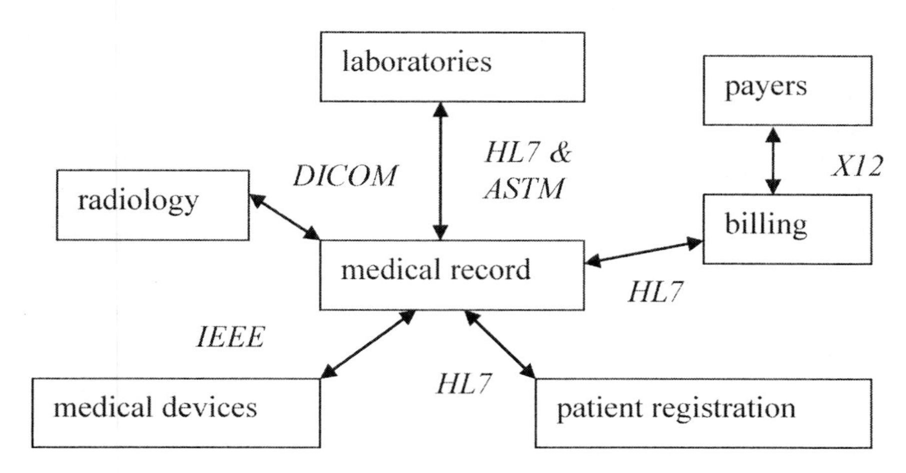

computer should be able to pass data to another computer and have it appropriately stored in a comparable field for 'Ear Exam'. Neither system, however, understands the meaning of the 'Ear Exam'.

- *Semantic interoperability* requires that the information can be used in an intelligent manner and takes advantage of both the structuring of the message and the codification of the data within the fields. Thus the 'Ear Exam' may have an attribute of 'Inflammation' with a value of 'positive' and this could trigger reactions in the receiving computer.

For optimal value, standards for semantic interoperability are needed.

Typically, standards are produced in large numbers, and entities pick or choose which ones to follow. Standards are only important when organizations adhere to them. A standard becomes binding when compliance is *mandatory* by legislation or when a party is contracted to work to it (Rada, 1993). Governments currently make some standards important by insisting on purchasing only products or services consistent with a certain standard. A yet more absolute way to make a standard important is for the government to mandate that organizations comply with the standard. The HIPAA Transaction Rule is powerful because the government has mandated that healthcare organizations comply with the standards indicated in the Rule.

Standards Organizations

The principal *stakeholders* with active involvement in standards are:

- **Providers and payers:** Providers and payers communicate healthcare data.
- **Government:** The federal and state governments are large payers and—in some cases—providers of healthcare. The federal government frames national healthcare policy, regulates the industry, and sets standards, as in the case of HIPAA. States also regulate and license providers and payers.
- **Standards development organizations:** These are defined later in this section.
- **Vendors:** Most healthcare organizations purchase their software from healthcare information systems vendors. Thus, interoperability standards depend on support from the vendor community.

Interoperability standards and how they work in the information value chain are critical business issues for vendors. Generally, hospital information systems vendors claim HL7 compatibility, and imaging vendors support DICOM standards.

A *standards development organization* is any organization that develops standards. However, the term 'standards development organization' is typically used to refer to an organization that has been recognized by some authority for its process. The process should be open to the public and should not only develop the standard but also maintain it over time. Health Level 7 (HL7) is the primary standards development organization for standards for system interfacing within provider organizations. Like HL7 in the clinical domain, ASC X12N is the acknowledged leader in the healthcare financial domain.

Each country typically has a standards development organization that helps coordinate the standards of that country. For the United States, that organization is the American National Standards Institute (ANSI). ANSI (ANSI, 2006):

... coordinates the development and use of voluntary consensus standards in the United States and represents the needs and views of U.S. stakeholders in standardization forums around the globe. ANSI oversees the creation, promulgation and use of thousands of norms and guidelines that directly impact businesses in nearly every sector.

The ANSI *Healthcare Informatics Standards Board (HISB)* was created within ANSI to help coordinate and promote adoption of standards relating to healthcare information system applications. HISB focuses on encouraging communication among existing standards development organizations in the healthcare domain.

The *American Society for Testing and Materials (ASTM)* is an ANSI-accredited standards development organization and has been developing standards since 1898. ASTM began doing healthcare informatics standards in the 1960s. ASTM's first healthcare standards addressed laboratory message exchange, properties for electronic health record systems, and health information security. *Health Level Seven (HL7)* is an ANSI-accredited standards development organization and in 1987 developed its first in a wide range of message format standards for patient registration, orders, and observations reporting.

Some healthcare standards organizations are not ANSI-accredited. The development of standards in the healthcare arena has not typically relied as extensively on formal standards development organizations as have some other industries. Initially, a clinical specialty group or professional association would identify a need for a standard in a specific area. The *College of American Pathologists* started developing a nomenclature of pathology in 1965. The College of American Pathologists first became an ANSI-accredited standards development organization in February 2000. In 1974, DHHS (which is not an ANSI-accredited standards development organization) promulgated the first Uniform Hospital Discharge Data Set. The American Medical Association's 'Current Procedures and Terminology' is a standard code set of medical procedures and is an example of a standard developed by a professional society that is not ANSI-accredited.

In an unusual approach to developing a medical standard that had strong practitioner input and was associated with an ANSI-accredited standards development organization, the American College of Radiology (ACR) and the National Electrical Manufacturers Association (NEMA) collaborated. ACR was not ANSI-accredited but NEMA was. ACR-NEMA identified a need in 1985 for standards for communicating biomedical images and created the *Digital Imaging and Communications in Medicine (DICOM)* standard.

The *National Council for Prescription Drug Programs (NCPDP)* first started developing standards in 1977 with the development of the Universal Claim Form (www.ncpdp.org). NCPDP's Telecommunication Standard is used to process over 1 billion claims per year. NCPDP achieved ANSI accreditation status in 1996.

Interoperability

High quality health care depends on comprehensive patient medical record information. While health care has adopted information technology for financial and administrative systems, it has made limited progress in utilizing information technology to support patient care. One impediment to the adoption of information technology is the lack of comprehensive *standards* for patient medical record information.

The U.S. *National Committee on Vital and Health Statistics* concluded that an adequate computerized patient record requires that clinically specific data are captured once at the point of care and that all other legitimate data needs are derived from those data. This requires *interoperability*.

Interoperability is the ability of products, systems, or business processes to work together to accomplish a common task. For a computer system, this means the ability of one computer system to exchange data with another computer system. Health care entities typically employ many different information systems. For example, a hospital may have a laboratory system from one vendor, a radiology system from another vendor, and a medical records system from a third vendor. Physicians affiliated with the hospital may have different systems in their offices. The physician will want information from the hospital in his office and information from the office in the hospital. He will be stymied by the incompatibility between the office and hospital systems. To achieve coordination among the components of the health care system, the components must first share a *common vocabulary* and then communicate to make decisions.

To achieve interoperability between different information systems, the healthcare delivery system has message format standards. About these standards, the National Committee on Vital and Health Statistics has said (NCVHS, 2000):

These standards have a high degree of optionality to accommodate the variability of workflow and availability of information in different care settings. This optionality creates the need for costly and time-consuming customization when implementing message format standards. In addition, vendors and providers have developed their own implementation guides that differ from the standards. Finally, there is little or no conformance testing of message format standards. Non-standard implementations result in the need for costly and time-consuming customization to allow information systems to seamlessly exchange data with one another. These customized solutions contribute to high cost of systems. Such high cost, in turn, restricts the broadest possible adoption of information systems by providers. If, by accelerating uniform message format standards development and implementation, the cost of these healthcare information systems can be lowered, their market acceptance would increase. This would contribute directly to improved quality of care, improved provider productivity, and reduced healthcare costs.

Related to interoperability is data comparability. Comparable data has the same meaning when shared among different parties. Lack of comparable data can directly impact patient care. For example, physical therapists use a pain scale that ranges from 1 to 4, while nurses use a pain scale that ranges from 1 to 10. Pain designated at 'level 3' means something different to the physical therapist than it means to the nurse. *Comparability* would make the meaning of that pain data consistent between the physical therapist and nurse. Standard healthcare vocabularies could be used to facilitate comparability of data. Information system vendors and healthcare providers sometimes create their own proprietary set of terms that are not comparable with other vocabularies. The use of national standard vocabularies would facilitate clinical data collection and interpretation across organizations. This use of standard vocabularies would also support the study of best practices and developmental of clinical guidelines.

Codes

Usability and expressiveness may conflict. The biggest challenge to using a medical vocabulary is to balance usability with the necessity to capture adequately rich information. For example, a physician may order vital signs to be taken at specific intervals, but different physicians may have different concepts of what *vital signs* means. The physician might say vital signs are temperature, pulse, respiration, and blood pressure. However, a sign like 'blood pressure' might be different if the patient is standing, sitting, or supine. The physician will not specify the full details each time of what 'vital signs' means. The various users of the concept must agree in advance as to exactly what is intended by the use of any potentially ambiguous concept, such as 'vital signs'.

Conceptual Models

A code is a representation assigned to a term so that it may more readily be processed. A simple listing of codes and the terms with which they are associated is a *code set*. For example, in the state postal code set, the code for Maryland is MD and for Virginia is VA.

Coding systems include code sets but have additional structure. The ASTM gives these criteria for good coding systems:

- Concepts are clearly defined and the concepts do not overlap with one another. Plus the set of concepts covers all the necessary concepts of the intended scope of the vocabulary.
- Structured relationships among the concepts facilitate the use of the concepts in indexing and retrieval.
- The coding system is designed so as to readily support refinement across time.

Librarians, biologists, philosophers, and others have studied the nature of coding systems for centuries. A coding system may be used to index documents, classify animals, or represent human knowledge.

One type of coding system is a *classification language*. The classic way to develop a classification language is to study members of the population (be they medical journal articles, organisms, or something else) to be represented by the language and to first determine the key concepts needed to describe the members of the population. Each key concept is associated with a key term. Given that several alternate key terms exist, they are represented as synonyms of one another and a definition for the concept is provided. To better understand the classification language, the key concepts are organized in a hierarchy. Each time a member of the population appears that raises questions about the ability of the language to adequately represent that member, then those developing the language need to consider whether the concepts appropriate to the new member map to existing concepts or require the generation of a more specific (narrower) concept than any already in the language or a more general (broader) concept than any already in use.

Diseases and Procedures

The code for diseases is the *International Classification of Diseases, 9th edition, Clinical Modification (ICD-9-CM)*. The complete ICD-9-CM is available for free from DHHS. ICD-9-CM includes one volume as an alphabetical index and another volume as a tree-structure in which concepts are located hierarchically by their associated code numbers. For example, in the alphabetical index one finds at 'nasopharyngitis' the following information:

- Nasopharyngitis (acute) (infective) 460
- Natal tooth 520.6
- Nausea 787.02

In the hierarchical index at the code 460 for nasopharyngitis, one finds:

- 460-519 RESPIRATORY SYSTEM DISEASES
- 460-466 Acute Respiratory Infections
- 460 Acute nasopharyngitis [common cold]
- 461 Acute sinusitis

ICD-9-CM is utilized to facilitate payment of health services, to evaluate utilization patterns, and to study the appropriateness of health care costs. ICD-9-CM also provides access to medical records for medical research and public health purposes.

ICD-9-CM is not always precise or unambiguous. However, there are no viable alternatives immediately. Many problems cannot be resolved within the current structure, but are addressed in *ICD-10-CM.*

Different coding systems are used for physician procedures and dental procedures:

- For dental procedures the *Code on Dental Procedures and Nomenclature* is available from the American Dental Association for a charge
- For inpatient hospital services 'ICD-9-CM, Volume 3 Procedures' is appropriate
- For physician services a combination of the *Current Procedural Terminology-4* (available from the American Medical Association for a charge) and the Healthcare Common *Procedural Coding System* (available for free from DHHS) is appropriate

The standard code set for drugs is the National Drug Code Directory from the Food and Drug Administration. The full Directory is available for free (*National Drug Code Directory*, 2006). The drug codes are also published in the *Physicians' Desk Reference* under the individual drug product listings. NDC is useful in retail pharmacy systems where bottles of pills are tracked. NDC identifies the manufacturer, the size of the bottle, and so on.

The standard use of codes harmonizes the sharing of information in the health care industry. However, codes can have the problem of being imprecise and ambiguous.

Decision-Making

Health-related decisions depend on scientific and other evidence. A system for finding and appraising scientific information to support health care is called *evidence-based medicine*. Evidence is, however, not sufficient for decisions. People also have preferences and constraints that may or may not be consistent with scientific evidence. Examples of evidence, preferences, and constraints follow:

- **Evidence:** Patient data, basic and clinical research, systematic reviews
- **Preferences:** Cultural beliefs, personal values, education, experience
- **Constraints:** Policies and laws, time, finance

The intersection (Tranfield et al., 2003) of:

- Evidence and preferences provides the knowledge for decision-making
- Evidence and constraints forms guidelines
- Preferences and constraints forms ethics

The intersection of the three represents everything that is considered in a healthcare decision. The next subsections explore the intersection of evidence and preferences as reflected in decision theory and utility theory.

Decision Theory

Intelligent systems in health care are best developed by thoroughly understanding the human decision-making and knowledge manipulating processes. This kind of study can result in new knowledge-based tools for practitioners but also may result in new insights about health care practice. Schwartz (1970) speaks of:

... the possibility that the computer as an intellectual tool can reshape the present system of health care, fundamentally alter the role of the physician, and profoundly change the nature of medical manpower recruitment and medical education .... The key technical developments leading to this reshaping will almost certainly involve exploitation of the computer as an 'intellectual,' 'deductive' instrument—a consultant that is built into the very structure of the medical-care system and that augments or replaces many traditional activities of the physician.

Approaches to this 'intelligent' type of medical computing originally emphasized the clinical algorithm or flowchart and applications of decision theory.

A *flowchart* is conceptually a simple decision making tool. A flowchart can represent the logic of a computer program. With the emergence of structured programming in the 1980s, variations on flowcharts, such as data flow diagrams, were introduced. Flowcharts remain vital to business analysts who seek to describe the logic of a process in a graphical format. Flowcharts are commonly found in project documentation and are widely used in education, health care, service industries, and other areas where graphical, logical depiction of process is helpful. In a clinical setting, a flowchart might encode the sequence of actions a clinician would perform for a patient. For example, a flowchart could represent all sequences of questions asked, answers given, procedures performed, laboratory analyses obtained and eventual diagnoses, treatments and outcomes for patients who present at the emergency room with severe chest pain. Deficiencies of the flowchart for encoding medical decision-making knowledge are its lack of compactness and perspicuity (Szolovits, 1982).

Decision theory is concerned with how decision-makers make decisions and how optimal decisions can be reached. Much of decision theory is concerned with identifying the best decision to take, assuming an ideal decision taker who is fully informed and rational. The practical application of this prescriptive approach is called decision analysis and is aimed at finding methods or tools to help people make better decisions. Software tools of this sort are called decision support systems.

An agent operates in an uncertain world, and choice under uncertain conditions is studied by decision theorists. The theory of expected value was developed in the 17th century and begins by assuming that someone faces a choice among a number of actions, each of which could give rise to more than one possible outcome with different probabilities. The decision method involves identifying possible outcomes and determining their values and their probability of occurring. By multiplying the value times the probability, one gets the *expected value*. The action is chosen that gives rise to the highest total expected value.

A simple example illustrates the role of probability and value in determining a decision. If a person has a choice of receiving:

- $1,500 with a probability of 1.0
- $4,000 with a probability of 0.25

then what should the person choose? The value of the first option is $1,500 times 1.0 which equals $1,500. The value of the second option is $4,000 times 0.25 which equals $1,000. The person should choose the first option because it has the higher *value*.

Utility Theory

Decision theorists have extended the notion of expected value to the notion of *expected utility*. The estimated utility of some action is based on the utility of its possible result(s). A simple example of the application of utility theory revisits the preceding example of a person offered two options for money. If a person has a choice of receiving

Table 5.1. Utilities of surgery given disease

Surgery	Disease	
	yes	no
yes	$2000	-$400
no	-$200	$200

- $1,000 with a probability of 0.99
- $3,000 with a probability of 0.34

then what should the person choose? The value of the first option is $1,000 times 0.99 which equals $990. The value of the second option is $3,000 times 0.34 which equals $1,020. While the second option has a higher monetary value, many people would prefer the first option. That first option appeals to people more than the second option because the extra money gained with option two (namely, $1,020-$990 = $30) has a higher risk that the person gets nothing. The utility of the first option is higher.

Another example of expected utility provides a *medical context*. Patients may present in the emergency room with symptoms of a disease d. The treatment for d may be a surgical procedure s. Of course, s has adverse effects too. Given that the diagnosis of d can only be made with certainty after surgical intervention, what should the probability of d be in order that performing s has more benefits than costs?

Consider a *2-by-2 table* that shows d and s and for which the utility measured in dollars of (see Table 5.1):

- s given d (the yes-yes condition) is $2000
- 'no s' given d (the no-yes condition) is -$200
- s given 'no d' is -$400 (the yes-no condition)
- 'no s' given 'no d' is $200

The probability for d, in order, that the patient should receive s can be obtained by first finding when the utility of s is equal to the utility of 'no s' (Warner, 1979). Abbreviate Utility as U and Probability as P. When does $U_s = U_{no\ s}$?

$U_s = \$2000 * P_d + (-\$400) * P_{no\ d}$
$U_{no\ s} = -\$200 * P_d + (\$200) * P_{no\ d}$

Thus, one wants to know when:

$\$2000 * P_d + (-\$400) * P_{no\ d} =$
$-\$200 * P_d + (\$200) * P_{no\ d}$

This can be simplified to:

$\$2200 * P_d = (\$600) * P_{no\ d}$

Since $P_{no\ d}$ equals $1- P_d$, the preceding equation becomes:

$\$2200 * P_d = (\$600) * (1- P_d)$

With further manipulation, one gets:

$\$2800 * P_d = \$600$

and then

$P_d = 0.21$

When the probability of d is greater than 0.21, then s brings more benefit than cost.

Determining actual values to include in a medical utility analysis is a non-trivial exercise. Consider the case of an appendectomy on a patient with appendicitis. The value of a decision is its benefit minus its cost The benefit is related to the number of *healthy days* remaining for the patient (Warner, 1979). For instance, the benefit might be partially captured by

('life expectancy'—'number of days lost from appendectomy and appendicitis') * (1—'immediate mortality of appendectomy')

The cost might be partly covered by:

'initial costs' + 'continuing costs' + 'lost income'

where

- 'Initial costs' include the typical professional fees and hospital expenses for the appendectomy
- 'Continuing costs' are the medications, doctor visits after discharge, and other such ongoing costs
- 'Lost income' is the patient's annual salary multiplied by the number of days in the year in which the patient will not work because of the decision

Since medical costs are typically measured in monetary units but benefits in 'days of good health', a way to translate between monetary units and days is needed. One way to do this translation is to assign a *monetary value* to each healthy day.

Continuing in the preceding fashion, one could determine the utilities under each of the combinations of disease present and treatment applied. From there one could determine the probability of disease that should justify that treatment. Furthermore, one could then experiment with the impact of a host of factors. For instance, a younger patient has a longer life expectancy and thus a different benefit than an older patient. This may mean that a procedure should be performed on a young patient that would not be *cost-effective* to perform on an older patient.

Expert Systems

The chief disadvantages of the decision theoretic approach are the difficulties of obtaining reasonable estimates of probabilities and utilities for a particular analysis. An *expert system* is a program that uses available information, heuristics, and inference to suggest solutions to problems in a particular discipline. The working of an expert system will be considered in detail so that the reader might develop a simple rule base. Famous systems will be reviewed, and challenges identified.

Model

Many medical expert systems are *rule-based.* Rule-based systems are based on rules of the form "if condition1, then action1." The condition may also be called the antecedent, and the action, the consequent. In general, the rule may have any number of conditions and actions, as in "if condition1, condition2, condition3, then action1, action2". The conditions might be joined together by logical connectives, such as AND and OR. The set of rules may be viewed as a network in which one rule R1 points to another rule R2 when an action of R1 is a condition of R2.

The rule-based system operates in an environment that provides facts or assertions to the system. For instance, if a condition is "patient has fever" and if the environment confirms that the "patient has fever", then the action occurs. The assertions plus the actions of rules might be called a *working memory* of the expert system.

The rule-based system has its content of rules and working memory but also, importantly, an inference engine. The *inference engine* examines the rules and working memory and determines what should happen. The system examines the rule's conditions and determines a subset whose conditions are satisfied by the working memory. This subset is called the conflict set. From this conflict set, one rule is activated. To the extent that the rule-based system mimics a human brain, the rules would be activated in parallel. However, most expert system technology activates rules in serial, and thus some conflict resolution strategy is needed to determine which rule to activate when more than one has its conditions satisfied by the current working memory. One such strategy chooses the rule with the most conditions from those that are in the conflict set—that rule might be considered

Figure 5.2. Rule firing process. To start, the rule base and working memory are populated. Next, the rules that could be fired are determined, and one of those rules is fired. Working memory is augmented, and the next set of possible rules to fire is determined.

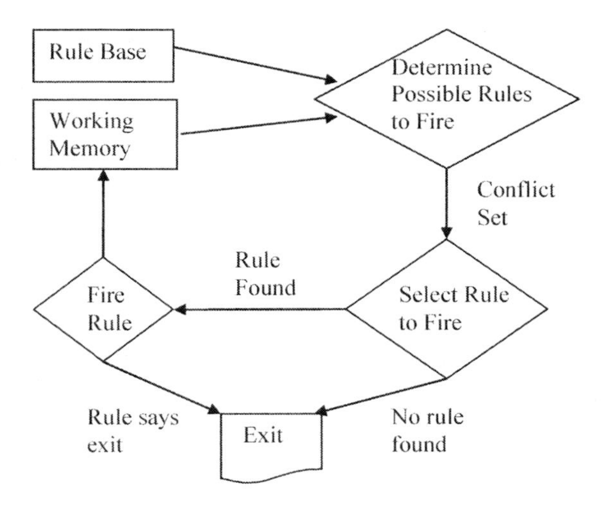

the most relevant rule to the current content of the working memory. The cycle of identifying a conflict set and firing a rule continues until either no more rules are satisfied or the firing of a rule causes some termination action of the system to be produced (see Figure 5.2).

A toy example of an expert system is provided for the case of the common cold. Say that the Rule Base is:

- **R1:** If 'nasal congestion' and 'fever' then diagnose 'common cold' and exit
- **R2:** If 'runny nose' and 'headache' then assert 'nasal congestion'
- **R3:** If 'temp greater than 100' then assert 'fever'

Say the Working Memory initially contains:

- Runny nose
- Temperature = 101.7
- Headache

The Expert System will work as follows:

1. Rules R2 and R3 are satisfied by working memory and are selected as possible rules to be next fired
2. Since R2 has more conditions, R2 is fired first
3. The assertion of 'nasal congestion' is added to 'working memory'
4. Rule R3 is now the only rule whose conditions are satisfied by 'working memory', and R3 is thus put into the set of possible rules to fire and is next fired
5. The assertion 'fever' is added to 'working memory'
6. Rule R1 is now satisfied and fired
7. The assertions of R1 include that the system should exit and thus the system exits

In this process of firing rules and adding assertions to working memory, the system could also return to the user with a question that could lead to information being added by the user to working memory.

The astute reader might have recognized that the toy example suggests incorrectly that all patients with fever and nasal congestion have the common cold. Medical practice deals usually in *uncertainty*. The common cold might be the most likely diagnose for the patient with fever and nasal congestion but the notion of 'most likely' was not represented in the previous example. To handle uncertainty, rule-based expert systems typically include weights on rules.

One approach to uncertainty is to associate a *certainty factor* between 0 and 1 with each assertion and each rule. This factor says how certain the fact or rule is, with 0 indicating extreme falsehood and 1 indicating extreme truth. Given that the rules and initial assertions in working memory have certainties associated with them, how does the expert system inference engine massage these factors through the processing of rules? In particular, two questions need to be addressed:

- How are the certainties of the rule's conditions combined into the rule's overall condition certainty?
- How is the output certainty determined from the combined input certainty and the rule certainty?

The typical answers to these questions do not have a provably correct interpretation in probability theory but have some pragmatic value. One of the simplest approaches follows (Winston, 1992):

- The minimum certainty associated with the rule's conditions becomes the certainty of the rule's overall input. This heuristic comes from the common notion that a chain is only as strong as its weakest link.
- The rule's output certainty is determined by multiplying the rule's certainty factor by the overall input certainty. This heuristic is based on the principle that the probability of two events occurring together is the product of the two probabilities that either occurs alone.

In the preceding 'common cold' example, the Rule R1 might be associated with a certainty of 0.7 to indicate that 70% of the time 'nasal congestion' and 'fever' are correctly diagnosed as being the 'common cold'.

An advantage of the simple, uniform representation of rule-based systems is that the system can reason not only with the knowledge in the rules but also about them. Thus, methods can be created to:

- Help acquire new rules from the expert user when the expert and program disagree
- Suggest generalizations of some of the rules based on their similarity to others

- Explain the knowledge of the rules and how they are used to the system's users (Shortliffe, 1991)

This *metareasoning* about rules also supports machine learning.

The hypothesis behind expert system work is that the rules of the expert system will support actions that are comparable to those that a *human expert* would produce. Traditionally, rule-based systems are only practical for problems for which knowledge relevant to the problem can be expressed as if-then rules and for which the number of rules needed is not very large.

Example Applications

The *MYCIN system* is arguably the most famous expert system developed for medicine. A physician who became interested in computing developed the program as a graduate student at Stanford University in the 1970s (Shortliffe, 1976). The subsequent

Figure 5.3. Rules from MYCIN (Adapted from Shortliffe, 1976). The first rule identifies streptococcus as a disease agent, while the second rule suggests a change in route of administration of a therapeutic antibiotic. The certainty factor for each rule is indicated in the 'then' clause.

A rule for diagnosis:

If

1. stain of the organism is gram positive,
2. morphology of the organism is coccus, and
3. growth conformation of the organism is chains,

Then

evidence suggests (with certainty 0.7) that the identity of the organism is streptococcus.

A rule for therapy:

If

1. route of administration of penicillin is oral and
2. a GI factor may interfere with the absorption of penicillin,

Then

evidence suggests (with certainty 0.6) that route of administration of penicillin is not adequate.

explosion of interest in rule-based expert systems often cited the MYCIN work. MYCIN supports the diagnosis and treatment of certain bacterial infections.

One *rule* from MYCIN for determining the bacterial type (Shortliffe, 1976) reveals very specific attention to laboratory data (see Figure 5.3). Another rule for helping determine therapy shows how therapy selection is also a complex process (see Figure 5.3). Both rules demonstrate the typical pattern described in the preceding subsection of several conditions and an action with a certainty factor associated with the rule.

Numerous *experiments* were done with MYCIN under rigorous conditions. The program needed to get precise input about the signs, symptoms, and laboratory values for a patient. The experiments assumed the patient had an infectious disease of the blood. Given these constraints, *MYCIN* was able to give more accurate diagnoses consistently than the average infectious disease expert.

In practice, MYCIN was not used. With government research funding, MYCIN was installed in various clinic settings, but doctors did not want to use it. The first interpretation of the researchers was that the system was lacking certain vital functions, like the ability to explain its behavior. The system was extended with ability to give to the physician the rules that had been most instrumental in any given diagnosis, and these rules were put into attractively understandable natural language. However, this additional feature did not increase the *usage* by practitioners.

Hundreds of medical expert systems, other than MYCIN or its extensions, have been developed. One direction of expansion was to cover as many diseases as possible. The *Internist-1* system for diagnosis of diseases in internal medicine was developed in the early 1980s at the University of Pittsburgh (Miller et al., 1982). The Internist-1 system included 500 diseases and 3550 findings. For each disease, a list of findings was defined and connected with this disease. The program proceeded through the findings on the patient and computed the likelihood that each disease was associated with the particular history, signs, symptoms, and lab values of the patient. Internist-1, like Mycin, proved competent in doing diagnosis. Experts did not perform better than Internist-1. However, the developers of Internist-1 were also unable to achieve significant usage of their system by practicing physicians.

Other infection disease expert systems were developed and *evaluated* after MYCIN. For one such expert system (Evans et al., 1999), physicians who used the system gave the correct diagnosis 94% of the time, whereas only 77% of the physicians who did not employ the expert system got the correct diagnosis. Physicians who used the expert system allowed less time to elapse between the collection of culture specimens and the ordering of antibiotics. Moreover, in response to a survey, most of the physicians said that use of the expert system improved patient care.

Health care organizations have used expert systems that can assist practitioners by issuing reminders, offering diagnostic and therapeutic options, and providing links to the literature. *Benefits* have been demonstrated. Clinicians who receive such expert system support respond faster to changes in their patient's condition (Safran et al., 1996). Expert systems for nurses have also been developed and have had beneficial effects. For instance, a nursing expert system to support the management of minor eye injuries improved nursing care (Martin, 2001).

Challenges

Encoding *human expertise* in the computer is amazingly difficult. The difficulty rests both on:

- A lack of understanding of how people know what they know
- Technical problems of structuring and accessing large amounts of knowledge in the machine

Often, in expert, medical decision-making much knowledge of the world comes into play. The following scenario (Gorry, 1976) illustrates the subtlety of the problem:

A middle-aged, female patient goes to her doctor and complains of chest pain. The following dialogue ensues:

Patient: This whole side of my chest hurts.

Doctor: Are you experiencing any irregular heart beats?

Patient: No, my heart beat is fine.

Doctor: You will be okay.

Patient: Is the problem with my heart?

Doctor: I do not know. However, I just had a thought. Are you lifting any sacks at the store?

Patient: Yes, I lift some sacks. However, only for women customers and usually only weighing about 50 pounds.

Doctor: I think your pain may be secondary to lifting those sacks.

The doctor builds on his understanding of the physiological basis of pain to identify a life style problem for the patient—namely, lifting heavy weights (Szolovits, 1982). The doctor knows the patient and her occupation, the common practices in her store, and the weight of typical sacks. A computer program would not get to this diagnosis nearly as quickly as the doctor did.

Representing the reasoning of the doctor is difficult. Reasoning becomes simpler if the structure of the representation reflects the structure of the reality. Early *representation languages* were based on the predicate calculus, in which each fact, or item of knowledge, was represented as a single expression in the language. Newer representation languages incorporate automatic mechanisms to make the simple, local deductions implied by the conventions of their knowledge representation scheme.

Expert systems have been developed for many medical, diagnostic problems and typically have been successful within a certain sense. Understanding this sense and its implications is vital to properly anticipating the future of expert systems in health care.

The history of medical expert systems is a long and rich one. Thousands of medical expert systems have been implemented and shown experimentally to manifest intelligence. However, by and large, these systems have not been practically used as intended. What is the explanation for this phenomenon? Clinicians must confront patients in intense, intimate, time-pressured, face-to-face, *belly-to-belly* events. Typically, the patient record is not digital. Even when significant portions of the medical record are digitized, the patient-physician encounter does not occur with a computer between the two people. The physician is collecting vital information from the patient in real-time and going through a heuristic and pattern recognizing diagnostic process that is almost instantaneous. To use the expert systems, the physician needs to take several steps that do not fit comfortably into the situation at hand. First the physician needs to be seated before a computer screen and entering data collected from the patient, then the physician must wait for the computer to determine what it can from the information available, and then the physician must assess the feedback and decide how relevant it is to the situation at hand. If the computer program only handles a narrow range of diseases, such as Mycin did, then the utility is of course substantially reduced. However, even at the first step of needing to enter data collected from the patient into the computer, the physician faces a barrier or a cost that proves greater than the benefit given the way the health care system operates. The physician can make a good enough conclusion on his or her own without the support of an expert system relative to the cost of using the expert system.

Interesting medical *malpractice* issues arise when considering expert systems. What if a physician follows the advice of an expert system, but the advice proves faulty for the particular patient? Is the physician or the provider of the expert system responsible? On the other hand, if the physician does not use an expert system, and someone can show that the physician made a decision that would have been better had the physician used an expert system, then is the physician guilty of malpractice for not using an expert system.

The reasons for the failure to use expert systems suggest the conditions under which expert systems will succeed. The data needed by the intelligent system should be on the computer from some previous process and should not create an extra demand on the health care professional at a critical time of patient care. For instance, pharmacy and laboratory systems may be receiving data online and processing it by computer before returning it to the health care practitioner. Some expert systems monitor the prescribed drug therapies and provide appropriate advisory messages when it detects potential adverse drug interactions. Another similar class of expert or knowledge-based systems looks at the blood values computed by machines in the pathology laboratory and provides interpretation as to what the diagnosis might be along with returning the raw data to the physician. Such programs require no *extra effort* from the physician to obtain and can be valuable aids to diagnosis. This is the area in which expert systems find the most utility.

Other AI Systems

The field of artificial intelligence can be divided into sub-disciplines including computer vision, robotics, natural language processing, neural networks, and expert systems. *Computer vision* uses complicated techniques and mathematical algorithms and can simulate what the human vision system is able to accomplish. Some examples of applications of computer vision in health care include (Armoni, 2000):

- An example of pathological diagnosis occurs when on-line cytological diagnosis is applied to the data supplied by a needle introduced into a suspected tumor.
- Radiological diagnosis occurs when the computer interprets a computerized axial tomogram of the brain and determines what disease, if any, is present.
- Recognition of the structure of materials can be achieved by comparing known examples of structures with new samples. For instance, mineral bone composition can be determined and osteoporosis assessed.

- Graph analysis of results of vision tests can lead to interpretation of vision tests and is a valid approach to interpretation of electroencephalograms.

Since health care professionals rely extensively on visual input to do their job, one should not be surprised at the increasing importance of vision processing systems in supporting health care.

Robotic behavior is very difficult to achieve in the general case. For example, although it seems that housework is simpler than precision welding, from the robot's point of view the housework is harder because it is less well defined. Medical robotic applications need a well-defined domain. In hip replacement, a robot assists in the entire process of planning, locating, directing, and performing the surgery. A 3-dimensional knowledge of the anatomy allows the robot to work with the surgeon and automatically do the required drilling and cutting at the optimal location. Industrial-type robots have been used in warehouses and manufacturing plants for years and have now arrived in health care. One system enables the computerized locating of drugs at pharmacies and conveying them to the party ordering the drugs.

Natural language processing can be applied in many aspects of health care. Physically disabled people can give instructions by voice to steer a wheelchair or operate electrical appliances. Radiologists can dictate radiological interpretations and have them automatically transcribed in the medical record by computer. The machine may require a vocabulary of 30,000 words, and the machine needs to adjust to the varying speech habits of different radiologists.

Robotics, vision processing, and natural language processing remain challenging areas because the human performance of the task is often difficult to replicate by machine. The sub-discipline of neural computing, by contrast, is not trying to reproduce the performance of people but rather to apply adaptive, statistical methods to data, and such methods are the forte of computer scientists. *Neural network computing* can be applied to statistical classification, signal processing, and image processing. Neural networks process numeric results of tests, signals from electrocardiograms, and images and may identify statistical correlations hidden from human view. They might recognize relevant facts for diagnosis from among hundreds of variables. In research projects, neural networks have proven able to improve diagnosis in several areas of medicine.

Intelligent systems will be increasingly used in health care, but the *precondition* for this use will be the digital availability of information. These insights about the importance of integrated systems to the ability of computers to provide intelligent support are not new insights but have been appreciated for decades (Rada, 1983). The problem is that achieving this digital availability is a slow process. The integrated health care information system is the key to the diffusion of intelligent systems. The integrated system cannot be under-estimated for its importance to the general utility of health information systems. As the ability to share information across applications and institutions grows, so does the ability of the computer to support health care.

The possible applications of *intelligent systems* are not limited to medical applications. Strategic information systems that are a component of administrative systems are a type of decision-support or intelligent system. In general, any part of a health information system can include extensions that incorporate further rules about how the organization works and further semi-automate decision-making, thus making that part of the system more intelligent. Intelligent systems can detect fraudulent claims processes, suggest optimal allocations of physicians to patients, and so on. Anywhere that knowledge and reasoning relevant to the health care enterprise can be somehow captured in the computer, the exercise of that knowledge and reasoning can be automated or semi-automated.

Research Systems

Knowledge-based systems give to and get from *research systems*. Research systems, in turn, include 'literature systems' and 'clinical research systems'. These systems put unique demands on a health information system.

Literature Systems

More than eighty percent of American adults who use the Internet have searched for health information online (Morahan-Martin, 2004). Ninety percent of physicians use the *Internet*. However, the most common uses of the Internet by physicians is non-patient related email. While physicians use the Internet to seek answers to medical questions, they most commonly turn to their peers for such answers (Ely et al., 2005).

Scientists, educators, and physicians seek information in many ways (Wood et al., 1997):

- Direct personal communication with peers and experts is frequently the easiest way to gain assistance in problem solving.
- Within large organizations, technical communications often take place through a gatekeeper. The gatekeeper is a person who maintains a high level of external communication and, through contacts, keeps colleagues informed of new developments.

- Attendance at meetings and conferences also serves to keep individuals informed of recent developments in specialized fields.
- The broadest and most comprehensive access to innovations and new knowledge, however, comes from an examination of the published literature.

For many years health care professionals relied on personal or institutional *libraries* of books and journals to which they turned when they needed literature. However, the sheer volume of written material makes the medical literature unusable without special auxiliary methods, including computer systems.

The *National Library of Medicine* (NLM) is the world's largest medical library. NLM indexes about 3,400 journals. These 3,400 journals are carefully chosen from the over 20,000 journals published each year to represent the premiere journals. The journal article index, and more, is today available in the database MEDLINE via the World Wide Web. MEDLINE has more than 10 million journal article references and abstracts going back to the early sixties. Through the Web at www.nlm.nih.gov health professionals, scientists, librarians, and the public do some 250 million searches of MEDLINE each year. There are increasing links between article references and full text.

Prior to the late 1990s people doing searches on MEDLINE paid a fee for each search. The American government that funds NLM had a principle that private enterprises should not be prevented from competing with government services and thus the services had to be charged at full cost to produce the service. However, by the 1990s and with the wide popularity of the Web, the government was persuaded that *free access* to a medical literature index was more important as a public service than was economic competition.

The information in MEDLINE is massive and could be exploited by numerous computer applications. NLM maintains a 100,000-concept thesaurus, called the Medical Subject Headings (MeSH), for indexing medical literature. This *thesaurus* itself is a valuable knowledge base of medicine. One important property of a thesaurus is that it indicates parent-child relationships. For instance, the concept 'cardiovascular disease' has a parent of 'disease' and a child of 'heart attack'. To query MeSH one might go to the NLM web site and then in the 'Search' menu select the 'MeSH' option, enter the term 'Management Information Systems' in the 'for' text box, and select 'go'. Once the term appears with its definition, if the user selects the term, then the user will be given its hierarchical position. The relationships are indicated in top-down order with indentations as in:

Information Systems
        Management Information Systems
                Ambulatory Care Information Systems

Figure 5.4. MEDLINE Article Index. This information from MEDLINE shows for a particular article these items: AU for author, TI for title, MH for Medical Subject Heading, AB for Abstract, AD for address of authors, and SO for source of article.

AU - Gupta A
AU - Masthoff J
AU - Zwart P
TI - Improving the user interface to increase patient throughput.
MH - *Efficiency, Organizational
MH - Human
MH - Inservice Training
MH - Radiology Department, Hospital/*standards
MH - *Radiology Information Systems
MH - *User-Computer Interface
AB - One of the main goals of a radiology department is to optimize patient throughput. We have observed a number of factors that reduce patient throughput, one of them being suboptimal system usage. In this article, we distinguish and discuss two ways to reduce suboptimal operation: improved design of the user-interface and active support for learning during system usage, i.e., during examinations. We outline the rationale for this by looking at the current situation and trends in radiology departments. We have based our work firmly on the principles of user-centered design. Observations, task modeling, user involvement, and prototyping have been undertaken.
AD - Philips Research Laboratories, Redhill, United Kingdom.
SO - Top Health Inf Manage 2000 May;20(4):67-77

where 'Management Information Systems' is the child of 'Information Systems' and 'Ambulatory Care Information Systems' is the child of 'Management Information Systems'.

Each article is indexed into about ten concepts from MeSH. This indexing creates an enormous semantic network atop the world's premiere medical literature and can be used by artificial intelligence programs to support information retrieval and decision-making (Rada et al., 1990). When a user performs a search on *MEDLINE*, the user can request to get various views of the information. Typical users will take the default, tailored view that gives only the essential information. However, extensive information for each article in the collection can be presented in a highly structured way (see Figure 5.4).

The NLM has created a special Web site, MEDLINEplus, to link the general public to many sources of consumer health information. *MEDLINEplus* is designed to help users find appropriate, authoritative health information. To do this, NLM provides access to information produced by the National Institutes of Health, a database of full-text drug information, an illustrated medical encyclopedia, and much more. MEDLINE*plus* contains pages that link to other web sites. The *selection guidelines* for links demonstrate high standards for quality and reliability. The service provided by MEDLINEplus competes with some commercial health information resources such as WebMD but has the advantages of being unbiased by any particular commercial concern and having the quality standards and long-term commitment of the government behind it.

With the growth of the Web, a new form of publishing has emerged, mostly removed from traditional scientific publishing. Some of this information may be flawed. For instance, Lissman and Boehnlein (2001) assessed sites on treatment of depression and found that only half mentioned any symptoms or criteria for depression and that less than half made any mention of medications, psychotherapy, or professional consultation as suggested treatments of depression. While sensational results may be widely publicized, their subsequent *retraction* sometimes receives little attention (Rada, 2005).

Numerous concerns exist about the quality of information outside journals. For instance, over half of authors of clinical practice guidelines endorsed by major medical societies received financial support from the pharmaceutical firms and that support might bias the reporting of results (Choudhry et al., 2002). Presenters at scientific meetings often have work that is preliminary (L. M. Schwartz et al., 2002), but that work may be sensationalized by the media. *Pharmaceutical firms* sometimes encourage the media to emphasize medical problems for which the firm is marketing a drug, and patients might then seek medication that they do not need (Woloshin & Schwartz, 2006). The point is that from the vast sea of continually appearing medical research results, the reader needs to exercise caution in the interpretation of the results.

Clinical Research

The goal of *clinical research* is to advance the state of medical science and thus to improve the practice of medicine. In many scientific disciplines, researchers can investigate problems by conducting controlled laboratory experiments. Ethical and practical concerns, however, limit experimentation in medical care. In general, clinical researchers must be content with observing interventions and the resulting outcomes as physicians try alternative therapies to help patients regain health (Wiederhold & Perreault, 1990).

Two of the central tasks of clinical research are data management and data analysis. The most scientifically desirable form of clinical research is the randomized *clinical trial* in which patients are randomly assigned to alternate groups, and are treated according to a study protocol. Investigators collect data and compare the results obtained from each group to determine whether patients who receive different interventions experience significantly different outcomes. One technique to minimize bias is called blinding. In single-blind studies, patients do not know which treatment they are receiving. They may, for example, be given a placebo instead of an active drug. In double-blind studies, neither patient nor researcher knows to which group the subject belongs, thus avoiding systematic bias in the way treatments are given or in the way results are reported. The blinding approach makes good sense from the research perspective but raises problems as regards patient rights-to-know. In any case, information systems are crucial to the successful implementation of a clinical trial.

Various types of professionals participate in the clinical research process:

- The physicians, nurses, and other health care providers who administer treatments and collect data
- The medical-records personnel who enter, store, and retrieve data
- The epidemiologists and statisticians who model the problem and analyze the data
- The patients themselves as subjects

Clinical researchers often use *database management systems* to help in the tasks of data entry, multi-user access to data, and long-term maintenance of stored information.

Clinical researchers use a variety of statistical techniques to analyze data. *Statistical packages* are collections of programs that can be invoked to perform calculations on data and generate reports. Statistical packages are well developed. The Statistical Package of the Social Sciences (SPSS at www.spss.com) and the Statistical Analysis System (SAS at www.sas.com) are two well-known packages.

Various computer systems offer specialized support for clinical research. One such system, called MEDLOG (www.medlog.net), is tailored for medical data management incorporating a Time-Oriented Design that supports tracking variables which are measured repeatedly over time. *MEDLOG* also provides a clinical data management system.

Questions

Reading Questions

1. What is the role of standards development organizations in the development of de jure standards and how does this differ from the role of those organizations that develop de facto standards?
2. Compare and contrast methods of putting knowledge in computers that rely on flowcharts, decision theory, databases, and rules?
3. Why were medical expert systems not wanted by practitioners?
4. How are vision and robotics systems used in health care?
5. What contributions has the National Library of Medicine made to health care information systems?
6. How are registries important in clinical research?

Doing Questions

You will need to teach yourself a little about using PubMed to do this assignment. There is an online tutorial. By way of background, a bibliographic citation is information that describes a specific bibliographic item. For example, the bibliographic citation for a book would include the book's title, author or editor, place of publication, year of publication. The bibliographic citation for an article would include the article's title, author, title of the magazine or journal, volume number, and page numbers of the article. Sometimes also referred to as a bibliographic entry, reference, or just as a citation. On PubMed, when you do a search for article citations and then display with the 'citation' option, you get not only the typical citation information but also the list of MeSH terms used to index the article.

1. Go to PubMed on the Web (use http://www.ncbi.nlm.nih.gov/entrez/query.fcgi).
2. Find the heading Management Information Systems in MeSH as a child of Information Systems (either in the Search Menu scroll to 'MeSH' or select 'MeSH Database' from the left-hand column and then search on the term).
3. Copy the list of children (immediate descendants only) of "Management Information Systems".
4. For each such child, retrieve one recent article citation for which that MeSH heading was one of the major index terms assigned to that article and for which

you can obtain the abstract via Medline also. (You can do the retrieval with "heading"[majr]).

5. Copy the citation for each article retrieved in step 4 into the appropriate place on your list. The citation must contain the journal name, date of publication, article title, author(s), abstract, and list of MeSH terms used to index the article. To retrieve the abstract and list of MeSH terms you should use the "Medline" option in the "Display" pull-down menu (this assumes you are using the interface that you would get by going from www.nlm.nih.gov).

Next, write anywhere from 100 to 400 words about latest trends in health care management information systems based on your 9 retrieved citations. Your coherent synthesis should include one sentence dedicated to extracting a message from each citation. That sentence will include a pointer to the citation in the American Psychological Association citation format of '(first author last name, date)' like '(Smith, 2004)'. These citing sentences constitute nine sentences of your essay and beyond that you only need a transition sentence here and there.

Finally, consider anomalies in MeSH. A well-designed thesaurus (and MeSH is a thesaurus) should ideally have all siblings of the same kind. For instance, if a taxonomy has "tree" as a heading, then I could accept that the children are "maple, pine, and oak" or "big, medium, and small" but not "maple, pine, and big". Explain what you see as an anomaly in the children of "Management Information Systems". One anomaly could be when a concept is both a sibling and a parent of another concept. Another kind of anomaly is illustrated in my example of mixing sibling types—my "maple, pine, and big" example (all children should carry salient properties of their parent in such a way as to be recognizably siblings of the parent).

References

ANSI. (2006). *Overview*. American National Standards Institute Retrieved October 2, 2006, from www.ansi.org

Armoni, A. (Ed.). (2000). *Healthcare Information Systems: Challenges of the New Millenium*. Hershey, PA: Idea Group Publishing.

Bali, R. (2005). *Clinical knowledge management: Opportunities and challenges*. Hershey, PA: Idea Group Publishing.

Benson, T. (2002). Why general practitioners use computers and hospital doctors do notPart 2: scalability. *British Medical Journal, 325*(7372), 1090-1093.

Choudhry, N., Stelfox, H., & Detsky, A. (2002). Relationships between authors of clinical practice guidelines and the pharmaceutical industry. *Journal American Medical Association, 287*(5), 612-617.

Ely, J. W., Osheroff, J. A., Chambliss, M. L., Ebell, M. H., & Rosenbaum, M. E. (2005). Answering physicians' clinical questions: Obstacles and potential solutions. *J Am Med Inform Assoc, 12*(2), 217-224.

Evans, R., Pestotnik, S., Classen, D., & Burke, J. (1999). Evaluation of a computer-assisted antibiotic-dose monitor. *Ann Pharmacother, 33*(10), 1026-1031.

Gorry, G. A. (1976). On the mechanization of clinical judgment. In C. Weller (Ed.), *Computer applications in health care delivery.* Miami, FL: Symposia Specialists.

Lissman, T., & Boehnlein, J. (2001). A critical review of Internet information about depression. *Psychiatric Services, 52*, 1046-1050.

Martin, L. (2001). Knowledge acquisition and evaluation of an expert system for managing disorders of the outer eye. *Computers in Nursing, 19*(3), 114-117.

Miller, R., Pople, H. J., & Myers, J. (1982). Internist-1, an experimental computer-based diagnostic consultant for general internal medicine. *N Engl J Med., 307*(8), 468-476.

Morahan-Martin, J. M. (2004). How Internet users find, evaluate, and use online health information: A cross-cultural review. *CyberPsychology & Behavior, 7*(5), 497-510.

National Drug Code Directory. (2006, March 10, 2006). U.S. Food and Drug Administration Retrieved May 8, 2006, from http://www.fda.gov/cder/ndc/

NCVHS. (2000). *Uniform data standards for patient medical record information: Report to the Secretary of the U.S. Department of Health and Human Services*. Washington, DC: National Committee on Vital and Health Statistics (NCVHS).

Rada, R. (1983). A direction for artificial intelligence in medicine. *ACM SIGBIO Newsletter, 6,* 6-8.

Rada, R. (2005). A case study of a retracted systematic review on interactive health communication applications: Impact on media, scientists, and patients. *J Med Internet Res, 7*(2), e18.

Rada, R., Carson, G. S., & Haynes, C. (1994). Standards: The role of consensus. *Communications of the ACM, 34*(3), 15-16.

Rada, R., Zanstra, P., Potharst, J., Barlow, J., Robbe, P. d. V., & Bijstra, D. (1990). Expertext for medical care and literature retrieval. *Artificial Intelligence in Medicine, 2*(6), 341-355.

Safran, C., Rind, D. M., & Davis, R. (1996). Effects of a knowledge-based electronic patient record on adherence to practice guideline. *M.D. Computing, 13*(1), 55-63.

Schwartz, L. M., Woloshin, S., & Baczek, L. (2002). Media coverage of scientific meetings: too much, too soon? *Journal American Medical Association, 287*(21), 2859-2863.

Schwartz, W. B. (1970). Medicine and the computer: The promise and problems of change. *New Engl. J. Medicine, 283*, 1257-1264.

Shortliffe, E. H. (1976). *Computer-based medical consultations: MYCIN*. New York: Elsevier.

Shortliffe, E. H. (1991). Medical informatics and clinical decision making: the science and the pragmatics. *Med Decis Making., 11*(4), 2-14.

Smith, J. (2000). *Health management information systems: A handbook for decision-makers*. Buckingham, UK: Open University Press.

Szolovits, P. (1982). Artificial intelligence and medicine. In P. Szolovits (Ed.), *Artificial intelligence in medicine* (Vol. 51, pp. 10-33). Boulder, CO: Westview Press.

Tan, J. (2001). *Health management information systems: Methods and practical applications* (2nd ed.). Sudbury, MA: Jones & Bartlett Publishers.

Tranfield, D., Denyer, D., & Smart, P. (2003). Towards a methodology for developing evidence-informed management knowledge by means of systematic review. *British Journal of Management, 14*(3), 207-222.

Warner, H. (1979). *Computer-assisted medical decision-making*. New York: Academic Press.

Wiederhold, G., & Perreault, L. E. (1990). Clinical research systems. In E. H. Shortliffe, L. E. Perreault, G. Wiederhold, & L. Fagan (Eds.), *Medical informatics: Computer applications in health care* (pp. 503-535). Reading, MA: Addison-Wesley.

Winston, P. H. (1992). *Artificial intelligence* (3rd ed.). Reading, MA: Addison-Wesley.

Woloshin, S., & Schwartz, L. M. (2006). Giving legs to restless legs: A case study of how the media helps make people sick. *PLoS Medicine, 3*(4).

Wood, F., Wallingford, K., & Siegel, E. (1997). Transitioning to the Internet: Results of a National Library of Medicine user survey. *Bulletin Medical Library Assoc, 85*(4), 331-340.

Chapter VI

Provider-Payer Transactions

Learning Objectives

- Assess costs of transactions
- Delineate the different parts of transaction and code sets standardization
- Analyze the alternatives for implementation of provider-payer transactions
- Construct a sketch of an X12 message based on Implementation Guide details and certain data content
- Describe different code sets and issues relevant to mapping terms from one code set to terms in another code set
- Distinguish "identifiers" from "code sets" and illustrate the complexities of creating a neutral identifier, but a rich associated file
- Differentiate whistleblowers from fraud investigators
- Demonstrate that controlling health insurance fraud is a higher-level concern than controlling health insurance solvency
- Construct a model for software for fraud control
- Construct relationships between software to support coding and software to support fraud detection
- Demonstrate that shared information among payers can increase the ability of fraud investigators to successfully, semi-automatically detect fraud

The key *financial transactions* in U.S. healthcare occur when the provider sends a claim to the payer and the payer adjudicates the claim. This chapter first explains the history of electronic data interchange (EDI) and then shows the powerful, cost-saving impact that it can have on healthcare. One bottleneck to EDI in healthcare has been the lack of standardization. This problem was addressed with a law passed in 1996, with which the healthcare industry was still grappling a decade later. The standardization of these transactions will be explored in detail in this chapter. After that, a different aspect of provider-payer transactions is examined, namely, the temptation to cheat and the role of software in combating fraud.

Standardizing Transactions

Standardizing transactions has practical value:

- Forms with erroneous data will be readily recognized and returned to the sender to fix
- Fraud surveillance will be facilitated
- Claims that need to go to multiple health plans can be automatically routed
- Eligibility inquiries should be readily answered automatically, and providers could thus avoid long delays and high costs of making eligibility inquiries by phone

The list of benefits to standardized transactions is long.

EDI

A business transaction is an interaction between two parties where one party agrees to do something for the other party in return for some kind of compensation. The goal of business-to-business e-commerce is to enable companies to perform business transactions electronically. Thus activities of human actors need to be transferred to the computer. When human actors are directly involved in a business transaction they have an understanding (often implicit) about the context of the transaction. E-commerce captures the context of the transaction from the real-world and brings it to the system level in a structured way (Biagi, 2004). Standards for business transactions strive for electronic *interoperability* between organizations (Stegwee & Lagendijk, 2001). Business transaction standards are a set of definitions, specifications, and guidelines that enable the interoperability of independent systems with respect to the joint execution of a specific class of business transactions.

Standardizing commerce is as old as culture. The invention of money was to abstract goods. For the use of electronic communication, history might go to 1910 when fifteen florists in Belgium banded together to exchange out-of-town orders for flower arrangements via telegraph. Their *Florists' Telegraph Delivery* group, now FTD Inc., was an example of standardizing commerce with electronic communication. A larger example of the use of telegraph in commerce occurred in 1948, when the Soviet Union cut off road, rail and barge access between Western Germany and the parts of Berlin that were controlled by the U.S., England and France after World War II. Western powers intervened to supply Berlin's inhabitants with the necessities of life by air. With aircraft landings at the rate of one every three minutes, cargo had to be loaded and off-loaded faster than accompanying paperwork could be completed and verified. Because of this, inventory lists were rarely up-to-date and ordering and expediting lists became of little consequence. Recognizing the need to standardize the paper manifests from different countries (and in different languages) and the need to communicate this information independently from delivery, a standard manifest system was developed that could be communicated via telex. From this standard manifest system, electronic data interchange (EDI) evolved.

By 1968, so many railroads, airlines, truckers and ocean shipping companies were using electronic manifests that they formed the Transportation Data Coordinating Committee to create cross-industry standards. In 1975, that Committee published its first EDI specifications. In 1978 this became the *Accredited Standards Committee X12* (ASC X12). Tasked with the development of EDI standards that would be acceptable across industries, X12 created standards for purchase orders, invoices, and requests for quotation.

Both users and vendors input their requirements to create a set of standard data formats that:

- Are hardware independent
- Are unambiguous and can be used by all trading partners
- Reduce the labor-intensive tasks of exchanging data, such as data re-entry
- Allow the sender of the data to control the exchange, including knowing if and when the recipient received the transaction

The EDI developers did not use then-current words and phrases, and what others were calling an electronic document, they instead termed a *transaction set.* That which might have been deemed a record, was named a data segment, and what seemed to others to be a field, was called a data element (Bass et al., 2002).

History

The healthcare transaction standards were stimulated by the anxiety about rising healthcare costs in the 1980s. Political debates at that time said that the nation's multiplicity of private insurers contributed to high costs and uninsured poor people. One movement called for universal health coverage funded by industry, and another movement called for elimination of the insurance industry to be replaced with a government-based healthcare system. Those in favor of the government-based system noted the *administrative waste* in the insurance industry and provided the following data (Morrissey, 2000):

- Twelve cents of every premium dollar goes into overhead and profits for insurance companies
- In the government-based healthcare system in Canada the insurance aspect of the operation only takes 1 cent on the dollar
- The healthcare providers in the U.S. spend about 20% of total revenues for billing and administrative costs because of the complexity of dealing with hundreds of insurers

Such data highlighted healthcare's *paper-based*, arcane methods of handling insurance claims and led to efforts to examine the obstacles to automating the process.

The 1991 Bush Administration called a group of healthcare industry leaders together to discuss how healthcare administrative costs could be reduced.The group was called the *Workgroup for Electronic Data Interchange (WEDI)*. The government asked WEDI to evaluate electronic claims standardized billing issues for the purpose of advancing electronic data interchange. However, leaders of the insurance standardization movement could not break from the vested interests and capital tied into the proprietary ways their organizations were exchanging information. No private insurer wanted to go first, but each said, "We'll follow."

The reluctance to standardize held for the *healthcare providers*. Despite arguments that standards could help trim days in accounts receivable and ease the financial pinch, providers saw the project not as a potential benefit but as another burden they could not afford. Providers did not want to be early adopters of a new and capital-intensive effort.

In 1993 the Clinton administration included standardized transactions in its blueprint for healthcare reform. The legislation, known as HIPAA, was finally passed in 1996. The legislation calls for the Department of Health and Human Services to create a transaction rule and that rule was finished in 2000. The rule specifies the format of transactions and the codes that will fill the fields in the forms.

Transactions

Electronic data interchange (EDI) has been important for decades. The prominent American standards development organization for EDI is the Accredited Standards Committee X12 (commonly referred to simply as X12). X12 specifies an envelope structure for messages. The information on the envelope is used in routing messages through the electronic networks. Various committees of X12 work on implementation guides to specify in some detail how the content of the envelope might be standardized to carry information most useful to a given industry.

The Healthcare Task Force of the Insurance Committee of X12 has developed several *implementation guides* that the federal government has mandated as the standard for healthcare. These implementation guides include:

- Enrollments of individuals in health plans (X12, 2000b)
- Eligibility inquiries (X12, 2000a)
- Claim submissions which appear as three distinct guides for dentists (X12, 2000d), professionals (X12, 2000f), and institutions (X12, 2000e)
- Claim payment advice (X12, 2000c)

For each implementation guide the transaction has a relatively simple hierarchical structure culminating in particular values from code sets or identifiers. The message is transmitted as a string of bits. X12 creates a language for authoring the message that people can understand and that is rigorous enough that a computer program can encode and transmit it and another computer program can receive and decode it.

X12 Details

Every X12 transaction occurs within an *envelope*. The envelope structure has four levels:

- The communications transport protocol is determined by the communications network transporting the transactions. This has no affect on the transactions themselves, and this information is never used by any application other than the network software.
- The interchange control header is used to determine how the translators will operate on the transactions when arriving, what X12 version to use, what characters are used for terminators, and so on.

- The functional group header is the first level of information that is application oriented. It is basically used to indicate what type of transaction is in the transaction set that followed. The primary use of this information is for routing data to the correct processing queues or systems for processing.
- The transaction set header is where actual application data begins.

Within a transaction set header are various data segments.

A *data segment* is an intermediate unit of information in a transaction set. It appears as:

- A segment identifier
- One or more data elements
- A segment terminator

A segment can be repeated in a transaction set.

Data elements are the smallest unit of information within a transaction. A data element may be mandatory to appear, may be optional, or may be conditional. A conditional element will appear, if, and only if, some specified, preceding data element is present.

The value that can go in a data element may be constrained by a *code set*. These codes may be internal to X12 or may be defined and maintained external to X12. For the internally developed codes, X12 maintains a data dictionary. For instance, the data dictionary includes a "provider code." The provider codes and their meaning include:

H Hospital

R Rural Health Clinic

AD Admitting

AS Assistant Surgeon

AT Attending

BI Billing

BS Billing Service

CO Consulting

CV Covering

HH Home Healthcare

LA Laboratory

ON On Staff

OP Operating

OR Ordering

OT Other Physician

When a transaction is actually prepared for transmission, it is placed into a *stream of characters*. Each data element is separated from the data elements before or after it with a special character, such as "*." For instance the transmission might include:

ITA * 1 * 1 * CA * 1.08 * CT * CB * 141151;

where ITA is the data segment initiator. The subsequent two 1's are data elements separated by "*." The segment is terminated with a ";." The symbols that will be used in a given message as separators of data fields and of segments are defined in the interchange control header.

The *data element* is the smallest named unit of information in the X12 standard. Each data element has a name, description, type, minimum length, and maximum length. For ID type data elements, the manual or guide provides the applicable X12 code values and their descriptions, or references where the valid code list can be obtained.

X12 has standard *conditions* designators. Data element conditions are of three types: mandatory, optional, and relational, as follows:

- **M – Mandatory:** The designation of mandatory is absolute as there is no dependency on other data elements.
- **O – Optional:** The designation of optional means that there is no requirement for a data element to be present in the segment. The presence of a value for a simple data element is at the option of the sender.
- **X – Relational:** Relational conditions may exist among two or more simple data elements within the same data segment based on the presence or absence of one of those data elements (presence means a data element must not be empty). Relational conditions are specified by a condition code and the reference designators of the affected data elements. A data element may be subject to more than one relational condition.

These define the circumstances under which a data element may be required to be present or not present in a particular segment.

The following first overviews the transactions and then summarizes the "270/271 Eligibility Request and Response Transaction" Implementation Guides (X12, 2000a). The transaction standards are related to one another (see Figure 6.1). For instance:

- The *834 Enrollment Transaction* contains demographic, eligibility, and plan information pertinent to the covered lives within an insurance plan (X12, 2000b). The health plan member completes an enrollment form and the information is entered into a member database or a payroll system. This information is forwarded to the health plan in an "834 Enrollment Transaction."
- The healthcare provider may request eligibility information from the health plan by using the *270 Eligibility Request Transaction*. The health plan returns the requested eligibility information to the provider using the "271 Eligibility Response Transaction."
- The *837 Healthcare Claim Transaction* contains the information required to submit a claim for payment or reporting purposes.
- The health plan returns an *835 Remittance Advice Transaction* to notify the provider of the benefit determination. The actual payment may be done using electronic fund transfer or by generating and mailing a check.

For situations where an "implementation guide" is not comprehensive, an entity can provide its own requirements and publish those in a "compendium guide."

Figure 6.1. Transactions among provider, payer, sponsor: The 270 is the eligibility inquiry, while the 271 is the eligibility information in reply. The 837 is the claim submission.

PROVIDERS	routing	PAYERS	routing	SPONSORS
Eligibility Verification	270 inquiry → ← 271 reply	Enrollment	←834	Enrollment
Claim	837 claim →	Claims Adjudication		
Accounts Receivable	← 835 payment advice	Accounts Payable		

Eligibility Details

The "270" is used to request information, and the "271" is used to respond with coverage, eligibility, and benefit information. The basic *flow* is for a requester (usually a provider) to ask a responder (usually a payer) about healthcare coverage eligibility and associated benefits:

1. A provider initiates a 270 transaction and routes it to a payer (see Figure 6.2)
2. The payer accepts the inquiry and prepares a response
3. The response is formatted into the 271 transaction that is sent to the provider

The requester is normally asking about one individual. Sometimes the responder is a third party administrator, or a utilization review organization, or a self-paying employer. However, in all cases, the basic flow is the same—a request sent and a response received.

The "270/271 Implementation Guide" is about 400 pages long. The "270/271 Transaction" has a *loop* inside a header and trailer which loop gives details of first information source, then information receiver, then subscriber, and finally dependent as follows:

Figure 6.2. Eligibility transaction workflow

PROVIDER	ROUTING	PAYER
Step 1 INITIATION prepare inquiry	→ Step 2 270 Transaction	Step 3 ACCEPT accept inquiry
Step 6 USE RESPONSE accept information	← Step 5 271 Transaction	Step 4 PREPARE RESPONSE

Transaction Set Header
Loop
Information Source
Information Receiver
Subscriber
Dependent (if needed)
Transaction Set Trailer

Seeing the completion of the fields for some specific examples gives an understanding of what exactly is entailed. The structure of the data segment for the *information source name* follows with the field name on the left and a sample value on the right:

Entity Identifier Code: PR
Entity Type Qualifier: 2
Name, Last or Organization: Blue Cross Blue Shield Illinois
Name, First:
Name, Middle:
Name, Suffix:
Identification Code Qualifier: PI
Identification Code: 12345

The results are transmitted as *alphanumeric strings* without any further structure. Thus, the "information source name" is transmitted as:

PR*2*Blue Cross Blue Shield Illinois****PI*12345~

Blank fields are indicated by *field separators* without any characters between them, as in "**." To continue the example and more fully indicate the way the data segments are completed, the "information receiver name" loop is completed as:

Entity Identifier Code: 1P
Entity Type Qualifier: 1
Name, Last or Organization: Welby
Name, First: Marcus

Name, Middle
Name, Suffix: MD
Identification Code Qualifier: XX
Identification Code: 123456789

The resultant data stream is:

1P*1*Welby*Marcus**MD*XX*1234567890~

The two loops have the same structure but different values. Given that both the sender and the receiver of the transaction are expecting the X12 messages, the computer can correctly parse these messages.

Codes and Identifiers

Key components for the values of the fields of the transactions are the codes. A code is a representation assigned to a term, and a listing of terms and their associated codes is a code set. The simple code sets are part of the implementation guidance coming from the standards organization, primarily X12 that developed the transaction standards. The *complex code sets* include the:

- *International Classification of Diseases, 9th Edition, Clinical Modification, (ICD-9-CM), Volumes 1, 2, and 3*
- *National Drug Codes* (NDC)
- *Code on Dental Procedures and Nomenclature*
- *Health Care Financing Administration Common Procedure Coding System* (HCPCS)
- *Current Procedural Terminology, Fourth Edition* (CPT-4)

Problems with the existing code sets are acknowledged (Chute et al., 1996).

Some of the fields in the transactions are filled with values from identifiers. In January 2004, DHHS published the final rule that adopts the national provider identifier (the NPI) as the standard unique health identifier for healthcare providers. Covered entities will use the NPI to identify providers in all standard transactions. The NPI is all numeric. It is 10 positions in length (9 plus a check-digit in the last position).

The employer identifier final rule was published in 2002. The rule specifies that the "employer identifier" is the employer identification number (EIN) assigned by the Internal Revenue Service. The EIN is the *taxpayer identifying number* and has nine digits.

At the moment, different entities use different methods of identifying individuals. When the public learned that the government was developing standard personal health identifiers, various protests ensued that were magnified by the media. In the end the government ordered a moratorium on work to produce a *personal identifier*.

Testing

Software exists for healthcare information systems that will generate the transactions in the appropriate form. For systems that generate transactions in other than *compliant forms*, other software might translate the information from the one format to the other.

Each organization should test that it is producing *valid transactions* that are meeting the specification requirements found in the X12N implementation guides. This process will require:

- Internal quality assurance testing
- Testing with a certification entity
- Additional assurance testing with selected trading partners

Trading partner level testing will also insure that connections are working properly, security is working properly, and other submission requirements are being satisfied as required by each entity.

Health plans must test the standard transactions with a large number of submitters, and providers must test with all their health plans. This testing could overwhelm both health plans and providers. A *third-party certification* could reduce the cost of testing.

The different levels of testing within transaction certification systems include:

- **Level 1:** Integrity testing, validation of X12 syntax
- **Level 2:** Requirement testing, testing for implementation of guide-specific syntax requirements
- **Level 3:** Balance testing, testing the transaction for balanced field totals, such as financial balancing of claims

- **Level 4:** Situation testing, the testing of specific inter-segment situations; for example, if the claim is for an accident, the accident date must be present
- **Level 5:** Code Set testing, testing for valid code set values to make sure the usage is appropriate for any particular transaction
- **Level 6:** Type of Service testing, specialized testing is required by certain healthcare specialties

This testing does not address the testing of the adjudication systems. These systems must be tested to ensure that data elements are not truncated or ignored, but such testing is outside the scope of the preceding six-level certification.

Reviewing a *transaction testing result*, one gains insight about transaction processing and about testing. The HIPAA auditor (www.applabs.com) gives error reports that pinpoint the location and nature of errors in EDI files. First the user selects input file(s). One file chosen as input is an 837I, which is a claim from an institution (see Figure 6.3). The partial results of the transaction test on this transaction show several errors (see Table 6.1).

Cost Savings

A considerable portion of every healthcare dollar is spent on provider-payer transactions, including:

- Filing a claim for payment from an insurer
- Enrolling an individual in a health plan
- Paying health insurance premiums
- Checking insurance eligibility for a particular treatment
- Requesting authorization to refer a patient to a specialist
- Responding to requests for additional information to support a claim
- Coordinating the processing of a claim across different insurance companies
- Notifying the provider about the payment of a claim

The cost of paper versus electronic transactions can be readily computed. Ten minutes on the phone to check eligibility compared to six seconds electronically adds up. An electronic remittance advice can be posted in a fifth of the time required for manual posting. While the savings in labor is significant, the biggest savings could come from *reduced bad debt*. With faster, more accurate eligibility inquiries and claims, the number of denied claims could be reduced significantly and impact

Figure 6.3. Actual complete transaction: The transaction is simply a sequence of lines of codes following a pre-agreed format—in this case an X12 837I format.

```
ST*837*987655~
BHT*0019*00*12345*19980202*2121*CH~
REF*87*004010X096~
NM1*41*1*HEALTHCARE PPO*NAME1*NAME2***46*1234~
PER*IC*JANE DOE*TE*123456789~
NM1*40*2*INSURANCE COMPANY*****46*962TT8R~
HL*1**20*1~
PRV*BI*ZZ*203BA0200N~
CUR*85*AFA~
NM1*85*2*GENERAL HOSPITAL*****XX*32322~
N3*125 VIRGINIA AVE~
N4*CALIFORNIA*CA*90210*US~
REF*LU*420456789~
PER*IC*NAME1*TE*123456~
HL*2*1*22*1~
SBR*T********CI~
NM1*IL*1*BOZARTH*LANCE*D***ZZ*123456~
N3*5707 FERN FLOWER DR~
N4*COLUMBIA*MO*65202~
DMG*D8*19980201*M~
REF*SY*123456789~
NM1*PR*2*KEY INSURANCE COMPANY*****PI*66783JJT~
HL*3*2*23*0~
PAT*01~
NM1*QC*1*BOZARTH*MAGGIE*B~
N3*5707 FERN FLOWER DR~
N4*COLUMBIA*MO*65202~
DMG*D8*19691125*F~
CLM*72255589*2593.69***11:A:1*Y*A*Y*Y*********Y~
DTP*434*RD8*19961222-19961224~
DTP*435*DT*199612220930~
DTP*096*TM*1630~
QTY*CA*2*DA~
REF*9A*6003E0332701~
HI*BK:643.03~
HCP*06*2040*553.69*252665599~
NM1*71*2*NORDSTRUM*HAROLD****XX*572999543~
PRV*AT*ZZ*363LP0200N~
LX*1~
SV2*11**949.68*UN*1~
SV4*12345~
NM1*71*2*ABCD CORP*****34*123456789~
PRV*AT*ZZ*203BA0200N~
SVD*CD*1123*HC:111*123*123*123~
SE*45*987655~
```

Table 6.1. Partial test results

Line No	Description
8	*PRV*BI*ZZ*203BA0200N*
8	"203BA0200N" specified at Provider Taxonomy Code (PRV03) is not a valid Health Care Provider Taxonomy Code
13	Value "LU" does not look like a valid Reference Identification Qualifier (REF01). If Identification Code Qualifier (NM108) has a value of "XX", then REF01 must be either EI or SY.
16	*SBR*T*******CI*
16	Insured Group Name (SBR04) is required when Insured Group or Policy Number (SBR03) is not present.

the gross proceeds of the practice on an annual basis to the tune of hundreds of thousands of dollars.

If one considers a small group physician practice, then one can illustrate simply enough the benefits to electronic transactions. The *calculation* basics are illustrated in a few lines of data:

1. Number of claims per week: 215
2. Average claim value: $191
3. Time to prepare a manual claim: 6 minutes
4. Time to prepare an electronic claim: 0.5 minutes
5. Staff cost per hour: $14
6. Manual cost per year: #1 * #3 * #5 * (1 hr/60 min) * (52 wks/yr) = $15,652
7. Electronic cost per year: #1 * #4 * #5 * (1 hr/60 min) * (52 wks/yr) = $1,304
8. Labor saving is #6 - #7 = $14,348
9. Bad debt now: 10%
10. Bad debt after automation: 5%
11. Annual savings from debt change: #1 * #2 * (#9 - #10) * (52 wks/yr) = $106,769

The labor savings from automation is about $14k. The savings from bad debt reduction is about $105k (see Table 6.2). Secondary to automation, the annual impact of

Table 6.2. Cost savings

General Practice Information	Your Information	Automated Process
Number of Visits Per Week	260	x
Average Claim Value ($)	$191	x
Number of Visits with Insurance/week	215	x
Staff Cost per hour ($/hr)	$14	x
Ave. number eligibility checks/week	33	x
Ave. number claim follow-ups/week	44	x
Ave. number referrals/week	25	x
Amount of time spent to (minutes)		
Obtain eligibility on a patient	11	0.5
Prepare a claim	6	0.5
Post a Payment	11	0.5
Obtain status of a claim	18	0.5
Referral check	13	2
Yearly Cost Estimates		
Eligibility Verification	$4,404.40	$ 200.20
Claims Preparation	$15,652.00	$1,304.33
Account Posting	$28,695.33	$1,304.33
Claim Status Follow-up	$9,609.60	$ 266.93
Referral Prepared	$3,943.33	$ 606.67
Total Estimated Yearly Costs	**$62,304.66**	**$3,682.46**
POTENTIAL YEARLY SAVINGS		**$58,622.20**
To look at the impact of reducing bad debt on your practice, enter your overall level of bad debt into the cell below in the first column. Then, enter a guess as to your bad debt after you were to do more eligibility inquiries, claim status inquiries, and referral checks. Enter that figure in the white cell below in the second column. Bad debt expense 5%=0.05.		
0.10		0.05
Increase in Potential Profits – Yearly		$106,769.00

bad debt reduction may easily exceed the annual impact of reduced labor costs. In the case where bad debt is reduced by 5% after automation, the income increases by 5%. In other words, the *annual gain* is the difference in the bad debt before and after automation times the weekly income times the number of weeks in the year.

A different perspective on costs considers the challenge of different formats that have historically plagued the management of provider-payer transactions in the U.S. To understand the costs of multiple formats, an analysis of the number of translations is presented. Assume there are formats A and B and messages have to be shared that might be in either format. A *translator* is needed from format A to format B and conversely. If there are four formats A, B, C, and D, then 12 translators are needed: A to B, A to C, A to D, B to A, B to C, B to D, ..., D to A, D to B, and D to C. The 12 can be computed from 4 times (4-1). In general, for n formats, n times (n-1) translators are needed. Thus, for 400 standards there would be needed 400 times 399 or approximately 160,000 translators.

Problems

Achieving compliance with the intent of the transactions rule has proven more difficult than initially envisioned. The intent was to reduce costs by standardizing the transactions. However, *transaction variability* has proven problematic. The sources of this problem are two-fold:

- The standards fail to cover some situations that need to be addressed, and thus entities are left in a quandary as to what to do. For instance, the standards do not adequately address the mode of the transaction or the acknowledgement of a claim.
- Entities are promulgating too many entity-specific requirements within a companion guide. They use situational and optional data elements in non-standard ways. In fact, some required data elements that have mandatory rules of use are used in non-standard ways. For example, some trading partners require the 837 to be submitted with the provider identification information (usually in the NM or REF segments) at the provider level (Loop 2000), the claim level (Loop 2300), and at the service level (Loop 2400), even though the provider has never changed. Standard use would only require the provider identification at Loop 2000 and any provider identification at Loops 2300 or 2400 as situational, if the provider were different at those levels.

This propagation of additional requirements that have not been outlined in the HIPAA-mandated implementation guides has caused abrasion among payers, providers, and the vendors that serve each (WEDI, 2005). This non-standard use of the transaction can play havoc with standard translators, testing systems, and other systems downstream.

The health transactions enterprise has a long history of introducing requirements in the transactions to accommodate particular workflow processes of each trading partner. In general, if a transaction exchange is not working and the transaction standard is in question by one of the trading partners, the use of the standard has been perverted and the non-standard work process has continued. To change this approach will require breaking old-style, well-working, well-rewarded habits in the industry. The transactions include a variety of optional data fields, enabling payers to customize claims to meet their business needs. This has resulted in providers and vendors not only having to follow requirements of the claim transaction implementation guides, but also hundreds of payer "companion guides" that show how individual payers want their claims formatted. HIPAA was implemented long after electronic claims were established, and the best intentions of the law ran into *established business practices* of health insurers. One senior executive in the health plan industry said (Goedert, 2005) that HIPAA was a great idea, it was just 25 years too late.

Fraud

The number one *white-collar* crime in the United States is healthcare fraud. Fraud is an intentional deception or a misrepresentation that the individual or entity makes knowing that the misrepresentation could result in some unauthorized benefit to the individual, or the entity or to some other party. The most common kind of healthcare fraud involves a false statement, misrepresentation or deliberate omission that is critical to the determination of health benefits payment.

The variety of fraudulent reimbursement and billing practices in the healthcare area is potentially infinite. The most common healthcare fraudulent acts include, but are not limited to (NHCAA, 2005):

- Billing for services, procedures, or supplies that were not provided
- The intentional *misrepresentation* of any of the following for purposes of manipulating the benefits payable:
  - The nature of services, procedures, or supplies provided
  - The medical record of service or treatment provided
  - The condition treated or diagnosis made

- The charges or reimbursement for services, procedures, or supplies provided
- The deliberate performance of unwarranted services for the purpose of financial gain

Fraud by *billing* for services not provided is easier to detect than fraud by misrepresentation of the patient condition. The following is an example of flagrant fraud (Thornton, 1999):

A physician previously convicted of fraud in another state begins a new life in Pennsylvania. He opens a clinical office using a corporate name not easily tied back to his prior life. He recruits patients who provide him with their insurance coverage information in return for a one-third share of the proceeds of his billings. Most patients appear at his office only to sign forms and pick up their share. Investigators retained by the local Blue Shield discover his history and obtain admissions from two patients about their arrangement. They refer the matter, together with signed witness statements, to the FBI and U.S. Attorney.

The ensuing investigation will take an average of eighteen months before return of an indictment. Bank subpoena returns show that in the meantime the doctor is netting $250,000 per month.

Imagine that a patient goes to the *dentist* for a routine examination. The dentist detects that a small cavity has appeared near a filling in a molar that already has one small filling. The proper treatment is another small filling for which the dentist would get paid about $200 by the insurance. However, if the dentist says that the cavity is large and convinces the patient to accept a crown on the tooth, then the dentist may earn $1,000 for doing the crown. How are the patient or the insurance company to know whether the cavity warranted a crown or not? Determining whether fraud has occurred in this case would require another dentist to see x-rays of the patient's tooth and perhaps re-examine the patient. Another dentist may hesitate to dispute the practice of a peer. The cost of such an investigation might exceed the difference in cost between the small filling and the crown and might breed ill-will for the insurance company among the providers, so an *insurance company* or other payer may hesitate to pursue this type of fraud.

False Claims Act

The False Claims Act dates back to the Civil War. Passed during the Civil War, the False Claims Act was intended to protect the Union Army from fraudulent suppliers who sold faulty war material to the government. In support of the False Claims Act, *Abraham Lincoln* wrote:

Worse than traitors in arms are the men who pretend loyalty to the flag, feast and fatten on the misfortunes of the nation while patriotic blood is crimsoning the plains of the south and their countrymen are moldering in the dust.

During the *Civil War* the government was so busy with the war that it did not have time to investigate fraud in bills sent to the government for the purchase of supplies. The False Claims Act asks citizens to report to the government any evidence of fraud. It allows a private individual with knowledge of fraud (a whistleblower) on the federal government to sue for the government to recover compensatory damages, stiff civil penalties, and triple damages.

If the false claim suit is successful, it not only stops the dishonest conduct, but also deters similar conduct by others. The *whistleblower* may receive a substantial share of the government's ultimate recovery—as much as 30% of the total.

Retaliation by the employer is prohibited. The False Claims Act punishes an employer for retaliating against an employee for attempting to uncover or report fraud on the federal government. If retaliation does occur, the whistleblower may also be awarded all relief necessary to make the employee whole, including reinstatement, two times the amount of back pay, litigation costs, and attorney fees.

Trends

In 1992, only seventeen healthcare fraud suits were filed. In 1992, *National Health Laboratories* settled a case with the U.S. Government for $110 million. In 1998, almost three hundred such suits were filed. The settlements made it apparent that recoveries in fraud cases had the potential to be of budgetary significance. That got the attention of Congress.

In the 1990s several state legislatures required joint efforts between state law enforcement agencies and private insurers to address healthcare fraud. In 1994, Pennsylvania established its Insurance Fraud Prevention Authority to serve as a conduit for insurers to fund specific investigators and prosecutors who work only on insurance fraud. For certain information-sharing activity, Massachusetts, Florida, Ohio and New Jersey have similar legislation. These laws are often quite specific in imposing obligations upon insurance companies to:

- Establish anti-fraud units with specified dollar budgets
- Deliver the results of their investigations to specific state law enforcement agencies

The *state law enforcement agencies* in turn provide immunity for the authors of such reports when they form the basis of state civil and criminal action.

The late 1990s witnessed a dramatic increase in federal funding to control fraud in the healthcare industry. As a direct result, the numbers of successful *prosecutions* rose dramatically. Many providers have reacted to the enforcement effort by devoting significant resources to compliance. In other words, the providers are making accurate billings. The Medicare program is benefiting by this trend, the "sentinel effect" of enforcement.

Threats of looming insolvency for *Medicare*, combined with protests from a public convinced of rampant fraud, spurred *Congress* into action. The Health Insurance Portability and Accountability Act (HIPAA) of 1996 contains tough, concrete provisions aimed directly at fraudulent practices. HIPAA significantly expands the False Claims Act. It lowers the bar for the definition of *fraud* itself (Thornton, 1999). HIPAA removes the concept of intentional from civil fraud, preserving it only for criminal acts. HIPAA increased:

- The percent of the award that could be paid to whistleblowers
- Returned the fines collected back into the Fraud and Abuse Control Program, which funds the investigations
- Created the *Medicare Integrity Program*, which contracts out the investigative work to the private sector

Billions of dollars are now annually paid in settlements on healthcare fraud.

Coding

In the course of treatment, physicians or other healthcare professionals insert diagnostic and treatment information into the medical record. This information is then classified or coded. Insurers and the government will then relate these *codes* to categorical *reimbursements*.

Pressure exists to recover the greatest reimbursement for an episode of care. If a healthcare provider says that patient with condition x was treated, then a lesser reimbursement may be possible than when a patient with condition y was treated, even when the treatments are the same in each case. The difference between x and y may be subtle and knowledgeable people might even argue whether the proper diagnosis is x or y. So the healthcare provider is motivated to say that the diagnosis is y. Of course, if the provider says this knowing that it is false, then the provider is *guilty of fraud*.

Reimbursement consultants and software packages can help providers increase reimbursement through *up-coding* or coding that is intended to earn the maximum revenue based on the available evidence. Some up-coding is accomplished by a few consultants who review charts and try to apply all available codes. If proper coding guidelines are not followed, then some simple checks of certain properties of the codes might betray those facilities that inappropriately utilize this strategy for maximizing revenue.

Given the practices followed by insurance companies and the government to combat up-coding, providers may also engage in "down-coding" or "under-coding":

- "Down-coding" occurs when the proper code is known and a deliberate decision is made to submit a claim for a lesser service in the belief that the proper code would subject the case to strenuous scrutiny. This scrutiny may require considerable effort by the provider to create copies of the medical record for the payer to study, and the payer may delay payment to the provider. Providers fear that their submitted code will be diverted for manual review and result in cash-flow problems.
- "Under-coding" occurs when physicians systematically report less work than they do, believing they can avoid a confrontation by not getting near the line. When physicians do not fully understand the coding rules and the anti-fraud regulations, "under-coding" may seem the safest route. The cynics believe the government does not investigate these cases because more accurate reporting would result in greater payments.

Those that systematically *under-code* might receive greater reimbursement when technology assists them in coding.

One insidious form of fraud is known as *unbundling of services*. A fictitious example follows. Suppose a patient has a soft tissue abscess. She goes to her physician, and he drains the abscess. The proper way to bill for the service according to Medicare guidelines is as a single procedure "Incision and Drainage of Abscess" costing $250 (see Figure 6.4). Instead, the physician decides to unbundle the bill into three procedures to get a higher reimbursement:

- "Local Anesthesia" costing $100
- "Surgical Procedure on Skin or Soft Tissue, Not Otherwise Specified" costing $200

Figure 6.4. Fraudulently unbundling

Correct Claim		
Procedure Code	Description of Procedure	Reimbursement
ID1234	Incision and Drainage of Abscess	$250

Fraudulent Unbundling of Claim		
Procedure Code	Description of Procedure	Reimbursement
ABC7890	Local Anesthesia	$100
GHI0011	Surgical Procedure on Skin or Soft Tissue	$200
XYZ5555	Wound suturing	$150

- "Wound Suturing" costing $150

Medicare is starting to use software to attempt to identify unbundling of services. Procedure and diagnosis codes are vital for this effort, as Medicare would be hard pressed to detect unbundling in narrative claims rather than in coded claims.

Coding Software

Tools are available to facilitate coding. Physicians can turn to vest pocket cards, paper templates, and computers for help in anticipating how much reimbursement might be received for a particular diagnosis or treatment. Functionality ranges from table lookups of published requirements to logic-based, real-time background monitoring and analysis of clinical documentation.

3M Corporation (www.3m.com) is a leader in healthcare coding for billing software. The *3M Coding and Reimbursement System* includes several standard references. There are many cross-references, which can make coding, and reimbursements more accurate and consistent. The system is designed to optimize revenue:

- Special prompts highlight explanations that can influence code choice
- Edits are incorporated into the software to help the coder arrive at the correct code
- A review process analyzes the record and highlights information that can be used to further enhance the code assignment

Analytic software that is contained in the 3M Coding and Reimbursement System:

- Manages the complex rules and terminology of coding.
- Helps determine the standard code for procedures and services provided for outpatients.
- Calculates reimbursement based on formulas that implement the appropriate national and hospital-specific variables. It utilizes Medicare inpatient and outpatient formulas and a variety of other reimbursement formulas.
- Helps coders uncover additional, often overlooked, secondary diagnoses or treatments.

3M's *coding compliance tool* audits and records each critical step in coding. The resulting "snapshots" allow the healthcare financial services unit to document exactly what coding problems have been found. The software has two interface options—it can work with a batch interface or can review coding concurrent with the coding session. The software provides edit messages that specify the nature of the compliance problem. The healthcare provider will have the information needed to influence individual coders and clinicians that caused the errors in the first place to take corrective action. For example:

- **Resource Edits:** Evaluate length of stay and charges to determine if they are consistent with clinical data
- **Clinical Edits:** Evaluate the clinical consistency of the coded data
- **Code Edits:** Evaluate the coding sequence and compliance with established coding rules

In order to cover the spectrum of compliance issues, Audit Expert Software incorporates the coding rules and guidelines of many organizations—the same guidelines the government inspectors use in their audits. As the software supports variations in coding to achieve different reimbursements, it legally and ethically toes a fine line between supporting the most accurate conclusions and those that are financially most beneficial.

Fraud Detection Software

Software can help detect fraud. For instance, Texas has the *Texas Medicaid Fraud and Abuse Detection System* (Cupito, 1998). The system produces a profile and a numerical score for each provider's risk of Medicaid fraud. The system provides lists of people whose behavior is different. Lists of suspects are given to fraud analysts and investigators for follow-up. The Texas fraud detection system uses statistical methods and logical rules. The system gathers information from many sources, and combines and analyzes it. One of the most important initial tasks is defining *features* to extract from raw claims data.

Typical fraud patrolling is done reactively. A deviant pattern of claims is detected, and an investigation is done as to whether that past pattern represented fraud. A proactive mechanism predicts future events. It might anticipate possible fraud and then investigate whether it was occurring. Or a proactive mechanism might alert investigators to anticipated deviations in data and let the investigators know that those deviations would not be expected to be fraudulent in nature and thus would not merit further attention. For instance, if a major, new, high-risk construction project begins near a small town that will lead to a higher rate of accidents in the short term, and then those patrolling the health reimbursement claims could be notified of this and could anticipate the change in claims patterns. With this proactive approach, the *fraud patrol* could focus its attention where problems were most likely to be.

The costs of fraud to the American healthcare system are enormous. The government has mounted various campaigns to try to stop fraud. Information systems can play an important role in supporting the fight against fraud.

Epilogue

Initially, only a handful of transactions were standardized, and they emphasized claims and payments. However, the transactions that were initially standardized are the tip of the iceberg. For the payer-provider relation more transactions will progressively cover other aspects of the communication between payers and providers.

Standardized transactions are the currency of quality management and the endowment for continuous quality improvement of patient care. Only by capturing clinical data from healthcare providers in a way that the data can be applied to healthcare decisions for individuals and to policy decisions for populations can the goal of high-quality, affordable healthcare be achieved. HIPAA's Administrative Simplification represents a major step towards such *standardization*.

Questions

Reading Questions

1. What are some of the historical precedents to EDI standards?
2. What is X12?
3. Demonstrate that shared information among payers can increase the ability of fraud investigators to successfully, semi-automatically detect fraud.
4. What motivates a whistleblower? Why did the False Claims Act encourage whistleblowing?

Doing Questions

1. Take the small entity spreadsheet and enter the appropriate formulas and data values into an Excel spreadsheet. Assume the values in the table are as given in the book (bad debt with manual transactions is 0.10 and with electronic transactions is 0.05). Now increase the value of the bad debt remaining after electronic transactions. Give the lowest value (to the hundredth place) for "electronic bad debt reduction" at which the:
    - Savings from bad debt reduction for going from manual to electronic transactions is less than
    - The labor savings for electronic transactions

    (Your value for bad debt reduction in electronic mode has to exist between 0.05 and 0.10.)
2. What is the fragile relationship between coding software that helps a provider assign codes that will earn fair compensation and fraud detection software that looks for incorrect assignments of codes? Compare and contrast the coding software used by healthcare providers and the fraud detection software used by the government in terms of the rules employed, the scale at which applied, and the extent to which the algorithms inside one system would be used inside the other system. If you can find any supporting information about either coding software or fraud detection software related to coding, please provide that evidence.

References

Bass, S., Miller, L., & Nylin, B. (2002). *HIPAA compliance solutions: Comprehensive strategies from Microsoft and Washington Publishing Company*. Redmond, WA: Microsoft Press.

Biagi, M.D. (2004). Transaction automation on the Internet: Open electronic markets, private electronic markets and supply network solutions. *International Journal of Electronic Business, 2*(6), 674-685.

Chute, C., Cohn, S.P., Campbell, K.E., Oliver, D., & Campbell, J. (1996). The content coverage of clinical classifications, for the computer-based patient record institute's work group on codes and structures. *Journal of the American Medical Informatics Association, 3*(3), 224-233.

Cupito, M.C. (1998). Paper cuts? HIPAA's new rules. *Health Management Technology, 19*(8), 34-39.

Goedert, J. (2005). Taking another look at HIPAA and I.T. *Health Data Management, 13*(10), 56-58.

Morrissey, J. (2000). N.J. pushes e-claims. By November 2001 all payers will have to do business with providers electronically. *Modern Healthcare, 30*(41), 28-29.

Stegwee, R., & Lagendijk, P. (2001). Health care information and communication standards framework. In R. Stegwee & T. Spil (Eds.), *Strategies for healthcare information systems*. Hershey, PA: Idea Group Publishing.

Thornton, D.M. (1999). Perspectives on current enforcement: Sentinel effect shows fraud control effort works. *J. of Health and Hospital Law, 32*(4), 493-502.

WEDI. (2005). *Bringing partners together: Successful EDI testing and validation practices*. Workgroup for Electronic Data Interchange. Retrieved May 2006, from www.wedi.org

X12. (2000a). *270/271: Health care eligibility/benefit inquiry and information response*. North Bend, WA: Washington Publishing Company for ASC X12 Insurance Subcommittee.

X12. (2000b). *834: Benefit enrollment and maintenance*. North Bend, WA: Washington Publishing Company for ASC X12 Insurance Subcommittee.

X12. (2000c). *835: Health care claim Payment/advice*. North Bend, WA: Washington Publishing Company for ASC X12 Insurance Subcommittee.

X12. (2000d). *837: Health care claim: Dental*. North Bend, WA: Washington Publishing Company for ASC X12 Insurance Subcommittee.

X12. (2000e). *837: Health care claim: Institutional*. North Bend, WA: Washington Publishing Company for ASC X12 Insurance Subcommittee.

X12. (2000f). *837: Health care claim: Professional*. North Bend, WA: Washington Publishing Company for ASC X12 Insurance Subcommittee.

Chapter VII

Information Networks

Learning Objectives

- Indicate how community health information networks support public health
- Indicate how health e-commerce networks are a type of community health information network with a focus on e-commerce
- Explain the status of supply chain management in healthcare
- Explore the use of the Web to empower patients to assume more direct responsibility and control over their healthcare
- Explain how the objectives of a National Health Information Network would serve the needs of healthcare

The connection of components of the healthcare system is a major step in improvement of the healthcare system. Through networking, different entities can better coordinate their efforts. This chapter on *information networks* examines some of the human, organizational aspects of networking and begins with e-commerce networks, goes to supply chain management, and then goes to community and consumer networks. Consumerism is often touted as a way that patients can improve the efficacy of the healthcare system by becoming proactive. Some national governments are trying to improve healthcare by creating national information networks.

Community Health Networks

Community healthcare encompasses all the services for the prevention of illness in the community. A comprehensive range of community healthcare services is seldom to be found in any single location. Maintenance of accurate birth and death records, protection of food and water supply, control of communicable diseases, abuses of alcohol and drugs, and occupational health safety are examples of community healthcare activities (Smith, 2000).

Community health information networks (CHINs) include a computer-based information system and focus on community health. Some people use the term "community health information network" to refer loosely to any information network connecting different entities in a community involved in healthcare and would thus consider an information network connecting a hospital and a health plan in one community to be a CHIN. However, this book prefers the more focused definition of CHIN that includes an emphasis on "community health." Information networks that are primarily supporting hospital-based treatment of disease would thus not be CHINs. Examples of community health information networks (CHINs) appeared already decades ago, but their prevalence and importance have grown.

A CHIN has three essential technical services:

- Linkage
- Information access
- Data exchange

CHINs may link local clinics, state and federal health agencies, hospitals, and other entities. A CHIN should address community health concerns and eliminate geographic and bureaucratic barriers to communication and information exchange for community health purposes.

To understand better the complexity of the community or public health sector one can consider the organizations responsible for it in the United States. The *Center for Disease Control* (CDC) is a federal agency charged with surveillance and control of diseases. State and regional health departments possess responsibilities in the promotion, protection, and maintenance of the health and welfare of citizens and often connect local health authorities with national agenda. The local health authorities are often under the jurisdiction of municipalities and implement such services as restaurant inspections and the collection of birth and death data. Various non-governmental organizations, such as the Heart Foundation or the Rotary Club, assume various voluntary responsibilities as regards fund raising, education, and various services for community healthcare.

The CDC initiated the *Information Network for Public Health Officials* (INPHO) in 1992. The ultimate goal of INPHO is to improve the health of Americans through more effective public health practice. The INPHO initiative addresses the serious national problem that public health professionals have lacked ready access to the authoritative, technical information they need to identify health dangers, implement prevention and health promotion strategies, and evaluate health program effectiveness. Among other services, INPHO helps public health practitioners have electronic access to health publications, reports, databases, directories, and other information. Dozens of states have participated in INPHO projects since 1993 under funding from CDC.

INPHO uses CDC WONDER (*Wide-Ranging Online Data for Epidemiological Research*) as an online, multi-way public information system. WONDER provides a single point of access to a wide variety of CDC reports, guidelines, and numeric public health data. WONDER simplifies access to public health information for state and local health departments, the Public Health Service, the academic public health community, and the public at large. WONDER supports public health research, decision-making, priority setting, program evaluation, and resource allocation (wonder.cdc.gov).

INPHO is only one of many examples of CHINs. Another set of CHINs was created through U.S. federal funding under the banner of the Target Cities Program of the 1990s (Smith, 2000). The *Target Cities Program* provided federal aid to enhance substance abuse treatment systems. Target Cities established in each of 20 major cities a Central Intake Unit to be the single point of access for clients who experience substance dependency or abuse problems. Central Intake Units provided standardized assessment and care management to the clients, referring them to providers of treatment, recovery, support and other services.

Despite the significant technological investments in some CHINs, the successes have not always met the expectations. The primary challenges are *people-related* rather than technical-related. A CHIN is primarily about knowledge management, and knowledge management efforts depend fundamentally on organizational management. Successful CHIN projects thus typically require, among other things, extensive training of the people in the participating organizations (Hinman et al., 2004).

Health E-Commerce Networks

Another common use of the term community health information network is for a network that supports e-commerce among providers and payers. This book prefers to call those networks *health e-commerce networks* (HENs). HENs are particularly compelling when providers and plans seek to standardize transaction requirements and reduce the cost of creating a common platform. Representative collaborations include (Noss & Zall, 2002):

- Wisconsin Health Information Network (WHIN)
- New England Healthcare EDI Network (NEHEN)
- HealthBridge of Cincinnati

WHIN subscribers pay on a per transaction basis. Among the functionalities provided by WHIN are:

- Eligibility and benefits verification
- Referral status and submission
- Claims status and submission
- Hospital administrative and clinical data
- Lab and radiology results
- Access to educational resources

WHIN provides access to eligibility information for over 100 payers and provides access to information at 15 Wisconsin hospitals. WHIN demonstrated cost reductions between $17,000 and $68,000 per physician practice through making electronic requests for information to hospital departments.

NEHEN was formed by six provider organizations, eight health insurers, and the Massachusetts medical society. NEHEN focuses on HIPAA-compliant transactions. The systems have most of their affiliated doctors' offices connected to the network. The participants use *EDI standards* that all accept. The network is used primarily for insurance eligibility transactions, which are settled in seconds. The system has been successful because the three competing care providers have agreed that standardization of payer information is mutually beneficial (Glaser et al., 2003). The cost per transaction for NEHEN is reported to be less than 5 cents, compared to the typical 35 to 50 cents for nonstandard electronic transactions. NEHEN has been able to achieve significant provider adoption and at least 70% of each hospital's eligibility transactions can be done online.

HealthBridge of Cincinnati started in 1997 as an independent not-for-profit organization between major payers and hospital systems in Cincinnati, Ohio. Access to HealthBridge is free to physicians. The project provides:

- Eligibility inquiry
- Secure messaging
- Clinical results from hospitals

The hospital sponsors of HealthBridge have provided significant clinical information to physicians, including laboratory and radiology reports. Access to payer information and systems is limited.

What factors determine the success of a HEN? Hospitals tend to have more access to capital and technology resources than individual physicians and have important clinical information. Payers are critical to providing administrative and financial transactions. Achieving a *critical mass* of payers in a market is important. WHIN and NEHEN have had significant payer participation from the outset.

To obtain initial participation in a HEN, it is critical that it have *credible sponsorship* within its local community. In the cases of HealthBridge and NEHEN, neutral entities were created by a broad base of sponsors within the local healthcare community.

Unless the architecture for the HEN is going to be built in-house, a reliable *technology partner* is critical to the success of the HEN. NEHEN has had a successful partnership with one of the largest healthcare IT vendors. WHIN has been less reliant on a single technology partner and has different vendors for different functionalities. HealthBridge has relied primarily on internal architecture development.

Enterprise Resource Planning

Enterprise resource planning systems (ERPs) integrate data and processes of an entity. The term ERP originally referred to utilization of enterprise-wide resources. One might argue that an ERP system would only need to provide functionality in a single package that would normally be covered by two or more systems. The ultimate application of an ERP system would cover all basic functions of an entity. The introduction of an ERP system to integrate existing applications reduces the need for interfaces between systems and has the potential to increase standardization and functionality and to reduce costs. Major components of an ERP system are supply chain management (SCM) systems and customer relationship management (CRM) systems. The next two subsections look at examples of SCM and CRM systems in healthcare.

Supply Chain Management

Through group purchasing, companies may achieve cost containment, improve the quality of goods purchased, and allow staff to focus their efforts on other activities. Goods and purchased services account for the second-largest dollar expenditure in the hospital setting. About 80% of every acute care supply dollar is acquired through *group purchasing*. However, the state of supply chain management is primitive in healthcare, as contrasted with the consumer goods or industrial manufacturing industries (Langabeer, 2005).

Purchasing for healthcare organizations must meet the needs of management, key business stakeholders, clinician partner preferences, and patients. The enormous push to achieve standardization has achieved only modest success. Purchasing in the typical hospital is an antiquated process in which multiple customers independently access suppliers, distributors, and hospitals (Rundle, 2000).

The biggest potential *benefit* of supply chain management for providers involves eliminating overpayments and reducing rework and manual processes. The benefits for suppliers lie in freeing sales representatives from administrative tasks, enabling them more time to sell, providing access to real-time sales information, allowing for better management of fill-rates and operational processes, and reducing the level of effort for labor-intensive administrative processes.

Customer Relationship Management

Customer relationship management (CRM) systems help entities manage their relationships with clients. Information stored on customers is analyzed and exploited. A CRM system should:

- Identify factors important to customers
- Provide customer support
- Track sales

Three fundamental components in CRM are:

- Automation of marketing, sales, and service
- Analysis of customer behavior
- Communicating with customers

CRM is important to profit and non-profit entities. Since some entities do not use the term customer, the term CRM might be re-interpreted as "constituent relationship management," "contact relationship management," or "community relationship management." In healthcare, the term CRM is also sometimes translated into the term *patient relationship management*.

CRM systems are used in the healthcare industry throughout the world (Alshawi et al., 2003; Calhoun et al., 2006; Raisinghani et al., 2005). A typical approach to CRM is to survey *patient satisfaction* and to address management steps to improve the results of the next survey (Zineldin, 2006). Data mining of Web information is an alternative way to learn what consumers think. In the financial sector, consumer views on particular investments have been assessed through the comments that those consumers make in online, discussion groups (Antweiler & Frank, 2004).

Many *online patient groups* are established by volunteers on free sites, such as groups.yahoo.com (Rada, 2006). However, some healthcare entities maintain patient online discussion groups. For instance, Joslin Diabetes Center runs an online diabetes discussion group for the public, and experts from the Center provide feedback online. Kaiser Permanente maintains numerous discussion groups moderated by Kaiser's professionals, but access is restricted to enrollees in the Kaiser Plan. Healthcare professionals in online moderator roles might address adverse events, among other things.

A pharmaceutical example of a CRM system follows. *Pharmaceutical companies* have vast stores of information amassed in their sales, marketing, and research organizations (Barret & Koprowski, 2002). At many companies, sales force automation programs are evolving from simple contact-management software to robust data warehouse applications. For example, Pfizer Inc., a $10 billion pharmaceutical firm, has a sales force automation program that enables 2,700 sales representatives to customize their sales pitches. Sales people can quickly provide doctors with highly detailed information about each product's effectiveness, side effects, and costs. The information is stored in an Oracle database that sales people access through customized territory-management software. Sales representatives no longer simply send call reports into headquarters to show which doctors they visited. Instead, they use data warehouse tools to assess whether managed-care contracts, which stipulate what drugs a doctor can prescribe, are being followed. They also maintain information about the status of accounts, customers' credit ratings, their last call to the company, and records of complaints.

Consumers

Healthcare and information systems trends combine to suggest a vision in which information systems are used to further control costs by bringing more players, particularly patients, more closely into the activities of healthcare. Healthcare in the U.S. has been provider-centered. This means:

- Authoritative decision-making from the doctor
- The provider is the source of all information
- Care is provided at the doctor's office or hospital
- Emphasis is on treatment

The Internet supports *consumer-centered* care. This means the provider and patient collaborate in decision-making, the consumer finds information from the Internet, care is provided at home, and the emphasis is on prevention.

Web Trends

Health is one of the top three categories of Internet users' interests. While health information for many is an episodic need, this could not be further from the truth for the 100 million individuals in the U.S. with chronic illnesses (as well as their families). People concerned about their health are some of the most active users of the Internet (Fox & Fallows, 2003), and such users gain health benefits (Murray et al., 2005).

Grove (1996) says the *strategic inflection point* of industries is the critical juncture where old models of conducting business are rapidly displaced by a new model, as a critical mass of cultural, regulatory, and technological change comes together. This may be happening now in medicine and has happened already in the financial markets.

The *financial industry* was at first skeptical of the individual investors' ability to manage their own portfolios. But the advents of the PC and the Internet have rapidly

Table 7.1. Healthcare on the Internet

Stage	Consumer Capability
1) Information Access	Medline, Disease Specific, Product Centric
2) Community	Support Communities, Treatment Alternatives, Quality Comparison
3) Personalization	Personalized News, Risk Profiling, Online Records
4) Transactions	Coverage Selection, Lifestyle Programs, Drug Authorizations
5) Services	Disease Management, Scheduling, Compliance Programs

and dramatically changed the face of investing. Will the healthcare industry enter an analogous transformation, as the confluence of the Internet and healthcare creates its own "strategic inflection point" for the industry (see Table 7.1)?

The Web allows *mass customization*. For example, information about specific health conditions can be provided at appropriate levels of understanding. Risk appraisal can also be done online. For example, personal health plans can be tailored to risks for heart disease. The Web can simplify routine transactions, such as prescription refills, scheduling office visits, and certain authorizations. For routine follow-up of specific problems, the Web sites that generate targeted e-mail might be helpful (Payne & Kiel, 2005).

Some software and services now support a *patient record online* that is largely maintained by the patient but also used by the physician and other healthcare professionals for entering certain information, like drug prescriptions. Since the patient has some control and responsibility of the record, one might expect the record to be generally more complete and to contain fewer errors. The patient should also be able to retrieve large amounts of information tailored to the patient's situation that the patient can browse and read in more leisurely fashion than when in the doctor's office. The patient would also have access to care guidelines and could actively participate in the management of treatments.

Examples

An example is provided of a Web system that supports patient-doctor interaction. *Aboutmyhealth.net* allows patients to online:

- Gather, view, and share physician medical records
- Communicate with physicians
- Order prescriptions and other healthcare products
- Manage diseases such as diabetes
- Assess wellness
- Receive context-specific health news and information

In one project with The Sisters of Providence Health System in Portland, Oregon, the patient initially sees a screen introducing the family medicine clinic. An example of the use of aboutmyhealth.net is provided based on a demonstration for a fictitious patient provided at aboutmyhealth.net.

The *fictitious patient*, "Linda Purcell," has asthma and acute sinusitis. When Linda logs on, the first screen she sees asks her to enter a user ID and PIN number. Then

Figure 7.1. Messages: In this schematic of a Web window onto the consumer medical record, the patient sees her incoming messages from the medical practice and specifics about refills.

Schematic of Web Screen for Patient Message Center		
Message Center		
Incoming Messages:		
Date	Subject	From
11/15/2006	Allergic Reaction	Southside Clinic
11/12/2006	Refill Request Confirmed	Southside Clinic
Request an appointment with:		
David Adams, M.D.	Southside Clinic	
Request a refill for:	Prescribed by	
Cotrimoxazole	Dr. Adams, Southside Clinic	
Proventil	Dr. Adams, Southside Clinic	
See your medication chart for more detailed information		
Send a message to your doctor's office		
David Adams, M.D.	Southside Clinic	

she sees a screen that offers her a choice of message center, doctors and charts, health news, and search. In the "Message Center" (see Figure 7.1) she can view communications from her physician, request an appointment, ask for a prescription refill, or send a message to the doctor.

When Linda moves to the *Doctors and Charts* section (see Figure 7.2), she can view a medical summary, a description of health problems, a medications list, allergies, weight data, blood pressure, and cholesterol data. She can also view and update registration information that includes her phone number, pharmacy, employer, insurance company, who has seen her chart, future appointments, and a printable wallet card. She can click on the health problems listed and get a summary of the problem, its diagnosis, and treatment. If she clicks on any of the medications she can receive instructions on taking the drug and contraindications. At any time, she can send a message to the physician's office.

A counterpart application allows physicians to create their own version of the medical record. With this *Web-based patient record program*, patients can receive prescriptions directly from their physicians over the Internet. Or patients can send their physicians a message, to which the physician can respond and then forward prescriptions to an online pharmacy. The patient can receive the medication in the mail, or retrieve it from a nearby pharmacy.

Figure 7.2. Doctors and charts: In this Web window of the consumer medical record system, the patient sees details of her medications and allergies.

Schematic of Web site for patient's view of medical record	
David Adams, M.D.	Southside Clinic
	My Medical Summary
My Medical Summary	**Personal Information**
Health Problems Medications List Allergies Height & Weight Blood Pressure Cholesterol	Linda Purcell 40 Rolling Road, Apt 12 Catonsville, MD 21228 Home phone 410-747-4445 Day phone 410-455-2645
Registration Info	**Health Problems** Asthma Acute Sinusitis
	Medication
Address & Phone Personal Contacts Pharmacy Employer Insurance Future Appointments Who has seen my chart Printable Wallet Card	Cotrimoxazole (Brand Names: Bactrim, Septra, Cotrim, Uroplus) 2 po twice daily 3d, 2 po once daily 4d
	Proventil (Generic name: Albuterol sulfate, Brand name: Novo-Salmol, Salbutamol) 2 puffs qid prn shortness of breath
	Allergies
	Aspirin Erythromycin

A "personal medical record" system that can be used either on a stand-alone computer or across the Internet is called CapMed (www.capmed.com). The CapMed system was developed by a neurosurgeon who used it with his patients. Denton (2001) provided 330 patients a copy of CapMed and their medical records as Denton had them in his office. One year later, he conducted a mail-in survey that posed a series of relevant yes-and-no questions regarding usage and invited narrative comment and anonymous responses. Patients:

- Intended to begin or continue keeping records
- Used CapMed on medical visits

- Would rather not store health information on the Internet
- Wished to use e-mail with the doctor's office
- Believed doctors do not keep full records
- Strongly believed individuals should keep their own records

In addition to gaining new information from informed patients, Denton established the technical feasibility of transferring information between doctor's office and personal health records.

E-Mail

E-mail usage has steadily increased. Perhaps a quarter of the U.S. population currently uses e-mail. In one study about half the patients had access to e-mail and about one-quarter were using e-mail to communicate with their healthcare provider. Guidelines for using e-mail in a clinical setting address two interrelated aspects: effective interaction between the clinician and patient and the observance of medico-legal prudence.

If a provider anticipates a need to contact a patient again soon with regard to test results or other follow-up, he or she should inquire about the patient's *communication preferences*. Prescription refills, lab results, appointment reminders, insurance questions, and routine follow-up inquiries are well suited to e-mail. It also provides the patient with a convenient way to report home health measurements, such as blood pressure and glucose determinations. Issues of a time-sensitive nature, such as medical emergencies, do not lend themselves to discussion via e-mail, since the time when an e-mail message will be read and acted upon cannot be ascertained. Sensitive and highly confidential subjects should not be discussed through most e-mail systems because of the potential for interception of the messages and the potential for transmission of messages to unintended recipients (Kane & Sands, 1998).

An extension of e-mail between two people is e-mail regularly exchanged among a group of people. Such groups are typically called online groups and may be supported by Web sites or specialized software. Online groups have become important in many areas of commerce, and patients are one of the most prominent participants in online groups (Edenius & Aberg-Wennerholm, 2005). Patient discussion groups typically focus on sharing empathy and information (Ebner et al., 2004). While patterns of participation tend to be highly skewed with most participants behaving as lurkers, patients will join and remain in groups based on some affinity that they feel to the group. Many patients who go online for help are well-educated (Gitlow, 2001) and may want to participate in a group with other well-educated people who want to engage in critical thinking. Patients with chronic conditions self-manage their illness, and participation in an online group is one way to engage in critical thinking about that management.

National Network

Evidence of the importance of information networks is reflected in the U.S. government creation in 2004 of the *Office of the National Coordinator for Health Information Technology* (ONCHIT). ONCHIT is to implement a vision for widespread adoption of interoperable electronic health records by 2015. Presidential Executive Order #13335 issued in 2004 created ONCHIT and charged it with four primary responsibilities:

- Serve as the senior advisor to the Secretary of DHHS and the President of the U.S. on all health information technology programs and initiatives
- Develop and maintain a strategic plan to guide the nationwide implementation of interoperable EHRs in both the public and private healthcare sectors
- Coordinate the spending of approximately $4 billion for health information technology programs and initiatives across the federal enterprise
- Coordinate all outreach activities to private industry and serve as the catalyst for healthcare industry change

Essentially, ONCHIT is to support the development of a nationwide health information network (NHIN). A NHIN is an Internet-based architecture that links disparate healthcare information systems together to allow patients, physicians, hospitals, community health centers and public health agencies across the country to share clinical information securely.

To gain broad input on the best mechanisms to achieve *nationwide interoperability*, the Department of Health and Human Services requested input. The request specifically asked for feedback on how a NHIN could be governed, financed, operated, and supported. Among the many opinions expressed, significant support emerged for the following concepts (DHHS, 2005):

- A NHIN should be a decentralized architecture built using the Internet, linked by uniform communications and a software framework of open standards and policies.
- A NHIN should reflect the interests of all stakeholders and be a joint public/private effort.

- A governance entity composed of public and private stakeholders should oversee the determination of standards and policies.
- A NHIN should be patient-centric with sufficient safeguards to protect the privacy of personal health information.
- Incentives will be needed to accelerate the deployment and adoption of a NHIN.
- Existing technologies, federal leadership, prototype regional exchange efforts, and certification of EHRs will be the critical enablers of a NHIN.
- Key challenges to developing and adopting a NHIN were listed as: the need for additional and better refined standards; addressing privacy concerns; paying for the development, operation of, and access to the NHIN; accurately matching patients' identity; and addressing discordant inter- and intra-state laws regarding health information exchange.

Other overarching concepts that were espoused by many of the respondents included:

- There is a need for some form of implementation and harmonization at a regional level
- Cooperation between the public and private sectors is essential for successful realization of a NHIN
- The NHIN should evolve incrementally and include appropriate incentives, coordination, and accountability to succeed
- The federal government plays a role in advancing a NHIN

The budget for ONCHIT has been far too small to finance the NHIN, but ONCHIT helps focus attention on the importance of a NHIN.

Questions

Reading Questions

1. Consider the lessons learned through the biographies of Lindberg and Barnett in Chapter 1 and compare those to the lessons learned in the implementation of Information Networks for Public Health Officials.

2. What services are offered by EDI vendors who connect providers and payers?
3. What are the trends for Web usage by consumers of healthcare?
4. Describe the features of a medical record system that is accessible over the Web and largely in the control of the patient.

Doing Questions

1. "Personal medical records" are medical records that are owned and controlled by the patient. Various synonyms exist, such as "consumer health record," but the basic point is that the patient or person or consumer has a copy and takes some responsibility that the record is maintained across time and across different providers and more importantly takes some responsibility for his/her health. How might the use of a personal health record be related to costs, data quality, and coordination issues raised in an earlier chapter?
2. How are standards for medical records relevant to the "personal health record?" Give an example of how a knowledge base might come into play to support the use of these personal medical record systems.

References

Alshawi, S., Missi, F., & Eldabi, T. (2003). Healthcare information management: The integration of patients' data. *Logistics Information Management, 16*(3/4), 286-295.

Antweiler, W., & Frank, M.Z. (2004). Is all that talk just noise? The information content of Internet stock message boards. *Journal of Finance, 59*(3), 1259-1295.

Barret, J., & Koprowski, S.J. (2002). The epiphany of data warehousing technologies in the pharmaceutical industry. *International Journal of Clinical Pharmacology, Therapy, and Toxicology, 40*(3), 3-13.

Calhoun, J., Banaszak-Hol, J., & Hearld, L. (2006). Current marketing practices in the nursing home sector. *Journal of Healthcare Management, 51*(3), 185-200.

Denton, I. (2001). Jr. healthcare information management. *Journal of HealthCare Information Management, 15*(3), 251-259.

Department of Health and Human Services. (2005, June 3, 2005). *HHS releases report on nationwide health information exchange*. Press Release. Department of Health and Human Services. Retrieved May 2006, from www.os.dhhs.gov/news/press/2005pres/20050603.html

Ebner, W., Leimeister, J.M., & Krcmar, H. (2004). Trust in virtual healthcare communities: Design and implementation of trust-enabling functionalities. R. Sprague (Ed.), *37th Annual Hawaii International Conference on System Sciences* (pp. 182-192). IEEE.

Edenius, M., & Aberg-Wennerholm, M. (2005). Patient communities, ICT, and the future: An exploratory study about patient communities and their status in the ICT-era. *International Telecommunications Society 16th European Regional Conference* (pp. 1-18). Porto, Portugal: International Telecommunications Society.

Fox, S., & Fallows, D. (2003). *Internet health resources*. Washington, DC: Pew Internet & American Life Project.

Gitlow, S. (2001). The online community as a healthcare resource. In D. Nash, M. Manfredi, B. Bozarth, & S. Howell (Eds.), *Connecting with the New Healthcare Consumer: Defining Your Strategy* (pp. 113-134). Gaithersburg, MD: Aspen Publication.

Glaser, J.P., DeBor, G., & Stuntz, L. (2003). The New England Healthcare EDI Network. *Journal of Healthcare Information Management, 17*(4), 42-50.

Grove, A. (1996). *Only the paranoid survive: How to exploit the crisis points that challenge every company and career*. New York: Bantam Books.

Hinman, A.R., Saarlas, K.N., & Ross, D.A. (2004). A vision for child health information systems: Developing child health information systems to meet medical care and public health needs. *Journal of Public Health Management and Practice* (Supplement), 91-98.

Kane, B., & Sands, D.Z. (1998). Guidelines for the clinical use of electronic mail with patients. *Journal of the American Medical Informatics Association, 5*(1), 104-111.

Langabeer, J. (2005). The evolving role of supply chain management technology in healthcare. *Journal of Healthcare Information Management, 19*(2), 27-33.

Murray, E., Burns, J., See, T., Lai, R., & Nazareth, I. (2005). Interactive health communication applications for people with chronic disease. *The Cochrane Database of Systematic Reviews,* (4), CD004274.

Noss, B., & Zall, R. (2002). A review of CHIN initiatives: What works and why. *Journal of Healthcare Information Management, 16*(2), 35-39.

Payne, V., & Kiel, J. (2005). Web-based communication to enhance outcomes: A case study in patient relations. *Journal of Healthcare Information Management, 19*(2), 56-63.

Rada, R. (2006). Membership and online groups. P. Isaias, M. McPherson, & F. Bannister (Eds.), *E-Society 2006: IADIS International Conference* (pp. 290-293). Dublin, Ireland: International Association for Development of the Information Society (IADIS) Press.

Raisinghani, M.S., Tan, E.-L., Untama, J.A., Weiershaus, H., & Levermann, T. (2005). CRM systems in German hospitals: Illustrations of issues & trends. *Journal of Cases in Information Technology, 7*(4), 1-26.

Rundle, R. (2000, February 28). E-commerce coming to health-care industry. *Wall Street Journal,* p. B4.

Smith, J. (2000). *Health management information systems: A handbook for decision-makers*. Buckingham, UK: Open University Press.

Zineldin, M. (2006). The quality of health care and patient satisfaction: An exploratory investigation of the 5Qs model at some Egyptian and Jordanian medical clinics. *International Journal of Health Care Quality, 19*(1), 60-92.

Chapter VIII

Regulation

Learning Objectives

- Predict the trends in government regulation of business in the U.S.
- Analyze the different types of regulations on healthcare relative to the costs they incur for compliance
- Design a corporate compliance program that balances the various forces that work for and against compliance

The use of innovative applications of technology in the highly regulated world of medicine requires compliance with various *government regulations* (Goldberg & Gordon, 1999; Health Information and Technology Practice Group, 2003). These regulations are intended to meet a public need. A "program" is defined in the dictionary as a system of projects intended to meet a public need. Thus, an organization's system of projects to achieve compliance with government regulations is called a compliance program. This chapter explores issues germane to compliance in the healthcare enterprise and begins with the history of government regulation of business.

Context

Government regulation of business is needed to protect citizens from unscrupulous businesses. This regulation requires first a *law*. However, citizens are seldom able to lobby successfully for laws without the help of business.

History

Beginning in *1764* the English government deliberately abandoned its policy of benign neglect towards the American colonists and imposed regulations. For instance, Americans needed to pay a stamp duty. The American Revolution led to a Constitution that encouraged free enterprise with minimal government intervention.

In 1800, only *300 civil officials* were employed in the nation's capital. The State Department consisted of the Secretary of State, a chief clerk, seven lesser clerks, and a message boy. The *Industrial Revolution* shook the foundations of American society. Purposive control of business in the name of the public good slowly became the American response to big business. The *Sherman Anti-Trust Act* of 1890 made illegal every contract that restrained free trade. The Act symbolizes the transition from a society in which government is regarded as the chief source of threats to individual freedom to one in which private economic power is an equal threat.

Since the late 1960s, regulations have appeared that effect corporate *internal operations*. The Occupational Safety and Health Administration, for example, may specify precise engineering controls that must be adopted by all industries. These regulations reach inside the production process. Management decisions are even more affected by applying the standards for equal employment opportunity in hiring, firing, advancement, and discipline of employees.

The new social regulations have added costs and burdens to business without adding to their ability to pay for these costs. While the public enjoys a safer environment and fairer working conditions, the *costs* for these gains has been high.

The 1980 election brought *Ronald Reagan* to the White House and a different approach to regulation. In his first presidential news conference, Reagan declared a crusade against "runaway government." He froze 172 pending regulations that had been left him by outgoing President Jimmy Carter. Reagan gave the *Office of Management and Budget* (OMB) primary supervisory responsibility over new regulations. OMB became a critic of customary approaches of regulatory agencies. For instance, OMB put pressure on the Environmental Protection Agency to make less stringent regulations to safeguard the environment. OMB questioned the scientific accuracy of EPA's reasoning and even the truthfulness of some of the EPA staff. OMB intervention, frequently in the name of cost-benefit analysis, blocked or altered many proposed regulations in a direction deemed acceptable to some major industrialists.

George Bush had served as vice president under Reagan, and when he became president, he continued the policies of Reagan. *Bill Clinton* was president from 1993-2001 and favored various forms of government regulation of business. In January 2001, George W. Bush became president and immediately froze Clinton's recommendations, not unlike Reagan froze Carter's recommendations.

American politics swings between friendship and hostility towards business. Sometimes regulatory policy is too rigid and excessively costly. Sometimes it is too lax. A *balance* is needed that allows business to prosper and the public to be protected against business excess.

Role of Business

Government regulation of business is partly a response to public opinion. However, government regulations typically require significant support of some businesses. The development of the *Pure Food and Drug Act* of 1906 illustrates this point. In 1883 Dr. Harvey Wiley, chief chemist of the U.S. Department of Agriculture, started a campaign against adulterated food. At the time, many basic foods were routinely mixed with additives and preservatives:

- Formaldehyde was used for preserving milk
- Hydrochloric acid was added to apple jelly
- Pork fat was mixed with butter

Wiley attempted to persuade Congress to take action, but Congress would not listen. Wiley enlisted the support of the:

- American Medical Association
- Pharmaceutical Manufacturers Association

How did Wiley manage to get these representatives of businesses to join his anti-business cause? They had *self-serving interests*:

- The Pharmaceutical Manufacturer Association provided crucial support because it would help eliminate competitors in the patent medicine business that were not members of the Association.
- The American Medical Association supported the measure to increase its monopoly on the treatment of disease.

While protection of the public is one result of the Food and Drug Act of 1906, the bill also disadvantaged certain businesses while helping others.

Associations

At least two types of organizations are pre-eminent in government regulation of the healthcare industry; namely, government and the industry. However, many other intermediary organizations also exist which play a key role. Associations of healthcare providers that self-regulate the industry are one such example of intermediary organization.

An *association* is an organization of persons having a common interest. Numerous associations are relevant to regulation and compliance. The Joint Commission on the Accreditation of Healthcare Organizations (JCAHO) and the National Committee on Quality Assurance (NCQA), as accrediting organizations, can contribute to the development of a common framework to guide the use of information systems in healthcare. JCAHO and NCQA tend to incorporate requirements from federal regulations into their standards and practices for evaluating healthcare organizations.

JCAHO and NCQA are created for and run by healthcare professionals. *JCAHO* and *NCQA* strive to reflect the preferences of healthcare professionals and at the same time to follow whatever laws and regulations apply to the professions. Thus their criteria for accreditation are a good indication of what is practical.

Cost of Compliance

Healthcare is one of the most heavily regulated businesses. Comparisons across industries suggest the following approximate *costs of compliance* (Conover, 2004):

- Airline 14%
- Manufacturing 2%
- Healthcare 25%
- Services 1%
- Telecommunications 20%

This data shows that the manufacturing and services industries spend relatively little to comply with government regulations, but the airlines, healthcare, and telecommunications industry spend about one-fifth of their budget to comply with regulation. Major categories of cost may be grouped according to:

- Access
- Costs
- Quality

Access regulations require healthcare providers to give care or other services for free. For example, hospitals that receive certain federal construction funds must care for some poor patients without charge; the term "hospital uncompensated care pool" refers to this situation. Another regulation affecting access is called the Emergency Medical Treatment and Active Labor Act (EMTALA). EMTALA was passed by the U.S. Congress in 1986 to ensure patient access to emergency medical care and to prevent the practice of patient dumping, in which uninsured patients were transferred, solely for financial reasons, from private to public hospitals without consideration of their medical condition or stability for the transfer. Even though its initial language primarily covered the care of emergency medical conditions, the law and the regulations it drove now apply to virtually all aspects of patient care in the hospital setting (Teshome & Closson, 2006).

Cost regulations are intended to control the cost of healthcare. Under cost-related regulations are fraud and abuse regulations, pharmaceutical price regulation (which in turn includes federal average wholesale price restrictions for Medicaid), and others. Cost control regulations tend not to raise the cost of healthcare, as indeed their purpose is to constrain the cost.

Quality regulations enforce quality. For instance, Medicare requires healthcare providers to be accredited or licensed. These Medicare conditions on eligibility of healthcare providers to be paid by Medicare have many purposes, but quality is arguably the central purpose. Another set of quality-related regulations comes from the Clinical Laboratory Improvement Act.

For a healthcare provider to comply with a regulation entails benefits and costs. For instance, a regulation that forces pharmaceutical companies to sell drugs at a lower price to healthcare providers is a benefit to some healthcare providers. Requiring a hospital to be licensed before getting paid entails a cost to the hospital. A tabular summary of the *costs and benefits* for healthcare providers (see Table 8.1) shows that compliance with:

- Access regulations inflicts a net cost of $8 billion per year
- Cost-containment regulations give a net benefit of $1 billion per year
- Quality regulations inflict a net cost of $18 billion per year

The next sections present first some details of regulations related to insurance and then some information about organizations and their role in compliance.

Table 8.1. Cost of health facilities regulation in billions of dollar. The broad categories are in bold and two examples are provided underneath each broad category. The costs of the examples do not sum to the cost of the broad category because they are only examples of the two highest cost categories rather than exhaustive. This table is adapted from Conover (2004).

Type of Regulation	Costs	Benefits	Net Cost
Access	**12**	**4**	**8**
EMTALA	4	2	2
Uncompensated care pool	7	2	5
Costs	**14**	**15**	**(1)**
Health care fraud and abuse	3	2	1
Pharmaceutical price regulation	8	10	(2)
Quality	**22**	**4**	**18**
Facility accreditation/licensure	14	4	10
Clinical Lab Improvement Act	3	0	3

Corporate Compliance Programs

Each corporation has its culture. A compliance program good for one corporate culture might not be good for a different corporate culture.

While a corporation will have an overall culture, inside a corporation there will exist numerous *subcultures*. For example, the legal department has distinctly different beliefs and customs from the billing department. An effective compliance program will address these differences and recognize natural alliances among certain subcultures.

For better or worse, corporations seldom approach compliance with the law in a generalized way. Rather compliance is approached on a piecemeal basis focused on separate areas of the law. One manager may be charged with compliance to OSHA, but that person would have little interaction with the person charged with compliance to HIPAA.

A typical *compliance program* may be viewed as involving four steps:

- Management commitment
- Education

- Implementation
- Control

An executive policy endorsement would be an appropriate sign of management commitment. Education for topics like privacy would go to all staff. Implementation is a complex process that begins with a gap and risk analysis and proceeds to detailed planning and execution. Control is the review of the results and must itself, like the implementation, be continual.

Tracking and documenting progress may be a crucial part of compliance. No matter how lofty the objectives or how laudable the work towards them, unless the work is documented, compliance is in doubt. One of the most significant compliance techniques is in the *internal review*. Usually such reviews will produce written reports intended for internal consumption and address problems that need to be remedied. Some regulations require such internal vigilance, documentation of information processing, documentation of training success, and so on.

Unfortunately, internal reviewers may take on the mantle of *enforcement officers* who want to make sure the company follows the rules. Groups responsible for internal reviews tend to become clearly established as a compliance constituency.

Any internal review group can find things that should be corrected. Furthermore, the group can be expected to want to bring attention to its successes by highlighting irregularities. The healthcare entity needs to be careful to both:

- Encourage internal review
- Assure that such review does not assume an independent political life inside the entity and thrive unfairly at the expense of other legitimate activities

Government intervention into healthcare operations has its upside and its downside.

HIPAA

The next two chapters of this book examine privacy and security. Those concerns have become important in the healthcare industry because of government regulation. The U.S. Congress determined in 1996 that the health insurance market should be given further federal goals and placed these in the Health Insurance Portability and Accountability Act (HIPAA). In effect, HIPAA established a federal floor for a degree of assurance that health status will render neither individuals nor their dependents *uninsurable*. However, HIPAA covers much more than insurance, as is typical of much legislation. During the legislative process, provisions may get added that seem politically convenient despite the original purpose of the legislation.

HIPAA covers a wide-range of topics that are not always related to one another. The Act calls for health insurance that is portable and accountable, and the acronym is the "HIPA Act" or "HIPAA." Despite this name based on portable and accountable insurance, the Act is particularly known for its emphasis on standardized transactions, security, and privacy—all three of which are placed under the heading of *Administrative Simplification* in HIPAA, although the "A" in "Administrative" is not represented in the acronym "HIPAA." The Administrative Simplification component of HIPAA calls for standardization of "identifiers and code sets" and "transactions" (as described in an earlier chapter), and after the politicians thought about the ramifications of the increased electronic communications, they decided to add provisions requiring regulation of privacy and security (Rada, 2003).

Questions

Reading Questions

1. Describe the history of government regulation of business in the U.S.
2. Illustrate how different corporations have different cultures as regards compliance with federal regulations.

Doing Questions

1. What lesson do you draw from the history preceding the Pure Food and Drug Act as regards the role of business in supporting the finalization of federal regulation of business? Imagine a piece of healthcare information systems legislation that you see having a challenging battle in congress and for which you can anticipate some businesses supporting it and some opposing it. Describe briefly the intent of the legislation and the opposing and supporting forces.
2. Make an analogy between the insight that some business needs to support a successful legislation and the observations about the nature of corporate compliance. If you were CEO of a large firm, what would you want to do and why regarding the distribution of authority between the corporate compliance unit and those units responsible for profit generation?

References

Conover, C.J. (2004). *Health care regulation: A $169 billion hidden tax*. Washington, DC: Cato Institute.

Goldberg, A., & Gordon, J. (1999). *Telemedicine: Emerging legal issues* (2nd ed.). Washington, DC: American Health Lawyers Association.

Health Information and Technology Practice Group. (2003). *Health information and technology practice guide* (2nd ed.). Washington, DC: American Health Lawyers Association.

Rada, R. (2003). *HIPAA @ IT Reference 2003: Health information transactions, privacy, and security*. Chicago: Health Information and Management Systems Society.

Teshome, G., & Closson, F.T. (2006). Emergency medical treatment and labor act: The basics and other medicolegal concerns. *Pediatric Clinics North America, 53*(1), 139-155.

Chapter IX
Privacy

Learning Objectives

- Integrate the various arguments about privacy into a theme of power
- Indicate the relationship of notices of privacy practices seen in everyday experience to the requirements of the Privacy Rule
- Distinguish situations in which an entity must give the patient an opportunity to object to the use of information from those situations in which the patient gets no such opportunity
- Apply the patient rights of access to develop scenarios in which a patient exercises such rights
- Breakdown the implementation requirements of the Privacy Rule, particularly as regards having a privacy officer, training staff, and documenting policies

Hippocrates was an ancient Greek physician whose writings not only had a great impact on the content of Greek medical thought but also on the privacy of patient information. He said (Staden, 1996):

About whatever I may see or hear in treatment, or even without treatment, in the life of human beings—things that should not ever be blurted outside—I will remain silent, holding such things to be sacred, and not to be divulged

Physicians take a variant of this oath to this day.

Political Struggle

Warren and Brandeis (1890) said:

In very early times, the law gave a remedy only for physical interference with life and property, for trespasses vi et armis. Then the "right to life" served only to protect the subject from battery in its various forms; liberty meant freedom from actual restraint; and the right to property secured to the individual his lands and his cattle. ...Gradually the scope of these legal rights broadened; and now the right to life has come to mean...the right to be let alone... and the term "property" has grown to comprise every form of possession—intangible, as well as tangible. ...Recent inventions and business methods call attention to the next step which must be taken for the protection of the person, and for securing to the individual what Judge Cooley calls the right "to be let alone." Instantaneous photographs and newspaper enterprise have invaded the sacred precincts of private and domestic life; and numerous mechanical devices threaten to make good the prediction that "what is whispered in the closet shall be proclaimed from the house-tops."

The contemporary concerns for *privacy* are not that an official will physically enter and search someone's house or that the newspaper will take photographs of private events. Rather the concern is for the use of records, particularly in computers.

Power

In the mid-19th century, three quarters of the adult population worked for themselves on farms or in small towns. Attendance at the village schoolhouse was not compulsory. Record keeping about individuals was limited and local in nature. Few individuals had insurance of any kind. A patient's medical record typically existed only in the doctor's memory. Now, by contrast, fewer than 10% of people are self-employed, and their employers often keep extensive records on them. Insurance is common, and medical care is institutionalized. Acquiring insurance or medical care requires the individual to divulge information, and usually leads to some evaluation of him based on information about him that some other *record keeper* has compiled.

What two people divulge about themselves when they meet for the first time depends on how much personal revelation they believe the situation warrants and how much confidence each has that the other will not misinterpret or misuse what is said. If they meet again, and particularly if they develop a relationship, their self-revelation may expand both in scope and detail. Throughout this process, each person may:

- Correct any misperception that develops
- Judge whether the other is likely to misuse the personal revelations

Should either suspect that the other has *violated the trust*, he can sever the relationship or alter its terms, perhaps by refusing thereafter to discuss certain topics. Such relationships are the threads of which the fabric of society is woven. The situations are inherently social and not private in that the disclosure of information about oneself is expected.

An individual's relationship with a *record keeping organization* has some of the features of individual face-to-face relationships, as it arises in an inherently social context, depends on the individual's willingness to divulge information, and carries some expectation of the practical consequences. Beyond that, however, the resemblance fades.

Typically, the organization decides what information must be divulged at what rate. The individual might theoretically take his business elsewhere when dealing with private organizations (but not when dealing with the government). Yet organizations tend to have similar *information gathering requirements*, the differences among them are poorly understood, and the individual often has little opportunity to meaningfully pick and choose.

Once an individual establishes a relationship with a *record keeping organization*, he loses some of the control that he has in face-to-face relationships and this control or power goes to the organization. The individual faces challenges in trying to:

- Check on the accuracy of the information the organization develops
- Correct any errors that may exist in the information
- Know the full extent of uses of the information
- Know the disclosures of the information
- Sever the relationship with the organization

Having power is in a certain sense the ability to invade someone else's privacy. Information, in the hands of people who know how to use it, is power. Privacy is first and foremost about power.

Balance

The social philosophy of *communitarianism* holds that a good society crafts a careful balance between individual rights and the common good (Etzioni, 1999). In a society that strongly enforces social duties but neglects individual rights (as does

Japan, for instance, when it comes to the rights of minorities), fostering individual rights might improve the balance. In the United States, individual rights are given high priority.

The challenge of balancing privacy and public good is particularly difficult in the context of specific historical and social conditions. Four criteria can be used to help determine whether an imbalance exists:

- First, a society should take steps to limit privacy only if it faces a well-documented and macroscopic threat to the common good. For instance, when many thousands of lives are lost, as with HIV, society faces a clear and major threat that may merit some infringement on privacy to manage.
- The second criterion is that the society tries first to use non-privacy threatening measures to remove the danger to the common good. For instance, when medical records are needed by researchers, the data should be collected as much as possible without identifying individuals.
- Third, to the extent that privacy-curbing measures are introduced, a communitarian society makes them as minimally intrusive as possible. For instance, the National Practitioner Data Bank allows a hospital that is considering whether to grant a physician the right to practice in the hospital to conduct limited background checks on the physician. The Data Bank discloses only high-level facts, such as that a physician's license to practice medicine was revoked, and does not give details of the violations. Because the hospital will know that a physician would not have had his license revoked for other than serious cause, the hospital does not need to know more detail.
- Fourth, measures that treat undesirable side effects of needed privacy diminishing measures are to be preferred over those that ignore these effects. Thus, if more widespread HIV testing is deemed necessary to protect public health, efforts must be made to enhance the confidentiality of the records of those tested.

Although the proceeding might include examples where invasion of privacy supports the public good, opposite examples exist.

The balances are complex and involve different types of entities and different types of good. To achieve harmony may require compromises. For instance, one kind of change that the government could help implement would be to reduce legal liability for errors in the record. A peaceful balancing of the power between individuals and organizations requires *mutual respect*. Organizations that share record keeping with individuals could be sheltered from legal battles each time an individual finds a discrepancy in the records. Rather the individual and the organization should work together to maintain good records.

HIPAA's Privacy Rule

HIPAA's Administrative Simplification first asks for standardizing electronic transactions between healthcare providers and payers. This standardization should increase the flow of electronic information and the ability of various organizations to take advantage of the information therein. To insure that the information is not misused, HIPAA also calls for security and privacy. This chapter presents the principles and related information of the *Privacy Rule*.

The Privacy Rule has two major purposes:

- To protect and enhance the rights of consumers by providing them access to their health information and controlling the inappropriate use of that information
- To improve the efficiency and effectiveness of healthcare delivery by creating a national framework for health privacy protection that builds on efforts by states, health systems, and individuals

The Rule may bring the patient closer to the healthcare process by more closely connecting the patient with the patient's record.

Applicable

The Privacy Rule only applies to health plans, healthcare clearinghouses, and healthcare providers that transmit health information in electronic form in connection with a HIPAA standard transaction. Thus, an *entity* needs to answer three questions:

1. Is it a health plan, clearinghouse, or care provider?
2. Does it transmit health information in electronic form?
3. Does it submit such health information in HIPAA transactions?

If the response to any of these questions is "no," then the entity does not need to comply with its requirements. If the response to all the questions is "yes," then the entity must comply with the Privacy Rule.

In the Privacy Rule, *health information* is any information, whether oral or recorded in any form or medium, that relates to the past, present, or future physical or mental health or condition of an individual; the provision of healthcare to an individual; or the past, present, or future payment for the provision of healthcare to an individual.

Individually identifiable health information is a subset of health information, including demographic information collected from an individual, with respect to which there is a reasonable basis to believe the information can be used to identify the individual. Protected health information means individually identifiable health information in a covered entity.

Notice of Privacy Practices

The Privacy Rule extensively describes a notice of privacy practices. *Health plans must provide the notice to all health plan enrollees* at the time of enrollment and to all enrollees within 60 days of a material revision to the notice. *Health plans* must notify enrollees no less than once every three years about the availability of the notice and how to obtain a copy. Health care providers must offer the notice to patients on their first encounter.

A healthcare provider with a *direct-treatment relationship* with an individual must make a good faith effort to obtain the individual's written acknowledgment of receipt of the notice. Failure by this provider to obtain an individual's acknowledgment, assuming it otherwise documented its good faith effort, is not a violation of the Rule. Other covered entities, such as health plans, are not required to obtain this acknowledgment from individuals, but may do so if they choose.

The notice must be in *plain language*. A covered plan or provider could satisfy the plain language requirement by:

- Organizing material to serve the needs of the reader
- Writing sentences in the active voice
- Using "you" and other pronouns
- Using common, everyday words in sentences
- Writing in short sentences
- Dividing material into short sections

Since the content of the notice should be communicated to all recipients, the covered entity should consider various means of communicating with various populations. Any covered entity that is a recipient of federal financial assistance is obligated under Title VI of the Civil Rights Act of 1964 to provide material ordinarily distributed to the public in the primary languages of persons with limited *English proficiency* in the recipients' service areas.

Entities must include prominent and specific language in the notice that indicates the importance of the notice. The header must read:

THIS NOTICE DESCRIBES HOW MEDICAL INFORMATION ABOUT YOU MAY BE USED AND DISCLOSED AND HOW YOU CAN GET ACCESS TO THIS INFORMATION. PLEASE REVIEW IT CAREFULLY.

This is the only specific language that entities must include in the notice.

Authorization

An *authorization* gives covered entities permission to use specified protected health information for specified purposes, which are generally other than treatment, payment, or healthcare operations, or to disclose such information to a third party specified by the individual.

Covered entities may use one authorization form for all purposes. The following are the core elements for a valid authorization (DHHS, 2000):

- A description of the information to be used or disclosed
- Identification of the persons or class of persons authorized to make the use or disclosure of the protected health information
- Identification of the persons or class of persons to whom the covered entity is authorized to make the use or disclosure
- Description of each purpose of the use or disclosure
- Expiration date or event
- Individual's signature and date
- Statement that the individual may revoke the authorization in writing
- Statement that treatment, payment, enrollment, or eligibility for benefits may not be conditioned on obtaining the authorization

Individuals may seek disclosure of their health information to others in many circumstances, such as:

- When applying for life or disability *insurance*
- In seeking certain *job* assignments where health is relevant
- In *tort litigation*, where an individual's attorney needs individually identifiable health information to evaluate an injury claim and asks the individual to authorize disclosure of records relating to the injury to the attorney

A *valid authorization* may contain additional, non-required elements, provided that these elements are not inconsistent with the required elements.

Uses and Disclosures

Uses and *disclosures* are foundational concepts in the Privacy Rule. Their meanings are (see Figures 9.1 and 9.2):

- "Use" means the employment, application, utilization, examination, or analysis of protected information within an entity that maintains the information
- "Disclosure" means the release, transfer, provision of access to, or divulging in any other manner of protected health information outside the entity holding the information (DHHS, 2000)

In short, "use" occurs inside an entity, and "disclosure" occurs outside an entity.

Figure 9.1. Use. Department X within the covered entity N is sharing protected health information (PHI) with another Department Y inside the same covered entity—this is 'use'.

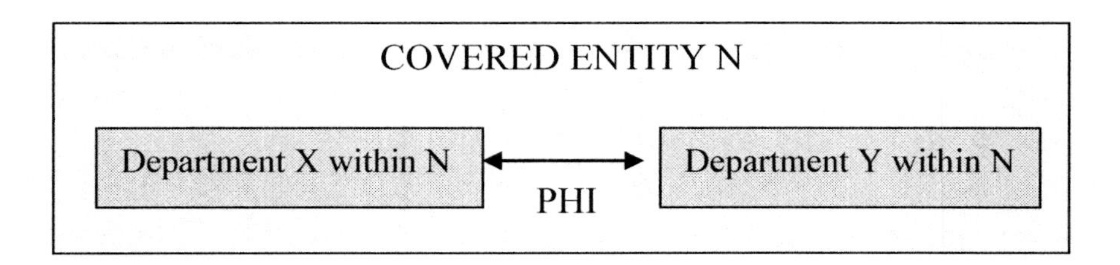

Figure 9.2. Disclosure. Covered entity N sends PHI to entity M—this is 'disclosure'.

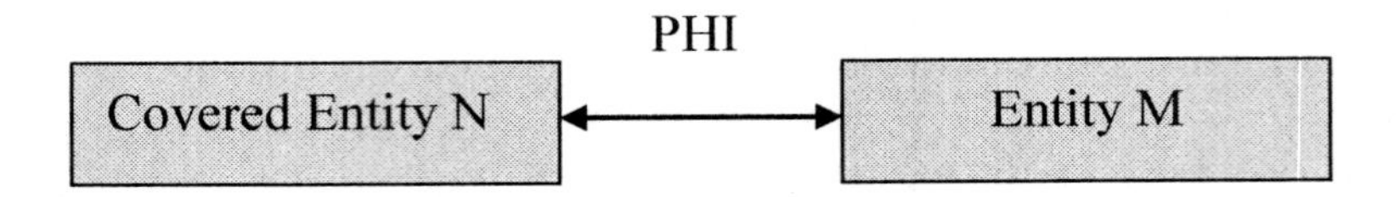

Minimum Necessary Standard

To maximize privacy one wants to *control information flow*. In some ways this control may be seen as minimizing the flow to that necessary. DHHS requires covered entities to implement policies and procedures for "minimum necessary" uses and disclosures. Implementation of such policies and procedures is required in lieu of making the "minimum necessary" determination for each separate use or disclosure. Covered entities can disclose protected health information for the treatment and payment activities of another covered entity or any healthcare provider, and for certain healthcare operations of another covered entity. Uses or disclosures for treatment purposes are not subject to the "minimum necessary" standard.

The *minimum necessary standard* has essentially three components (DHHS, 2000):

- "First, it does not pertain to certain uses and disclosures including treatment-related exchange of information among healthcare providers;
- Second, for disclosures that are made on a routine and recurring basis, such as insurance claims, a covered entity is required to have policies and procedures for governing such exchanges (the rule does not require a case-by-case determination); and
- Third, providers must have a process for reviewing non-routine requests on a case-by-case basis to assure that only the minimum necessary information is disclosed."

The policy must generalize the rules about the flow of information. Entities should establish policies and procedures to limit:

- The *amount of protected health information* used or disclosed to the minimum amount necessary to meet the purpose of the use or disclosure
- Access to protected health information only to those people who need *access* to the information to accomplish the use or disclosure

Such limiting of access, of course, means that the flow of information is constrained.

An entity should have an *organizational manual* that indicates the functions of the entity. People perform certain functions. This mapping of people to functions is integral to implementing the minimum necessary standard.

The Privacy Rule states (DHHS, 2000): "The policies and procedures must be based on reasonable determinations regarding the *roles* that require protected health information, and the nature of the *health information* they require, consistent with their job responsibilities. For example, a hospital could implement a policy that permitted nurses access to all protected health information of patients in their ward while they are on duty…For any type of disclosure that is made on a *routine*, recurring basis, an entity must implement policies and procedures that permit only the disclosure of the minimum protected health information reasonably necessary to achieve the purpose of the disclosure. Individual review of each disclosure is not required.

Large entities face tougher requirements than small entities. For example, a *large enterprise* might be expected to remove identifiers in disclosed information, while a solo *physician's office* would not. The solo office might be expected to limit disclosures to only relevant pages of the medical record.

The Privacy Rule does not require that all risk of incidental use or disclosure be eliminated. The Privacy Rule explicitly permits certain incidental uses and disclosures that occur as a result of a use or disclosure otherwise permitted by the Privacy Rule. An *incidental use or disclosure:*

- Is a secondary use or disclosure that cannot reasonably be prevented
- Is limited in nature
- Occurs as a by-product of an otherwise permitted use or disclosure

For example, a provider may instruct an administrative staff member to bill a patient for a particular procedure, and may be overheard by one or more persons in the waiting room. Assuming that the provider made reasonable efforts to avoid being overheard and reasonably limited the information shared, an incidental disclosure resulting from such conversation is permissible under the Rule.

Business Associate

Under normal circumstances, an authorization is required to share *protected health information* (PHI) with non-covered entities. However, under two conditions, PHI can be sent to a non-covered entity without an authorization from the patient—those two conditions are:

- The PHI will be used for certain healthcare serving purposes (detailed in the Privacy Rule)
- A business associate contract is agreed between the covered entity sending the PHI and the non-covered entity receiving the PHI

A business associate uses protected health information of a covered entity. In more detail, a business association occurs when the right to use or disclose the protected health information belongs to the covered entity, and another entity is using or disclosing it to perform a function on behalf of the covered entity (DHHS, 2000). "Business associate" services include (but are not limited too) legal, actuarial, management, accounting, consulting, administrative accreditation, data aggregation, and financial services. Examples of relationships that should include a business associate contract are a consultant that performs utilization reviews for a hospital and an independent transcriptionist that transcribes for a physician.

De-Identification

The Privacy Rule applies to "individually identifiable health information" and not to de-identified information. The statute defines *individually identifiable health information* as certain health information (DHHS, 2000):

- Which identifies the individual
- With respect to which there is a reasonable basis to believe that the information can be used to identify the individual

De-identified information may be valuable for various purposes.

The de-identification method can use a statistically sound technique or the Safe Harbor specifications. In further detail:

- For the *statistically sound technique*, an expert determines that the risk is very small that the information could be used by itself or with other available information to identify a subject of the information. The covered entity must also document the analysis that justifies the determination.
- The other method is the *safe harbor method,* by which a covered entity removes certain types of identifiers.

The Privacy Rule says (DHHS, 2000): "The safe harbor allows age, some geographic location information, and some demographic information to be included in the de-identified information. All dates directly related to the subject of the information must be removed or limited to the year, and zip codes must be removed or aggregated (in the form of 3-digit zip codes) to include at least 20,000 people. Extreme ages of 90 and over must be aggregated to a category of 90+ to avoid identification of very old individuals." The rule lists several specific identifiers that have to be removed, including telephone numbers, e-mail addresses, social security numbers, and full-face photographs. The safe harbor involves a minimum of burden and conveys a maximum of certainty that the rules have been met with an easily followed, cookbook approach.

To some the de-identification safe harbor of the Privacy Rule is too restrictive. DHHS addressed this concern by permitting the creation and disclosure of a *limited data set*. The use or disclosure of any such limited data set is restricted to research, public health, and healthcare operations purposes only. The limited data set could include the following identifiable information: admission, discharge, and service dates; date of death; age (including age 90 or over); and five-digit zip code.

Psychotherapy

The general principle is that all information is equally sensitive. The Privacy Rule generally would not require covered entities to vary the level of protection of protected health information based on the sensitivity of such information. *Psychotherapy notes* are an exception.

"Psychotherapy notes" document conversation during a counseling session led by a *mental health professional*. Such notes can be used only by the therapist who wrote them, have to be maintained separately from the medical record, and can not be involved in the documentation necessary for healthcare treatment, payment, or operations.

Minimum Necessary

The mapping of people to functions is integral to implementing the minimum necessary standard. An entity must implement policies and procedures to identify the:

- Persons or classes of persons in the entity's workforce who need access to protected health information to perform their duties
- Categories of protected health information to which such persons or classes need access
- Conditions, as appropriate, that would apply to such access

People are grouped or classified according to the functions they serve. In other words, people fill *roles*. Information is also categorized. Then roles are mapped to information categories. Entities must implement policies and procedures to limit access to only the identified persons, and only to the identified protected health information.

The policies and procedures must be based on reasonable determinations regarding the *roles* that require protected health information, and the nature of the *health information* they require, consistent with their job responsibilities. For example, a hospital could implement a policy that permitted nurses access to all protected health information of patients in their ward while they are on duty. A health plan could permit its underwriting analysts unrestricted access to aggregate claims information for rate setting purposes, but require documented approval from its department manager to obtain specific identifiable claims records of a member for the purpose of determining the cause of unexpected claims that could influence renewal premium rate setting.

For paper records, traditional methods may adequately limit disclosure. For example, if a health researcher wants access to parts of paper medical records, the covered entity might allow the researcher to review the records *on-site* and to abstract the information relevant to the research. By limiting the physical distribution of the record, the covered entity would have effectively limited the scope of the disclosure to the information necessary for the purpose (DHHS, 2000). Limiting disclosure is easier with electronic records than with paper records. Technological mechanisms are an important contribution of technology to personal privacy. For instance, covered entities could configure their record systems to allow selective access to different portions of the record, so that, for example, *administrative personnel* get access to only certain fields, and *medical personnel* get access to other fields (DHHS, 2000).

The Rule on Transactions and Code Sets helps define a common language for healthcare information systems. The minimum necessary standard presents recipes for decision-making. This combination of common language and *decision-making* is the basis of coordination.

Coordination theory says that organizations strive as a top objective to be coordinated (Malone, 1987). Coordination depends first on a common language and then on decision-making. Decision-making depends on an organizational manual and a role hierarchy. The organizational manual describes all the standard processes of the organization. The role hierarchy describes the various roles in the organization and the functions associated with each role. Roles operate on documents in processes that achieve the goals of the organization.

The Rule on Transactions and Code Sets plus the Rule on Privacy are closer than anything else in the United States to a *national plan* for a coordinated healthcare information system. Such a national plan has long been advocated by certain people as the key to improved efficiency and effectiveness in the American healthcare system. However, prior to now no one has had simultaneously the will to create such a plan and the *power* to implement it.

More De-Identification

Once de-identified, a record is no longer protected by privacy rules and the entity can do anything it wants with the record—sell it, broadcast it, study it. Furthermore, *de-identification* can be a unifying concept and mechanism.

Federal Approaches

The *Federal Committee on Statistical Methodology* (1978) recommended different approaches to de-identifying tabular data and microdata:

- Tables can be further divided into two categories: tables of frequency data and tables of magnitude data. For either category, data can be presented in the form of numbers, proportions or percents.
- A microdata file consists of individual records, each containing values of variables for a single person.

Several methods of protecting frequency data in tables have been developed. These include cell suppression, controlled rounding and the confidentiality edit. The Committee was unable to recommend one method in preference to the others.

Many decisions concerning the *disclosure limitation methods* used for microdata are based on precedents and judgment calls. The only rule is to remove all directly identifying information, such as name, and limit the amount of information that is reported from other identifying variables (Hurkens & Tiourine, 1998).

The Office of Management and Budget (Interagency Confidentiality and Data Access Group, 1999) released a *checklist* to help agencies accomplish de-identification. The checklist consists of a series of questions that are designed to assist an agency's disclosure review board to determine the suitability of releasing either public-use microdata files or tables from data collected from individuals under an assurance of confidentiality. This checklist is based on one used at the U.S. Bureau of the Census.

The checklist should be completed by a person who has appropriate statistical knowledge and is familiar with the microdata file or tabular material in question (i.e., branch chief, survey manager, statistician, or programmer). While this implies a familiarity with survey and statistical terminology, those without such *background* will nonetheless be able to understand much of what it intends to accomplish.

In addition to helping an agency's *disclosure review board* determine the disclosure potential of proposed data releases, the checklist has other uses:

- It can serve an important educational function for program staff that completes the checklist
- It can provide documentation when an agency is considering release of related data files and tabulations
- It can be useful in defending legal challenges to an agency's decision to withhold data

The checklist can be adapted by other organizations and used by them to review materials of varying levels of confidentiality.

A part of the checklist focuses on *geographic information* because it is the key factor in permitting inadvertent identification. In a demographic survey, few respondents could likely be identified within a single state, but more respondents—especially those with rare and visible reported characteristics—could be identified within a county or other geographic area with 100,000 or fewer persons.

The risk of *inadvertent disclosure* is higher with a publicly released data set that has both detailed geographic variables and a detailed, extensive set of survey variables. The risk is also often a function of the quality and quantity of auxiliary information (data from sources external to the data being released). This auxiliary information may be difficult to assess for its disclosure risk. Coarsening a data set by dropping survey variables, collapsing response categories for other variables, or introducing noise to the data are techniques that may reduce the risk of inadvertent disclosure.

Anonymity and Bin Sizes

De-identifying data does not guarantee that the result is anonymous (Sweeney, 2002). Anonymous data cannot be manipulated or linked to identify any individual. While the Privacy Rule officially talks about de-identification, in fact, the intention is to require the development of *anonymous data* rather than de-identified data.

A major difficulty in providing anonymous data is that unique values may be *relative*. For example, if a record notes that the person described is an Asian, 5-year old girl in a city and someone happens to know that that city has only one Asian, female, 5-year old, then the child's identity has been uniquely determined despite no traditional unique identifiers having been provided.

Measuring the degree of anonymity in released data is difficult. The Social Security Administration has a general rule that any subset of the data that can be defined in terms of combinations of characteristics must contain at least five individuals: the larger the bin size, the more anonymous the data. As the *bin size* increases, the number of people to whom a record may refer also increases, thereby masking the identity of the actual person.

The precise expression of anonymity is simply the probability of identifying a person given the released data and other possible sources. This *conditional probability* depends on frequencies of characteristics (bin sizes) found within the data and the outside world. Unfortunately, this probability is very difficult to compute since what is known about the outside world is not possible to precisely characterize.

The *motivation* to re-identify released data is a factor. For example, if data maps each record to 10 possible people and the 10 people can be identified, then all 10 may be contacted in an effort to locate a certain person. Some medical files are quite valuable, and in these cases, the minimum bin size must be increased.

Flexible

A system could dynamically modify values to be released based on the role of the requester. The *Datafly System* (Sweeney, 1997) maintains anonymity in medical data by automatically aggregating, substituting and removing information as appropriate. Decisions are made at the time of database access, so the approach can be incorporated into role-based information access within or outside an institution. The end result is a subset of the original database that provides minimal linking since each record matches as many people as the user had specified.

Every value in each field will occur at least as many times as the bin size. For instance, in a database of bin size 2, every row will match at least one other row. In addition, the user also provides a profile of the person who receives the data by estimating on which fields the recipient might link outside knowledge. Thus each field has associated with it a *profile value* between 0 and 1. 0 represents full trust of the recipient, and 1 represents full distrust of the recipient. If the recipient is the patient's caretaker within the institution, the patient has agreed to release this information to the care-taker, so the profile for these fields should be set to 0 to give the patient's caretaker full access to the original information. When researchers and administrators make requests that do not require the most specific form of the information, the corresponding profile values for these fields should warrant a number as close to 1 as practical.

The Datafly System was used to access a pediatric medical record system. Datafly processed all queries to the database over a spectrum of recipient profiles and anonymity levels to show that all fields in medical records can be meaningfully *generalized*. Diagnosis codes have generalizations using the International Classification of Disease (ICD-9) hierarchy. ZIP codes are generalized by dropping significant digits.

Privacy Surrendered

Privacy is surrendered in some situations. Entities may use protected health information without individual authorization for certain categories of uses to permit and promote *national healthcare priorities*. Entities are permitted to use or disclose an individual's protected health information, such as for research purposes or for certain marketing purposes.

Research

The Privacy Rule allows entities to use information for research without individual authorization provided that the *researcher's protocol* has been approved by an Institutional Review Board (IRB). Absent such review, the information can only be used with the patient's prior authorization.

An IRB uses the following criteria to decide whether or not to grant a *waiver* of patient authorization:

- Use or disclosure of protected health information involves no more than minimal risk to the privacy of the individual
- Research could not practicably be conducted without the waiver
- Research could not practicably be conducted without access to the protected health information

Obtaining IRB approval in some institutions is difficult.

Marketing

Any covered entity must obtain the individual's authorization before using protected health information for *marketing*. However, DHHS has defined "marketing" so as to allow certain "marketing communications." Certain activities, such as communications made by an entity for the purpose of describing the products and services it provides, are not marketing.

The marketing provisions allow the use of health information for *commercial communications* that some consider marketing. For instance, the regulation permits pharmacies to receive money from drug manufacturers to data-mine patient prescriptions and to send to targeted patients letters encouraging them to switch to the manufacturer's brand of drug. These communications are not necessarily based on a determination of what is medically best for the patient but are sent due to financial incentives. Since this activity is not defined as "marketing" in the Privacy Rule, pharmacies do not have to obtain the patients' authorization. The authorization requirement applies to materials that encourage the purchase or use of products and services that are not related to healthcare. Furthermore, in the above scenario, pharmacies never have to give patients an opportunity to be removed from the mailing list. Nor do they have to tell patients that the drug company is paying them to send the letters.

Access to Information

A person has a right to his or her medical record.

Right of Access

The definition of the right of access is linked to the definition of a *designated record set*. A "record" is "any item, collection, or grouping of protected health information maintained, collected, used, or disseminated by a covered entity." Designated record sets are any group of records that are used, in whole or in part, by or for a covered entity to make decisions about individuals. This information includes, for example, information used to make healthcare decisions or information used to determine whether an insurance claim will be paid. Two examples follow:

- For health plans, designated record sets include, at a minimum, the enrollment, payment, claims adjudication, and case or medical management record systems of the plan
- For healthcare providers, designated record sets include, at a minimum, the medical record and billing record about individuals maintained by or for the provider

Records that otherwise meet the definition of designated record set and which are held by a business associate of the covered entity are part of the covered entity's designated record sets.

Individuals have a right of access to any protected health information that is maintained in a designated record set. This right of access applies to health plans, healthcare providers, and healthcare clearinghouses that create or receive protected health information. Covered entities must provide *access* to individuals for as long as the protected health information is maintained in a designated record set. Despite the requirement to provide access, physicians maybe reluctant to share records, as they see less benefit in this sharing than the patients do (Ross et al., 2005).

An entity may deny access to protected health information when the *physical safety* of an individual is endangered. DHHS intends narrow exceptions to the right of access and expects entities to employ these exceptions rarely, if at all. Covered entities may only deny access for the reasons specifically provided in the Rule.

Provision

If an entity accepts a request, it must provide the access requested. Individuals have the right both to *inspect* and to *copy* the record. For copies, an entity may only charge for the labor and supply costs of copying.

Entities may not charge any fees for retrieving or handling the information or for processing the request. The inclusion of a *fee for copying* must not impede the access of individuals. The fee for copying must leave this option as a practical one for all individuals. Access should normally be provided within 30 days of the request.

Accounting of Disclosures

An individual has a right to receive an accounting of disclosures of protected health information made by an entity in the *six years* prior to the date on which the accounting is requested. However, this account is only for exceptional disclosures.

Examples of disclosures that may have occurred without a patient-signed authorization and that the covered entity should record for an "accounting of disclosures" are a report of:

- Gun shot wounds to police
- Child abuse to social services
- Positive tuberculosis test result to a public health agency

The entity must act on the individual's request for an accounting no later than 60 days after receipt of such a request. The entity must provide the first accounting to an individual in any 12-month period without charge.

Administration

DHHS requires that each affected entity *assess* its own needs and devise, implement, and maintain appropriate privacy policies, procedures, and documentation to address its business requirements. How each privacy standard will be satisfied will require business decisions by each entity. Entities of a similar type are encouraged to work together to establish best practices for that entity type.

Entities should develop a *privacy compliance program*. Although certain hospital departments, such as medical records, may have privacy policies, the Rule requires the institution as a whole to adopt privacy guidelines for all employees and departments. Covered entities are required to:

- Designate a privacy officer
- Document their policies and procedures relative to privacy
- Provide employees with training on health information privacy
- Implement safeguards to protect health information from intentional or accidental misuse
- Provide a means for individuals to lodge complaints about the organization's information practices and maintain a record of any complaints
- Develop a system of sanctions for employees and business associates who violate the organization's policies

The Rule touches many aspects of the healthcare operation.

Staff and Training

Covered entities are required to designate a *privacy official* who is responsible for the implementation and development of the entity's privacy policies and procedures. Entities must also designate a contact person to receive complaints about privacy and provide information about the matters covered by the entity's notice. Implementation may vary widely depending on the size and nature of the entity, with small offices assigning this as an additional duty to an existing staff person, and large organizations creating a full-time privacy official.

DHHS requires covered entities to develop and document their policies and procedures for implementing the requirements of the Privacy Rule. Entities must modify in a prompt manner their policies and procedures to comply with changes in relevant law. The policies and procedures must be maintained in writing. Entities must retain any required documentation for at least *six years* (the statute of limitations period for the civil penalties) from the date of the creation of the documentation.

An entity must *train* all members of its workforce on the policies and procedures with respect to protected health information, as necessary and appropriate for the members of the workforce to perform their function within the entity. A covered entity must provide training that meets these requirements:

- To each member of the covered entity's workforce by no later than the compliance date for the entity
- Thereafter, to each new member of the workforce within a reasonable period of time after the person joins the entity's workforce
- To each member of the entity's workforce whose functions are affected by a material change in the policies or procedures required by this subpart, within a reasonable period of time after the material change becomes effective

Entities are responsible for implementing policies and procedures to meet these *training requirements* and for documenting that training has been provided.

Complaints

Entities must have a mechanism for receiving *complaints* from individuals regarding the health plan's or provider's privacy practices. They must receive complaints concerning violations of the covered entity's privacy practices, not just violations of the rule.

The health plan or provider does not need to develop a formal appeals mechanism, nor must "due process" or any similar standard be applied. Additionally, there is no requirement to respond in any particular manner or time frame. The entity is, however, required to maintain a *record of the complaints* that are filed and a brief explanation of their resolution, if any.

The entity could implement the complaint mechanism based on its size and capabilities. For example, a *small practice* could assign a clerk to log written or verbal complaints as they are received. One physician could review all complaints monthly, address the individual situations, and make changes to policies or procedures as appropriate. The clerk would log results of the physician's review of individual complaints. A large entity could choose to implement a formal appeals process.

Sometimes an individual not otherwise involved in law enforcement uncovers evidence of wrongdoing, and wishes to bring that evidence to the attention of appropriate authorities—this is a whistleblower. *Whistleblowers* may use protected health information. An entity would not be held in violation because a member of its workforce or a business associate appropriately discloses protected health information that such person believes is evidence of a civil or criminal violation.

All covered entities must develop and apply sanctions for failure to comply with policies or procedures of the covered entity or with the requirements of the Privacy Rule. All members of the workforce who have regular contact with protected health information should be subject to *sanctions*, as would the entity's business associates.

Enforcement

Individuals have the right to file a complaint with DHHS if they believe that a covered entity has failed to comply with the Privacy Rule. Because individuals would have received notice of the uses and disclosures that the entity could make and of the entity's privacy practices, they would have a basis for making a realistic judgment as to when a particular action or omission would be improper. The notice would also inform individuals how they can file such *complaints*.

The DHHS procedures are modeled on those used by DHHS's Office for Civil Rights. DHHS requires complainants to identify the entities and describe the acts or omissions alleged to be *non-compliant*. Individuals must file such complaints within 180 days of those acts or omissions. The requirements for filing complaints are as minimal as possible, to facilitate use of this right. DHHS would also attempt to keep the identity of complainants confidential.

The second method of enforcement is *compliance review*. DHHS may conduct compliance reviews to determine whether the covered entity or business associate is complying with the rules.

The Department of Health and Human Services (2006) has published a HIPAA *Enforcement Rule*. That Rule adopts the complete regulatory structure for implementing the civil money penalty authority of the Administrative Simplification part of HIPAA. It completes the structure begun when the Privacy Rule was issued in 2000 and expanded by the interim procedural enforcement rules issued in 2003. That Rule covers the enforcement process from its beginning, which will usually be a complaint or a compliance review, through its conclusion. A complaint or compliance review may result in informal resolution, a finding of no violation, or a finding of violation. If a finding of violation is made, a civil money penalty will be sought for the violation, which can be challenged by the covered entity through a formal hearing and appellate review process. These rules apply to covered entities that violate any of the rules implementing the Administrative Simplification provisions of HIPAA.

The most significant exposure from HIPAA's Privacy Rule may result from HIPAA establishing a minimum floor for the protection of health information. A party that fails to implement the HIPAA Privacy Rule would risk tort lawsuits for breach of the *common law right of privacy*. Plaintiffs in those suits may point to the HIPAA Privacy Rule as the minimum reasonable level of protection. This Rule then becomes the "test" for adequate privacy to be applied to all entities and all health information—not just the information and parties specifically covered by the HIPAA rules (Britten & Melamed, 2001).

Example Implementation

Achieving compliance with the Privacy Rule has been taxing of covered entities. Entities have tried where possible to build on existing efforts. An example follows for *Carilion Health Systems*. Located in Southwest Virginia, Carilion Health System is an integrated delivery system of seven owned and three managed hospitals, long-term care facilities, and a health plan. Executive level awareness occurred first. In 2000 a privacy team was formed. The membership of the team was chosen to represent those areas of the entity most impacted by and whose participation in compliance was particularly critical (Rada et al., 2002).

Carilion next reformatted and reorganized the Privacy Rule. For example, one listing of rule components shows where documentation is required. Another early undertaking was to document the flow of protected health information. A data collection sheet was designed to help identify the areas within the organization that collect or use protected health information, where the information comes from, who uses the information, how it is stored, and where it goes. While seemingly a massive undertaking, creation of this *inventory* progressed well, using a combination of interviews and allowing unit managers to complete the inventory on their own. Completed data collection sheets were shared among like units, so that only differences needed to be recorded.

The components of the Privacy Rule were then assigned to individuals who were responsible to analyze the entity's situation relative to the requirement. In many cases, the entity was doing what the regulation required, but it was not recorded anywhere. To avoid a completely new set of policies and procedures just for HIPAA, the practice folded into the existing organizational manual the HIPAA requirements where possible to avoid duplication of effort and the creation of a redundant, *unwieldy organizational manual*. At Carilion, the organizational manual contained three components that needed amending:

- Information security and privacy
- Confidentiality of patient information
- Patient rights and responsibilities

To deal with HIPAA an entirely new component of the organizational manual was also created and called "Minimum Necessary Standard and Level of Access for Patient Information." While the privacy team proceeded with its work, the entity's internal audit unit contacted each department within the entity to document any internal deviations from the entity-wide organizational manual in the handling of protected health information.

Many *tools* are being developed to support compliance with the Privacy Rule. For instance, open source software is available to de-identify pathology reports (Beckwith et al., 2006). Tools for removing identifiers from radiological images in PowerPoint presentations are available (Yam, 2005).

Information Warfare

Privacy is not an issue that can be ignored. Legal or political action might provoke diverse reactions. One particularly intriguing, though also frightening, reaction involves *information warfare*.

What is it?

Information warfare is all operations conducted to exploit information to gain an advantage over an opponent, and to deny the opponent information which could be used to an advantage (Armistead & National Security Agency, 2004). The *taxonomy* of information warfare includes propaganda and espionage (Kopp, 2000):

- Propaganda is the use of information to confuse, deceive, mislead, destabilize, and disrupt an opponent, while
- Espionage divines secrets from an opponent and prevents the opponent from doing the same

Other views of information warfare provide further classifications. Shwartau (2001) defines three classes of information warfare:

- Class 1 is personal and includes the study of all sources of information about an individual
- Class 2 is corporate and concerns business or economic interests
- Class 3 is global and affects national interests

Another taxonomy focuses on the intent of the perpetrator. The *hacker* is deemed to be curious but not intentionally destructive. The cracker intends to do harm. The "power projectors" want to change the economic or political order.

Professional groups have been formed to wage information war. Typical *roles* in an information warfare group include:

- Analyst of existing information
- Software engineer to develop new programs for attacking or protecting information
- Attacker who actually goes into the field and steals or destroys data
- Camouflager that hides the activities of the information warfare unit

Information warfare can be serious business.

Health Implications

What does information warfare have to do with healthcare? Various scenarios are next sketched of *healthcare information warfare*.

Under the HIPAA privacy rule, covered entities would have to obtain the patient's authorization before the entity could use or disclose the patient's information for marketing purposes. Health insurers, benefits management administrators, and managed care organizations have the greatest ability and economic incentive to use protected health information to determine how to market services to patients. As regulations reduce the access to identified patient information, these organizations will need to look for ways to get de-identified data that supports marketing or will need other strategies for acquiring the information that they feel they need to compete in the marketplace. They will have incentive to acquire information that is hidden from them, and an information conflict situation exists. An organization's marketing and public relations departments often engage in *legitimate espionage* and can be expected to explore the options enabled by the Internet.

While some organizations want private information to support marketing, others might highlight their respect for private information as part of an advertising (or propaganda) campaign. Healthcare providers and payers might compete with one another for clients on the basis of how well they provide privacy and security. Thus a hospital x that had more patient-friendly privacy policies for patients than hospital y might expect on that basis to have more *satisfied customers* than y. Under normal market pressures, this should lead to benefits for x.

The laws or regulations about chains of trust among business associates also create a potential for dissatisfied parties to take action. If healthcare provider x buys medical equipment from supplier y and then x does not renew the contract with y, y might look carefully for evidence of information practices of x that would make x vulnerable to legal prosecution. More generally, one can imagine that an entity x that was in competition with an entity y might support the bringing of harmful evidence about y to the fore. Thus x might directly or indirectly support individuals who had rightful claims against y. Business x might attempt to nurture individual patients of a healthcare provider y to scrutinize y's privacy provisions or x could appeal to the employees of y. *Whistleblowers* are supported by the Privacy Rule. Thus an employee of business y who discovers some privacy violation has protection against reprisal from y.

The various situations under which information is withheld or shared reflect a range of information pressures in the *healthcare terrain*. The new highways and byways of the Internet redefine the healthcare terrain and introduce new pressures. Information traffic jams become increasingly common as the number of speeding travelers increases.

Conclusion

DHHS published a draft version of the Privacy Rule in 1999, and between 1999 and 2003 enormous debate occurred about the pros and cons of the Privacy Rule. Compliance with the Privacy Rule was mandatory as of 2003. Healthcare entities invested massive resources in achieving compliance, which included such time-consuming steps as training all employees and giving all patients a Notice of Privacy Practices. Maintaining compliance is also *costly*.

The hope by some had been that the Privacy Rule would usher a new era of electronic medical records and healthcare communication because people would now feel that privacy was assured. However, the impact of the Privacy Rule seems in many ways to have been otherwise. Healthcare professionals have been taught that the Privacy Rule makes severe restrictions in what can be done with patient information. Patients seem to have relatively little interest in exercising their right to access. The net impact seems to be largely that of another regulation taxing the healthcare system. For instance, the medical research community fears that important research is being compromised by well-meaning institutional review boards that are overly strict in their interpretation of the Privacy Rule (Feld, 2005). The challenge is to have the *benefits of compliance* exceed the costs.

The Privacy Rule limits the circumstances in which an individual's health information can be used. The use of health information is made relatively easy for healthcare purposes and more difficult for purposes other than healthcare. The Privacy Rule is based on five principles:

- **Boundaries:** An individual's healthcare information should be used for health purposes and only those purposes, subject to a few carefully defined exceptions
- **Security:** Organizations ought to protect health information against misuse
- **Accountability:** Those who misuse personal health information should be punished, and those who are harmed by its misuse should have legal recourse
- **Public responsibility:** Federal law should identify those limited arenas in which public responsibilities warrant authorization of access to medical information, and should allow but constrain uses of information in those contexts.
- **Consumer Control:** Patients should be able to see what is in their records, get a copy, correct errors, and find out who else has seen them.

On the first four principles, there is consensus in the large. Yes, boundaries should be secure. Yes, those who are responsible for boundaries and security should be held accountable. Yes, exceptions occur when the public good is at stake. However, the fifth principle of "consumer control" is not part of the tradition of American healthcare.

Questions

Reading Questions

1. What is the role of power in privacy?
2. Compare and contrast uses and disclosures.
3. What is de-identification?
4. How is the minimum necessary requirement related to workflow management?

Doing Questions

Exercise 1

Indicate three different, generic reasons for which a patient might want (you could imagine yourself as the patient) to exercise the "right of access" provisions relative to a healthcare provider? Describe each reason in one or two sentences to explain why the patient wants a copy of the record. For example, if the question had been about getting access from a health plan, then one reason might be that the patient is seeking further information about what the health insurance company has paid the provider because the patient wants to know what proportion of the services that the patient is receiving from the provider have already been paid by the health insurance company (call this the "bill checking circumstance"). Please note that there is not a right or wrong answer, but you need to demonstrate insight about the issues by making plausible arguments for positions that you take.

Consider how an information system might have different features in order to satisfy different patient circumstances for access and briefly describe [less than 200 words] for each of your preceding three "reasons for access" some special features that an information system to serve that reason might have. [Guide: for example, a system to provide a person something from the health plan about billing might also want to extract the related billing records from the provider and explanations of the policies on reimbursement of the health plan and provide all three of these simultaneously].

Exercise 2

Recall the HIPAA Privacy Training requirement. Design and implement a simple online privacy training system. Submit your entire assignment as one zip file containing, at least, the following seven html files:

1. index.htm (the introductory page with links to everything else and user manual embedded)
2. chief.htm (the chief training and quiz)
3. staff.htm (the assistant training and quiz)
4. disclosures.htm (exceptional disclosures training and quiz)
5. requests.htm (requests training and quiz)
6. businessassoc.htm (business associates training and quiz)
7. sysadmin.htm (system administrator manual)

You are only expected to use HTML. Among other things, you will develop quizzes. To implement a HTML form to which the user can respond, you may use the "mailto" option. The "mailto" link will send the quiz answers to the privacy officer. This is the FORM line to use.

<FORM METHOD="POST" ACTION="mailto:address"ENCTYPE="text/plain">

The multiple-choice quizzes can be entered as ‘selections’, for example:

<p>
A disclosure for which purpose needs to be recorded:
<SELECT NAME=”filename1” SIZE=4>
<OPTION SELECTED>for treatment, payment, or health care operations
<OPTION>made with patient authorization
<OPTION>covered by a business associate agreement
<OPTION>Public Health
</SELECT>

In order that the grader knows which quiz is being answered, the "select name" field for each question should begin with the name of the file for the training and end with 1 for question 1 and 2 for question 2. Thus for the first question in the chief.htm file the select name would be ‘chief1’.

You should also ask each trainee to identify him or herself (in case the e-mail from which the message comes is not revealing enough) with something like:

Name: <input type="text" name="traineename" size=64 maxlength=64>

Your submission has two major content components:

- Chief and assistant basic training
- Completing tables

For each major component, training is accomplished by giving the trainee an essay and then a two-question multiple-choice quiz. In particular, develop a small training essay (about 200 to 2,000 words) and a two-question multiple-choice quiz that is to train a person how to maintain the contents for each of the following tables:

- Exceptional disclosures
- Requests for access, amendment, and accounting of disclosures
- Determining and contracting with business associate contracts

Put on the introductory screen a link to each of those preceding "table" training materials.

Provide a manual for system administrators who need to install and maintain your system. For instance, this manual should explain how to change the e-mail address in the mailto link of the quiz form so that the appropriate person receives the quiz answers. The answers to the quiz should also be provided in this system administrator manual. This manual should also be an html file.

Develop an introductory page that has two major parts:

- Each link will take the user to the relevant training essay and quiz. One part will invite each person to choose his or her role of chief or assistant and the other part will provide links to the training on the maintenance of the tables.
- The introductory page will also include a "user" manual that explains what is expected of the trainee and how to proceed.

Include an e-mail link to the privacy officer.

References

Armistead, L., & National Security Agency. (2004). *Information operations: Warfare and the hard reality of soft power (Issues in twenty-first century warfare)*. Sterling, Virginia: Potomac Books.

Beckwith, B., Mahaadevan, R., Balis, U., & Kuo, F. (2006). Development and evaluation of an open source software tool for de-identification of pathology reports. *BMC Medical Informatics Decision Making, 6*(1).

Britten, A., & Melamed, D. (Eds.). (2001). *The HIPAA handbook: What your organization should know about the federal privacy standards*. Washington, DC: American Accreditation HealthCare Commission.

Department of Health and Human Services. (2006). Part III, Department of Health and Human Services, Office of the Secretary, 45 CFR Parts 160 and 164, HIPAA Administrative Simplification: Enforcement; Final Rule. *Federal Register, 71*(32), 8389-8433.

Department of Health and Human Services. (2000). Standards for privacy of individually identifiable health information, 45 CRF Parts 160 through 164, Department of Health and Human Services. *Federal Register, 65*(250), 82461-82510.

Etzioni, A. (1999). *The limits of privacy*. New York: Basic Books.

Federal Committee on Statistical Methodology. (1978). *Report on statistical disclosure and disclosure-avoidance techniques*. Washington, DC: U.S. Department of Commerce, Office of Federal Statistical Policy and Standards.

Feld, A. (2005). The Health Insurance Portability and Accountability Act (HIPAA): Its broad effect on practice. *American Journal of Gastroenterology, 100*(7), 1440.

Hurkens, C., & Tiourine, S. (1998). Models and methods for the microdata protection problem. *Journal of Official Statistics, 14*(4), 437-447.

Interagency Confidentiality and Data Access Group. (1999). *Checklist on disclosure potential of proposed data releases*. Washington, DC: Office of Management and Budget.

Malone, T. (1987). Modelling coordination in organizations and markets. *Management Science, 33*, 1317-1332.

Rada, R., Klawans, C., & Newton, T. (2002). Comparing HIPAA practices in two multi-hospital systems. *Journal of Healthcare Information Management, 16*(2), 40-45.

Ross, S.E., Todd, J., Moore, L.A., Beaty, B.L., Wittenvrongel, L., & Lin, C. (2005). Expectations of patients and physicians regarding patient-accessible medical records. *J Medical Internet Research, 7*(2), e13.

Schwartau, W. (2001). *Cybershock: Surviving hackers, phreakers, identity thieves, Internet terrorists and weapons of mass disruption*. Berkeley, CA: Thunder Mouth Press.

Staden, H.V. (1996). In a pure and holy way: Personal and professional conduct in the Hippocratic Oath. *Journal of the History of Medicine and Allied Sciences, 51*, 406-408.

Sweeney, L. (1997). Guaranteeing anonymity when sharing medical data, the Datafly System. In D. Masys (Ed.), *Annual Conference of the American Medical Informatics Association* (pp. 51-55). Washington, DC: Hanley & Belfus.

Sweeney, L. (2002). Achieving k-anonymity privacy protection using generalization and suppression. *International Journal on Uncertainty, Fuzziness and Knowledge-Based Systems, 10*(5), 571-588.

Warren, S., & Brandeis, L.D. (1890). The right to privacy. *Harvard Law Review, 4*(5).

Yam, C.-S. (2005). Removing hidden patient data from digital images in PowerPoint. *American Journal of Roentgenology, 185*, 1659-1662.

Chapter X

Security

Learning Objectives

- Recognize that the Security Rule covers only electronic protected health information
- Develop a risk analysis
- Understand the requirements for a security officer and for staff training
- Plan for administrative safeguards to include management, workforce, access, and contingency plans
- Plan for technical safeguards that address encryption but focus on audit and access
- Plan for physical safeguards that include facility access and media controls
- Describe a model of security in terms of real-world policy, computer models, and technical mechanisms
- Develop a role-based access control model that indicates several roles and their permissions for a healthcare entity
- Design a system for encrypting communications for a healthcare entity that includes a public key infrastructure

Privacy and security of health information is a global concern. However, this chapter will focus on approaches to security in the United States. In particular, the federal regulation of security in the form of the Security Rule will be studied. The HIPAA *Security Rule* details the system and administrative requirements that a covered entity must meet in order to assure that health information is safe from people without authorization for its access. By contrast, the Privacy Rule describes the requirements that govern the circumstances under which protected health information must be used or disclosed with and without patient involvement and when a patient may have access to his or her protected health information. The implementation of reasonable and appropriate security measures supports compliance with the Privacy Rule.

Introduction

Security of healthcare information systems is substandard. The solution to the problem is not the acquisition of a new technology but the improvement of an organization's *workflow*. A security framework shows that human policies come first and then drive a computer policy that in turn uses technical mechanisms.

The Problem

Security is inadequate. How many hospital-based organizations have developed at least minimally adequate health information security structures to date? In the private sector such information is hard to reliably obtain. If a hospital knows that its information systems are easily breached by hackers, then will the hospital announce that information to the public? Probably not. Experts estimate that the majority of private healthcare organizations have *inadequate security* (Dechow et al., 2005).

The federal government is sometimes more forthcoming with its own internal analyses than the private sector is. The Government Accounting Office under the direction of the U.S. Congress has performed various security audits of federal government agencies. In a report to the U.S. Congress from the *Government Accounting Office,* the title tells the story (Government Accounting Office, 2000a): "Information Security: Serious and Widespread Weaknesses Persist at Federal Agencies." An audit of the *Veterans Health Administration* (VHA) speaks more precisely to the problems with healthcare information. A September 2000 report about the VHA contains the following (Government Accounting Office, 2000b):

Access control and service continuity problems are placing financial and sensitive veteran medical information at risk of inadvertent or deliberate misuse, fraudulent use, improper disclosure, and/or destruction. ...we found additional access control and service continuity problems at these facilities and serious weaknesses at the VA Maryland Healthcare System. Similar security problems also persist throughout VHA and the department. One reason for the VA's continuing information system control problems is that it had not established an effective, integrated computer security management program throughout the department...it remains important for VA to develop detailed guidance to ensure that the key program elements we highlighted in our October 1999 report—periodically assessing risk, monitoring system and user access activity, and evaluating the effectiveness of information system controls—are fully addressed and implemented consistently across the department. Consequently, we are reaffirming our October 1999 recommendation for VA to develop detailed guidance in these areas... Moreover, VA's ability to continue to develop and implement an effective computer security management program is in jeopardy because VHA had not yet...

Computerized information is integral to the fabric of the healthcare enterprise. Yet healthcare computing systems are not secure enough for their crucial roles.

Workflow

Security is related to dependability. Security is something that secures, and secure means *dependable*. The work required to achieve security is intimately connected to many other operations of the organization. Maintaining a dependable information system requires that:

- Each person knows what information he is to see and what he is to change
- The system does not allow him to see or change anything else

Security involves managing *workflow*. Yet, security is often viewed as a technical issue, such as of a firewall in the computer network or a token card used to gain access to a computer terminal. The truth of security is far from this technical solution and closer to the essential concerns of running the organization.

Policy is more important than technology. The following extracts from an interview illustrate the importance of *policy over technology*. The interviewees are Douglas Fieldhouse and Albert Shar of Technology Services, University of Pennsylvania Health System, Philadelphia. The interviewer Mark Hagland (1998) asked "what tools offer the most promise for the future?"

Fieldhouse replied:

There are lots of great tools out there. Unfortunately, most people don't know what they need yet. The firewall you decide you require really depends on your own security policy; it's an instrument of your policy. If you don't have a current, up-to-date security policy, you're not going to know what products you need. A lot of my peers are in similar situations. We had to get something, and the policies and procedures were not forthcoming, and so we just went out and got the best, most flexible products out there we could. Unfortunately, we're working reactively.

Shar added:

Let me take an even more cynical view. The firewall technology is one more piece of technology that can really be exceptional if used properly. This should be used based on the policy that's determined. But what's happening is, just because we have a firewall, people end up believing that that's equivalent to a security policy, which it's not. Secondly, it's an abdication of responsibility, because the technologists—and that's what we are—essentially determine the policy de facto, and frankly without the input in terms of what the business needs are. I see that in some cases, some of the things we've done have actually had a negative impact on security. For example, because we had a firewall in our organization, and people couldn't get to electronic information that needed to be available, it was relatively easy for a doctor to get a modem and hook up to the medical record system and go around the system. And that was motivated by the desire to do better medicine. In other words, whenever we're not responsive to a business need in terms of the technology that we're implementing, it has sort of the opposite effect of what we're trying to achieve.

Computer security policies must reflect the *real-world policies* of the organization. One computer security policy begins with a decomposition of the data in the medical record (Pangalos, 1995):

- The data are divided into administrative information, non-medical historical information, social information, personal demographic information, non-personal demographic information, insurance information, billing information, diagnosis, examination request, examination result, treatment data, and use of special materials
- The staff are divided into head doctor, responsible doctor, on-duty doctor, head nurse, nurse, paramedical staff, registration staff, and financial staff

The computer security policy maps staff categories to data categories. One can readily see that such computer security policies require an intricate model of how the healthcare organization itself functions. A workflow management system would support the scheduling of operations by people on data. Such a system would be the essential ingredient of a secure system in which viewing or modifying data is only done at the right time by the right people.

Security is not Y2K. Yet, many healthcare organizations are likening the security problem to the Y2K problem and asking the Y2K team to solve the security problem.

The security problem is not like the Y2K problem. The *Y2K problem* was essentially a technical problem. The security problem is essentially a policy and management problem. A healthcare organization's security problems are more administrative than technical.

Security Framework

Tasks must be authorized. The National Research Council (2002) defined security as:

... the protection of information systems against unauthorized access to or modification of information, whether in storage, processing, or transit, and against the denial of service to authorized users or the provision of service to unauthorized users, including those measures necessary to detect, document, and counter such threats.

Achieving information system security involves activity at multiple levels, of which one breakdown gives (see Figure 10.1):

Figure 10.1. Security policy. The diagram shows the progression from an organizational policy, to a computer policy, to a computer model, to mechanisms.

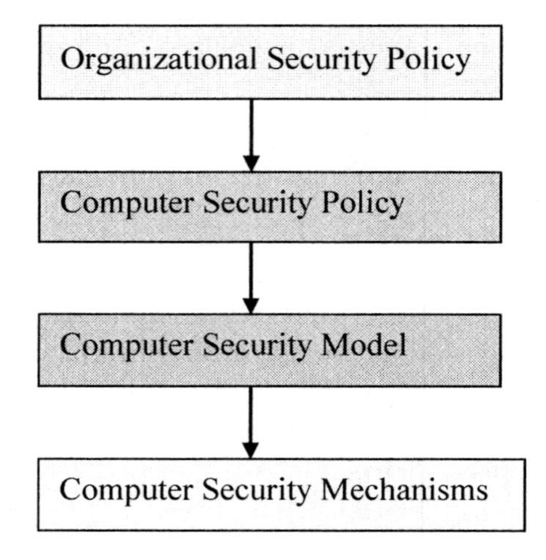

- *Organizational policy*
- *Computer security policy*
- *Computer security model*
- *Computer security mechanisms*

The goals of an organization combined with its environmental circumstance dictate the organization's security policy. This *organizational policy* regulates how an organization manages, protects, and distributes resources to achieve its security objectives. If an organization has no explicit security policy, then policy assumptions guide its actions.

Computers support people. A computer security policy must faithfully represent the organizational security policy. It must also consider threats that are not identified per se in the organizational policy but are intrinsic to computer operations, such as the threat of a computer virus. A *computer security policy* is expressed in a natural language such as English. The organization should make the computer security policy as precise as possible. Since natural language in complex cases is often ambiguous, organizations may designate who is to interpret the policy.

A computer security model restates the computer security policy in a formal or mathematical way and thus reduces the ambiguity. Such a model guides the design of the security aspects of computing systems. The designers need an unambiguous statement of what the policy means, and the model provides this.

Computer *security mechanisms* provide the trusted computing base and extensively use cryptography. Cryptography allows encoding of messages so that people who see the message cannot understand it unless they have an appropriate key. Sharing these keys becomes a complex matter which itself can lead to organizational policy.

Computer Security Policies

Computer security policies are categorized in various ways, of which one popular way uses the following three concepts (National Research Council, 1991):

- **Confidentiality:** Controlling who gets to read information
- **Integrity:** Assuring that information is changed only in a specified and authorized manner
- **Availability:** Assuring that authorized users have continued access to information and resources

Figure 10.2. Security relationships. Availability depends on confidentiality and integrity and together these support the assurance of quality (Adapted from National Institute of Standards and Technology, 2001).

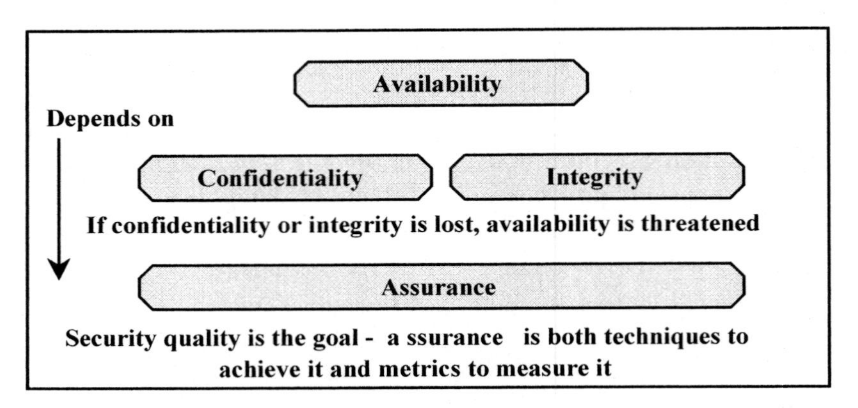

Availability depends on confidentiality and integrity (see Figure 10.2).

Confidentiality receives much attention. The most fully developed policies are those that have been developed to ensure confidentiality. The Department of Defense computer security policy is based on *confidentiality levels*. Every piece of information has a security level. A person is cleared to a particular security level and can see information only at that, or a lower, level.

Integrity policies have not been studied as carefully as confidentiality policies. Separation of duties in the changing of computer information is an example of an integrity policy. If one person can enter an order for a certain radiation to be administered to a patient, then a different person may be required to approve the order.

Availability is little understood. What causes a system to become unavailable and how can this be prevented? People do not understand availability disasters, but can address recovering from a disaster. A *contingency policy* is the extent to which most organizations currently have an availability policy. These contingency policies typically specify backup procedures and schedules so that an information system can be restored after a catastrophic loss.

Computer security concepts are wide-ranging. The description of confidentiality, integrity, and availability is far from an exhaustive accounting of the major concepts of computer security policy. Different people for different purposes view computer security policy differently. For example, two important concepts that are orthogonal to the three just described are:

- **Resource control:** Controlling who has access to computing resources exclusive of information
- **Accountability:** Knowing who has had access to information resources

Resource control includes the physical access to the components of the information system. Accountability is supported by audit trails, and, in turn, supports confidentiality, integrity, and availability.

Life Cycle

The *life cycle* of compliance begins with awareness. A gap analysis determines where an organization needs what kinds of changes to become compliant. Risk analysis considers the various threats to security and then suggests the remedies that are most cost-effective. Implementation and training must be followed by quality control.

Gap Analysis

The entity must determine the current status of its security protection – the baseline. Then this *baseline* must be compared to the requirements to determine the gap. The baseline assessment *inventories* an organization's current security environment with respect to policies, processes, and technology. The scope will drive how this should be done. If the assessment is tailored to the HIPAA Security Rule, the baseline assessment design can be driven by the regulatory framework.

Defining which security components can be reviewed once because they are standardized throughout an organization will help *avoid duplicate analysis*. For example, the wide area network does not need to be assessed in each part of the organization, since it should be the same across parts. However, capturing varying practices distinct from system capabilities is important. For example, standard password assignment procedures do not mean that adherence is consistent in different parts of the organization.

A *security configuration management inventory* includes documentation of hardware and software assets. An organization wants to understand this inventory in order to know its potential vulnerabilities and determine what existing security capabilities reside in the assets.

The measurement criteria suggested as part of the gap analysis could include rankings of current readiness weighed against requirements. A simple *five-point scale* could be used that identifies the organization's status relative to each requirement as follows:

1. No identified process or control
2. Informal or partial process or control
3. Process or controls implemented for many required HIPAA elements
4. Process or controls fully implemented for all required HIPAA elements
5. Process or controls exceed required HIPAA elements

Gap details should be captured. For instance, saying an organization has only partial or informal controls is not *sufficient detail* to help determine how the gap would ultimately be filled. Instead, a detailed statement is appropriate, like "the mainframe environment has the necessary control, but the following remote sites are inadequate because of certain reasons."

The gap analysis needs to involve the entire organization. Participants in the gap analysis should represent the entire organization and will need to include representatives from all lines of business and all support offices. Key support offices include legal, internal audit, information technology, training, human resources, facilities management, and risk management. Typically, many of these participants will already be part of the *cross-functional security team*.

Risk Analysis

Risk analysis follows gap analysis. No matter how well a system is designed, vulnerabilities remain. Users, whether normal or hostile, may trigger or exploit these vulnerabilities. Such vulnerabilities become risks, and organization must determine how much effort to invest in preventing what *risks*.

Determining *organizational risk* depends on an organization's definition of risk adversity and the criticality of its data. Both of these are organization-specific and require examining an organization's mission and business strategy. The process of determining organizational risk involves (Hellerstein, 1999):

1. Looking at the type of data an organization has
2. Determining who the likely candidates are for intercepting that data
3. Determining the level of capital resources to target the problem

The main goal of risk analysis is to help with selecting cost-effective safeguards. Risk analysis involves estimating the potential losses from threats, and how much the safeguards could reduce them. Risk analysis often measures risk in terms of annual, monetary loss expectancy. Safeguards can affect the annual loss expectancy by affecting the likelihood of the threat, or its impact, or both. A risk analysis involves the following steps (Summers, 2000):

1. Identify the assets and assign monetary values to *assets*..
2. Identify the *threats* and the vulnerabilities. Estimate the likelihood of each threat. For each asset vulnerable to the threat, estimate the impact of the threat.
3. Calculate the *exposure* of each asset to each threat, in the absence of any additional safeguards.
4. Identify potential safeguards and estimate how much they reduce the exposures. Estimate the costs of the safeguards and determine *cost-effective safeguards*.

Even considering only cost-effective safeguards, their total cost may well exceed the available funds. The organization must decide how to allocate its resources among the potential safeguards.

The Security Rule requires risk analysis. A thorough and accurate risk analysis would consider "all relevant losses" that would be expected if the security measures were not in place (National Institute of Standards and Technology, 2002). *Relevant losses* would include losses caused by unauthorized uses and disclosures and loss of data integrity that would be expected to occur absent the security measures.

Smaller entities, which deal with smaller amounts of information would have smaller physical facilities, smaller work forces, and therefore, would assume less risk. The smaller amount of risk involved means that the response to that risk can be developed on a *smaller scale* than that for larger organizations.

Risk Analysis Example

An example of risk analysis is presented for Georgetown University Medical Center's *kidney dialysis unit*. The site has dialysis machines in one facility with three remote facilities connected to the dialysis machines via an Internet link. A risk analysis will assess the current information security and propose improvements (Meissner et al., 1997).

Threats affect data integrity and confidentiality. A threat may have a *frequency of occurrence*. *Expected loss* refers to a threat's potential for damage. Both these features may have a value of low, medium or high.

For data integrity, the expected loss from a threat to data is rated "high" when the data is important to patient care. For confidentiality, the expected loss depends on the extent to which the person who seeks access intends to abuse confidential information. A hacker who will not use the information incurs a low confidentiality loss.

Data integrity can suffer from: alteration, input error, or software failure, call these Threat1, Threat2, and Threat3. For the case of the renal dialysis facilities, a description and the threat frequency and expected loss of each event are presented:

- **Threat1, Alteration:** Someone might be able to modify patient information stored in any of the computers either by accident or maliciously. Frequency: Low; Expected Loss: Medium
- **Threat2, Input error:** Entering information manually is error prone, but most data is automatically entered from monitoring equipment. Frequency: Low; Expected Loss: Medium
- **Threat3, Software failure:** Software could malfunction. Frequency: Low; Expected Loss: High

The threat frequency and expected loss for sources of breach of patient confidentiality are (call these Threat4,...,Threat7):

- **Threat4, Data interception:** Data is intercepted in transit between devices and computers. Frequency: Low; Expected Loss: High
- **Threat5, Password management problems:** Frequency: High; Expected Loss: Medium
- **Threat6, Unauthorized building access at off-site archive:** Frequency: Low; Expected Loss: Medium
- **Threat7, Inadequate system access control procedures:** Frequency: Low Expected Loss: Medium

The preceding seven threats are illustrative and not an exhaustive catalog of possible threats.

Countermeasures at the electronic dialysis unit can reduce the threats to security. Costs are ranked on a scale of 1 to 7 where 1 is the least expensive and 7 is the most expensive. The countermeasures follow in the form of a description of the countermeasure, its estimated cost, and the breakdown of components of the cost:

1. Increase security awareness training for all staff. Cost: 3 (time for staff and trainer, training supplies)

2. Use of encryption during transfer between devices. Cost: 2 (software, installation)
3. Control access to telemedicine application. Cost: 2 (software, implementation)
4. Enforce password management practices. Cost: 2 (inconvenience to personnel)
5. Install virus protection software. Cost: 1 ($100: cost of the software)
6. Better access control for off-site archive. Cost: 1 (cost of lock, minor inconvenience to users)
7. Upgrade to new operating system. Cost: 6 (cost of upgrade, installation)

The above seven countermeasures (they will be referred to as Countermeasure1,..., Countermeasure7) are evaluated by considering their cost, which threats they diminish, and by how much. To do this, the threats themselves are assigned a severity according to their frequency of occurrence and expected loss (see Table 10.1).

For each countermeasure and each threat, the percentage by which that countermeasure can reduce the threat is estimated. The impact of that countermeasure on the threat's overall contribution to entity security is the percentage reduction multiplied by the threat's severity. To determine a countermeasure's overall contribution to *severity reduction*, one simply adds together its impact on each individual threat. The overall cost/benefit value of a countermeasure is its cost divided by its total severity reduction.

Table 10.2 shows the reduction of a threat's severity achieved by the countermeasures. It lists the threats on one side and the countermeasures on the other side. In the cells between a threat and a countermeasure, a percentage indicates how much the countermeasure reduces the threat. At the bottom of the table is the sum of threat reductions for each countermeasure. For example, countermeasure1 mitigates threats 1, 2, 3, and 5 by 50%, 20%, 70%, and 70%, respectively. Threat1's severity is reduced by 50% (a contribution of 1 to the overall security reduction because

Table 10.1. Severity of threats

			Frequency
Expected Loss	Low	Medium	High
Low	1	2	3
Medium	2	4	6
High	3	6	9

Table 10.2. The cells of the table for the intersection of a Threat (T1-T7) and a Countermeasure (C1-C7) indicate the per cent reduction of the threat by the countermeasure. The column marked Severity indicates the Severity of the Threat. The row labeled Y/N shows a decision of whether or not each countermeasure should be recommended based on a cost/benefit ratio of 0.6.

Countermeasures versus Threats								
		Countermeasures						
Threat	**Severity**	**C1**	**C2**	**C3**	**C4**	**C5**	**C6**	**C7**
T1	2	50		90	20			
T2	2	20						
T3	3	70		90		70		
T4	3		100					90
T5	6	70			70			70
T6	2						90	
T7	2			100				100
total severity reduction		7.7	3	6.5	4.6	2.1	1.8	8.9
cost of counter-measure		3	2	2	2	1	1	6
cost/benefit		0.39	0.67	0.31	0.43	0.48	0.56	0.67
Y/N		Y	N	Y	Y	Y	Y	N

the threat was 2). Threat2's severity is reduced by 20%, and a 0.4 contribution to overall threat security is thus made by countermeasure1's impact on threat2. One continues in this fashion to compute that countermeasure1 overall reduces security threats by 7.7. That sum of 7.7 is entered in the row showing total severity reduction. The greater the *total reduction in severity*, the greater is the perceived benefit from the countermeasure.

Various approaches can be taken to these results. For instance, an organization could start implementing the countermeasures whose *cost/benefit ratio* was lowest – meaning their cost was low and their benefit high, relatively speaking. For the example of *Table 10.2* that would mean to begin with countermeasure3, whose cost/benefit ratio was 0.31, and after that to implement countermeasure1, whose cost/benefit ratio was 0.39. Countermeasure3 was to control access, and countermeasure1 was training.

An alternative approach is to choose a cut-off point and implement all countermeasures whose cost-benefit ratio is below the cut-off. A subjective choice is made of a cut-off point below which countermeasures are worth implementing. In this case,

0.6 might be the reasonable *cut-off point* and means that countermeasures whose cost/benefit ratio is below 0.6 will be implemented. In the example of *Table 10.2*, countermeasure2 and countermeasure7 would not be implemented.

Information Security Officer

The Security Rule says that responsibility for security should be assigned to a *specific individual* to provide an organizational focus and importance to security. The assignment should be documented and responsibilities would include:

- Management and supervision of the use of security measures to protect data
- Conduct of personnel in relation to the protection of data

The following material about information security officers is not from the HIPAA Security Rule but is general guidance. Security initiatives require organization-wide involvement, championed by both the CEO and CIO. The "owner," however, can be a corporate information security officer. The information security officer identifies the impact on the *information security program* of changes in the patient, business, and computer systems environments in the healthcare industry and specifically within the organization. Based on an awareness of the industry and organizational needs, the information security officer should direct the information security program. The scope of this responsibility encompasses the organization's information in its entirety.

The information security officer has authority and *responsibility* for:

- Implementing and maintaining a process for defining the organization's goals and objectives for information security
- Determining the methodology and procedures for accomplishing the goals of the information security functions
- Proposing information security policies to senior management and establishing standards and programs to implement the policies
- Determining which security incidents and findings will be communicated to senior management
- Determining the adequacy of risk assessment and the appropriateness of risk acceptance
- Determining information ownership responsibilities or when ownership decisions must be escalated

- Making personnel and administrative decisions in the supervision of the information security and computer access control administration staff, including hiring, termination, and training
- Controlling the use and expenditure of budgeted funds
- Preparing a quarterly status report for the chief executive officer

The information security officer requires these *skills and abilities*:

- Ability to organize and direct educational programs for all levels of staff on information security topics
- Knowledge about the organization structure, methodologies, and culture
- Ability to direct projects and participate in teams
- Knowledge of current technical and procedural techniques in information security
- Knowledge about state and federal regulations, accrediting organizations and healthcare industry standards, and litigation avoidance issues relative to information security matters
- Ability to establish liaisons with internal and external constituencies with respect to information security matters

The information security officer has a mix of responsibilities that requires both technical and managerial abilities.

Other staff supports the information security officer. There does not appear to be a specific relationship between the size of the organization and the *number of information security staff* required. The complexity of the organization, the status of the information security program, and the rate of change in the organization structure, systems and networks are significant factors in determining the information security staff required. The information security function may be a part-time assignment for one person or a full-time assignment to a large staff. The information security unit is typically assigned to the chief information officer but may be assigned to any senior manager in the organization, if that manager will provide the most effective reporting arrangement. Regardless of the size of the information security unit, the information security function must be an organization-wide function and not limited to a specific department or person. Many of the security administration functions will be distributed throughout the organization.

Training

The Security Rule requires training of the workforce. Security training would typically be incorporated in other existing training activities; for instance, it could be part of *employee orientation*. The amount and type of training that is appropriate depends on the entity's situation.

The Security Rule requires *security updates*. Security advisories or reminders should be periodically distributed to affected users, including contractors. Convenient delivery methods include e-mail, flyers and an Intranet site. Security reminders might include warnings on current risks such as latest viruses, social engineering, new technical vulnerabilities, and risks and countermeasures specific to the covered entity. The definition of periodic is left to each covered entity, but one reasonable frequency might be twice per year.

Quality Control

The gap analysis and risk analysis are steps in an organization confirming its *objectives* and assessing its compliance with its objectives. The Security Rule asks an organization to make a plan and stick to it. The details of the plan are left very open, but the high-level objectives are indicated. An organization must begin by assessing its position relative to the security standards, plan how to achieve its objectives, work to the plan, and document its work. Again the documentation must conform to the standard and the behavior of the people must conform to the documentation (see Figure 10.3).

Figure 10.3. Mapping documents and behavior

		documents relative to standard	
		good	**bad**
behavior relative to documents	**good**	documents conform to standard and people follow documents	documents do not follow standards but people follow documents
	bad	documents conform to standard but people do not	documents do not follow the standard or are missing and people do not follow them

Figure "Documents to Behavior": This 4x4 table has columns which indicate the quality of the documents and rows which indicate the behavior of people relative to the documents.

Security Rule

The U.S. Health Insurance Portability and Accountability Act (HIPAA) mandated that the U.S. Department of Health and Human Services (DHHS) publish and enforce a Security Rule. The Security Rule was published in the *Federal Register* in February 2003 and compliance was mandatory by April 2005. Many consultants found work as HIPAA security experts, and much new equipment was purchased in an attempt to be Security Rule compliant.

The covered entities of the Security Rule are the same as those of the Privacy Rule. Within covered entities, HIPAA's security provisions apply to electronic protected health information. *Electronically protected health information* (EPHI) is PHI that is transmitted by electronic media or maintained in electronic media.

In general, DHHS adopts standards already developed by standards development organizations. However, DHHS decided that previously existing *security standards* were inadequate. To have something adequately technology-neutral and scaleable, DHHS developed its own Security Rule.

The Security Rule has administrative, technical, and physical standards. These standards are elaborated in implementation specifications. The Security Rule establishes two types of implementation specifications (DHHS, 2003):

- **Required:** The entity is required to implement exactly the specification
- **Addressable:** The entity may assess whether the specification is reasonable and appropriate in the context of the entity's environment

If an entity determines that any addressable safeguard is reasonable and appropriate, it must implement that specification. If the entity determines that an addressable implementation specification is not a reasonable and appropriate answer to its security needs, then the entity must document why. At this stage, the entity could implement any equivalent alternative security measure. If an entity determines that it can meet the standard by doing nothing, the entity may do so The Security Rule simply requires that the entity document its rationale for its decision. To repeat, the covered entity may choose one of three options:

- *Implement the specification*;
- *Implement an alternative* security measure to accomplish the purposes of the standard
- *Not implement anything* if the specification is not reasonable and appropriate and the standard can still be met

In keeping with its results-based approach, the rule has heightened emphasis on internal risk analysis and risk management as the core elements of the security management process. Cost of security measures is a significant factor to be considered in security decisions. The decision about the *reasonable and appropriate* nature of an addressable specification rests on the covered entity and is based on its overall technical environment and security framework. This decision may rely on a variety of factors, including the results of a risk analysis, measures already in place, and the cost of implementing new measures.

Administrative Safeguards

Regardless of how much technology is used to lock or secure information, the way the people work with one another and with information ultimately has the greatest impact on security. The security policy has to come before the technical decisions are made. If the technology is in place before a security policy is, then the organization has the added difficulty of *retrofitting its technology* to suit its policy.

Management and Awareness

The HIPAA Security Rule provides guidance in its section called *Administration* that applies both to the life cycle of compliance and to security policies. The Security Rule's *Security Management Process* standard has four implementation requirements:

- Risk analysis
- Risk management
- Sanction policy
- Information system activity review

Risk analysis and management were described in the preceding "Life Cycle" Chapter. Sanctions would be relative to the policy of the entity, and *information system activity reviews* would regularly monitor activity.

The Security Rule has a standard for *awareness* with four addressable implementation specifications (DHHS, 2003):

- "Security reminders. Periodic security updates.
- Protection from malicious software. Procedures for guarding against, detecting, and reporting malicious software.
- Login monitoring. Procedures for monitoring login attempts and reporting discrepancies.
- Password management. Procedures for creating, changing, and safeguarding passwords."

Security reminders were covered in this book under "training" in the life cycle of compliance. The other specifications are described next.

Procedures for handling viruses should be known by all employees. System administrators should *monitor login* attempts. Users should be aware of the importance of having passwords that are at least eight characters long, which are safeguarded, and are changed regularly.

Workforce Security

The workforce security standard includes the following implementation guidelines (DHHS, 2003):

- **Authorization or supervision:** Implement procedures for the authorization or supervision of workforce members who work with EPHI or in locations where it might be accessed
- **Workforce clearance procedure:** Implement procedures to determine that the access of a workforce member to EPHI is appropriate
- **Termination procedures:** Implement procedures for terminating access to EPHI when the employment of a workforce member ends

The implementation specifications are addressable. What is appropriate for one entity will not be for another. For example, a clearance may not be appropriate for a solo doctor whose only assistant is his wife.

Authorization or supervision requires that workforce members be *supervised* or have *authorization* when working with or around EPHI. *Termination* procedures should minimize the chance that former employees use their employer's information for personal gain. No specific termination activities, such as changing locks, are required.

Information Access

Confidentiality means controlling who gets *access* to information. An organization should maintain policies and procedures for granting different levels of access to healthcare information. This involves policies for establishing access, authorizing access, and modifying access.

For *information access management*, entities need policies and procedures for authorizing access. Specifications include (DHHS, 2003):

- **Access authorization (Addressable):** Implement policies and procedures for granting access to EPHI, for example, through access to a workstation, transaction, program, process, or other mechanism
- **Access establishment and modification (Addressable):** Implement policies and procedures that, based upon the entity's access authorization policies, establish, document, review, and modify a user's right of access to a workstation, transaction, program, or process

Restricting access to those with a need for access is vital. DHHS does not specifically identify roles and privileges. This standard is consistent with the Privacy Rule (minimum necessary requirements for use and disclosure of protected health information).

In the next example, a policy is based on who is in a renal dialysis unit. A more elaborate policy for Partners HealthCare System is then presented and followed by an example from long-term care.

The security policy in the Georgetown University Medical Center renal care clinic provides patient information to appropriate people (Group, 2005). For instance, patients have the right to review their own information. Because patient records might be seen by anyone in the dialysis unit, only *authorized personnel* may enter the unit. Authorized personnel include the patients and unit staff. Family members of patients who assist patients for dialysis must leave the unit when the patient leaves. A member of the regular unit staff must accompany all persons with temporary access during their entire stay.

Partners HealthCare System was established in 1994 as the corporation overseeing the affiliation of Brigham and Women's Hospital, Massachusetts General Hospital, and North Shore Medical Center. In *Partners' information access management policy*, staff may see or modify patient information anytime they are involved in that patient's care. In further detail (Group, 2005):

- Emergency care staff may suddenly become involved in patient care and need *emergency access*.
- *Staff in support departments*, such as labs and "volunteer services," need access relevant to their responsibilities. Laboratory technicians might need the results of laboratory tests. Volunteers might need to know the patient's bed location but not other information.

Partners Healthcare System requires special security measures for certain clinical problems. For instance, records pertaining to sexually transmitted diseases are handled with more restrictions than non-sensitive information.

Another example of access models comes from the *long-term care industry*. The roles in a typical long-term care facility include:

- A facility's certified nursing assistants provide the basic care.
- The dietary director oversees meal preparation. Cooks and dietary aides provide the hands-on meal preparation and delivery.
- The director of activities develops and organizes a monthly calendar of events. Most nursing homes have maintenance personnel and a small laundry and housekeeping staff. The business office generally includes an office manager, receptionist and several clerical personnel.

The diagram of roles to information (see Figure 10.4) indicates how the facility might organize the assignment of people to the information they are allowed to access.

Incidents and Contingencies

Reporting and responding to incidents are both integral to a security program. The Security Rule includes a standard for *security incident procedures*. A *security incident* is the attempted or successful unauthorized access to information or interference with information system operations (DHHS, 2003).

A *contingency plan* protects data during crises when the usual security measures may be ignored. Each entity needs to determine its own risk in the event of an emergency and the extent to which its response needs to be complex or simple. For example, locking backup diskettes in a desk may work for a doctor's office, but not for a hospital.

Figure 10.4. Roles to information. The functions of the medical clinic are depicted in the upper tree—three major functions of 'front office', 'medical care', and 'back office' are shown. The roles of the people are shown at the bottom of the diagram. Each person in a role is expected to use certain types of information. The dashed line goes from the role to the information for which it is responsible.

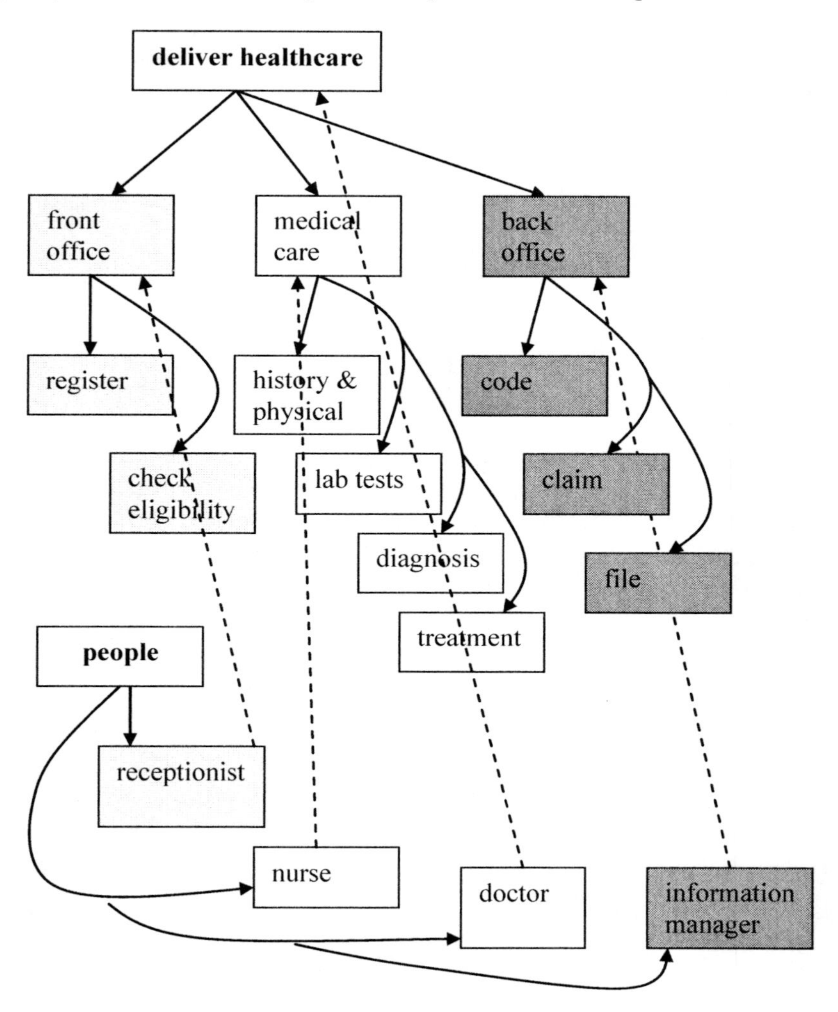

Business Associate

Covered entities have certain responsibilities relative to their business associates. The covered entity is subject to *sanctions* if it has knowledge of a business associate's wrongful activity and fails to address the wrongdoing. Next, the definition of a business associate and scalability are addressed.

The Security Rule supports the *Privacy Rule* and refers to the Privacy Rule for the definition of a business associate. The Privacy Rule allows the covered entity to send for certain "healthcare-serving" purposes "protected health information" to a non-covered entity without patient authorization. However, the two entities must have a "business associate contract" to protect the information.

The Security Rule requires, of course, different provisions in the business associate agreement from what was prepared for the Privacy Rule. The agreement is designed to confirm the business associate's commitment to provide security for EPHI. A covered entity is not in compliance with the Security Rule if the covered entity knew of a practice of the business associate that constituted a *violation* of the business associate's obligation under the contract, unless the covered entity took reasonable steps to end the violation.

Technical Safeguards

The Security Rule has five standards under the heading of *Technical Safeguards*, and the majority of the implementation specifications are "addressable" (meaning not required). The Security Rule technical specifics cover access control, audit, integrity, authentication, and transmission.

Integrity

Integrity entails policies, procedures, and tools to protect EPHI from improper alteration or destruction. The integrity standard has exactly one implementation specification and that specification is addressable – the data authentication specification. *Data authentication* means that an organization can corroborate that data in its possession has not been altered or destroyed in an unauthorized manner.

The Security Rule states that very little is required to achieve integrity. Storing information on magnetic disk, which is a common way to store information on computers, is considered adequate data authentication. The Rule specifically says:

Error-correcting memory and magnetic disc storage are examples of the built-in data authentication mechanisms that are ubiquitous in hardware and operating systems today.

Other examples of how data corroboration may be assured include the use of a check sum, a message authentication code, or a digital signature. The risk analysis process will address what data must be authenticated and how.

User Authentication

Person or entity authentication means implementing procedures to verify that a person or entity seeking access to EPHI is the one claimed. Whenever an operation is invoked, the computer uses *authentication* to determine whether the requester is trusted for that operation (American Society for Testing and Materials, 1996). If so, the computer allows the operation to proceed; otherwise it cancels the operation. Authentication mechanisms include:

- A password system
- A biometric identification system
- A personal identification number (PIN)
- Telephone callback

The prevalent means of entity or user authentication in healthcare systems is the entry of passwords.

Authentication can be tied to a person's body:

- *Biometric user authentication* identifies a human through a measurement of a physical feature of the individual
- *Behavioral action user authentication* identifies a human through a measurement of a repeatable action of the individual

Some administrators and practitioners are attracted to the possibility of biometric or behavioral authentication because it obviates the need to remember keys or passwords.

Access Control

Compliance with the *access control* standard means access to EPHI is only for those persons or software programs that have been granted access rights. The standard's "implementation specifications" are (DHHS, 2003):

- Unique user identification (Required). Assign a unique name or number for identifying and tracking user identity.
- Emergency access procedure (Required). Establish (and implement as needed) procedures for obtaining necessary EPHI during an emergency.
- Automatic logoff (Addressable). Implement electronic procedures that terminate an electronic session after a predetermined time of inactivity.
- Encryption and decryption (Addressable). Implement a mechanism to encrypt and decrypt EPHI." File encryption is one way to deny access to information in that file.

The first two specifications are explained next.

If a computer workstation is on the hospital ward and anyone who comes to the keyboard and screen can enter the system without identifying him or herself, then unique user identification is missing. *Unique user identification* is typically obtained by giving each user an identifier, such as their last name, and requiring the user to login with that identifier.

Once a user has been authenticated, ensuring that the current user is still the authenticated user must be addressed. Minimizing the opportunity for an unauthenticated user to utilize another's access can be supported through the use of automatic logoff after a stated period of inactivity or when the authenticated user accesses the system from another terminal. The logon and logoff processes should be quick. Various forms of inactivity lockout other than *automatic logoff* are permissible.

Access controls are necessary under *emergency conditions*, although they may be different from the normal. For example, if the computer has crashed in a doctor's office and the doctor cannot access the laboratory values on the doctor's computer, then a procedure should be in place to get the laboratory values, such as by contacting the laboratory and having the values faxed.

Audit

Audit controls entail hardware, software, or procedural mechanisms that record and examine activity in information systems that contain or use EPHI. The Security Rule points to two publications of the National Institute of Standards and Technology for further information about audit (National Institute of Standards and Technology, 1996, 2001).

In the extreme case, an entity would record each operation that is invoked along with the identity of the subject and object. For *medical records*, audit policies could be elaborate, though the Security Rule does not require it. For example, the computer system on which a patient record is maintained might:

- Record the date and time of each entry to a record
- Record the identity of each person who makes an entry
- When an error is corrected in a patient record, the system might preserve both the original entry and the correction
- The identity of the person making each correction and the date and time of correction might be recorded by the computer in the same manner as this information is recorded for original record entries

The sophisticated auditing mechanisms described in the immediate foregoing are *not required* by the Security Rule. The rule does not require the entity to be able to produce an audit trail of views or changes to a specific data record within its information systems. The entity does not need, for example, to be able to identify all the users who viewed a given patient's lab results.

For further insight on the Rule's auditing requirement, one might look to the NIST standards that the Rule cites. NIST says that a system's audit trail is a collection of audit records containing data about attempted violations of the security policy or changes to the security state of the system. When required, applications should be able to generate these audit records. This notion of *auditing security violations* or changes to the security state of the system is far more limited than auditing of each user action.

Modern operating systems often have *built-in facilities* to log security relevant events. However, tools for such auditing are also available as separate packages from third parties, sometimes as freeware. If some systems do not have auditing tools, the entity might consider acquiring and using such tools for those systems.

Transmission

Transmission security means that when EPHI is transmitted from one point to another, it must be protected in a manner commensurate with the associated risk. The Security Rule's "transmission security" standard has two implementation specifications:

- **Integrity controls (Addressable):** Security measures to ensure that electronically transmitted EPHI is not improperly modified without detection until disposed
- **Encryption (Addressable):** A mechanism to encrypt transmitted EPHI when appropriate

Integrity of transmission can be achieved with check sums. With a check sum, a string of transmitted digits is followed by another digit that indicates some attribute of the preceding digits. If the initial string is modified, then the check sum digit may no longer properly characterize the initial string and the transmitters can signal that a corruption in the data has occurred. Transmitting with check sums is routine in modern digital telecommunications. Another approach to data integrity in transmissions is electronic signatures.

Another type of protection of transmitted data is *encryption*. For the Security Rule, encryption is optional based on individual entity risk analysis. Non-judicious use of encryption can adversely affect processing times and become both financially and technically burdensome. Covered entities are encouraged, however, to consider use of encryption technology for transmitting EPHI, particularly over the Internet.

If entity e1 sends something encrypted with method m1 to entity e2 but e2 uses method m2 to try to decrypt the message, then miscommunication occurs. Without an agreed encryption method among entities, encryption is not practical.

DHHS is committed to the principle of technology neutrality, as rapidly changing technology makes it impractical and inappropriate to name a specific technology. Specification of an algorithm or specific products would be inappropriate. No specific (or minimum) cryptographic algorithm strength is recommended. For instance, the Centers for Medicare and Medicaid Services (CMS) have an Internet Security Policy, which requires certain encryptions. However, the *CMS Internet Security Policy* is the policy of a single organization and applies only to information sent to CMS, and not between all covered entities.

Physical Safeguards

The Security Rule includes standards for physical safeguards for facility access controls, proper workstation use and physical security of workstations that access EPHI, and device and media controls.

A "facility" is the physical premises, including the interior and exterior of a building. The *facilities access control standard* requires covered entities to implement policies and procedures that limit access to facilities that contain EPHI. These specifications could be very costly to implement, since they affect the *day-to-day flow* of people and information. In public buildings, provider locations, and in areas of heavy pedestrian traffic, sign-in procedures might be implemented for visitors, and escorts might be provided where appropriate. However, one should weigh the cost of such procedures against the expected benefit.

Access control to *physical resources* is in some way more cumbersome than access to software resources. The software is capable of semi-automating the access decisions based on data and rules. For physical access, this can be partially accomplished by providing people with identity cards that can be read by sensors at locked doors. The doors unlock if the person has been categorized as authorized to enter the door.

The Rule requires a covered entity to implement policies and procedures specifying the proper functions and the manner in which they are performed at *workstations* that contain EPHI. The workstation use policies and procedures should also address the physical location and surroundings of workstations. For instance, a policy may say that only patient care staff is to access the workstations on the hospital ward.

In the extreme case, a security advocate might request that every workstation be in a locked room to which only carefully screened, authorized users have access. However, in the healthcare environment this is not practical. Workstation physical security may rely more on *social conventions* than on physical mechanisms. A social convention would be that staff are alert to the presence of any stranger "behind the counter" and promptly check whether the stranger has appropriate authorization. Success with this kind of social security is a function of training and management.

Computer Models

The policy principles of the real world continue to hold for the computing world, but the scope of computer policy changes. First, the real-world security policy must be automated faithfully. This means that it must be specified *unambiguously* -- an ambiguous policy may work for people but will not for computers. Second, policy choices must be made about the computing situation itself, such as how users identify themselves to the computing system.

Label and Access

The earliest computer security modeling work was stimulated by the development of time-sharing systems in the 1960s. The early systems were developed and used at universities and so reflected the rather permissive policies of universities. The 1970s and 1980s saw a shift toward work reflecting military needs. In the late 1980s, another shift occurred toward business needs.

Two salient model types appeared from 1960 to now. One model is the *label model* or *information flow model* in which information is labeled and access depends on the label on the information. The other is the *discretionary access control model* in which a rule is developed for each combination of person, object, and operation to specify what operation that person can perform on that object.

Labels are ordered in the label model. A typical example is public, secret, and top secret with the obvious ordering. *Labels* are assigned to information and also to people. Thus, a document might be public, secret, or top secret. A person's label is often cited as the person's level of clearance. When a person identifies himself to a computer system, the computer ensures that he never sees information at a higher level than his clearance.

The label model is easily illustrated. The label model has long been used in Department of Defense computer security policies. For instance, a document labeled "secret" might only be read by people with the rank of lieutenant or higher. A document labeled "top secret" might only be read by people with the rank of colonel or higher. In the medical arena, the security level of a patient test report for a certain disease might be defined according to the possible social impact of an unauthorized disclosure about a patient with that disease. Thus test results for AIDS might be marked "top secret," while test results for "sore throat" might be marked "secret."

Tufts Health Plan in Massachusetts has 236 million rows of detail data about claims, membership, provider, pharmacy, and employer. It uses label-based access control. Two hundred of Tufts two thousand employees use the warehouse for various purposes, such as claims analysis and retrieval of member information for specific transactional purposes (Hagland, 1997). Data in the warehouse is carefully segregated at the row level for access by staff and business partners, and audited regularly using audit trails. With extremely sensitive patient record information, involving plan members with HIV or who have had psychiatric care for example, Tufts has developed a *data vault*. There are only two people in the organization who have access to that data vault. This method of controlling access is a combination of identifying data by security-risk level, and severely restricting the people who have access to certain types of data. If the number of people needing to access the data is reasonably small and static and the data relatively easily labeled, then this labeling approach is practical.

Permission to write entails refinements to the label model. The same medical data often has to be treated differently by different users. For instance, a nurse should be able to read the doctor's prescription but not to change it, whereas the doctor can also change the prescription. The label model has generally assumed that whenever a user could read an object that the user could also modify the object. To distinguish reading from writing privileges requires introducing refinements to the flow model. A more complicated version of the flow model has *subjects* that can initiate operations and *objects* that simply contain data, such as a piece of paper. Flow from object to subject is a read operation, and flow from subject to object is a write operation. A subject can only read from an object at an equal or lower level. A subject can only write to an object at an equal or higher level. Thus a subject can contribute potentially highly secure information to an object but only to an object at least as secure as any the subject can read. Notice that a subject in being entitled to write to a higher-level object is not entitled to read any part of that object (other than ostensibly the part that the subject is writing).

The label model can be further enhanced. A label on data can describe the security level of the data and other *categorizations*. For instance, for a label on a medical record another category might reflect that the medical record is associated with a certain ward in the hospital. Only the responsible doctor in the appropriate ward is granted access to that data.

A label model provides mandatory access control. Although not logically required, the label model policy has generally been viewed as *mandatory* in that neither users nor programs in the system can break the flow rule or change levels. No real system can strictly follow this rule, since, for instance, procedures are needed for declassifying data.

Discretionary access control adds flexibility. The discretionary access control model is based on the idea of stationing a guard in front of a valuable resource to control who has access to it. This model organizes the system into objects, subjects, and operations. *Operations* specify the ways that subjects can interact with objects. The objects are the resources being protected. A set of rules specifies for each object and each subject what operations that subject can perform on that object. There are many ways to express the access rules, of which the most popular is the access matrix. The access matrix has a row for each subject and a column for each object. In the access matrix, the cell corresponding to subject s and object o specifies the rights that subject s has to object o. A right represents a type of access to the object, such as read or write. A row of the access matrix corresponds to a *capability list*—the list of all the rights of a subject. A column of the access matrix corresponds to an *access control list*—the list of all the rights held by subjects to some object (see *Figure 10.5*).

Role-Based Access Control

Models to increase efficiency may introduce hierarchies and exploit inheritance properties. For instance, a role might be defined and several people might be assigned to the role. The operations for that role are *inherited* by the people in the role without requiring explicit assignment of an operation to each person. This is the basis for role-based access control.

With role-based access control (RBAC), access rights are grouped by roles (Ferraiolo, 2000). Role models vary by organization. One model (see Table 10.3) calls for a doctor to see everything and other staff to see only patient name (Barkley et al., 1999). Roles can be modified without modifying the privileges for individuals because the individuals inherit the privileges of their role. Users are assigned to roles based on their job responsibilities, but these assignments can be dynamic.

Figure 10.5. Access matrix. Three objects and five subjects are depicted in this matrix.

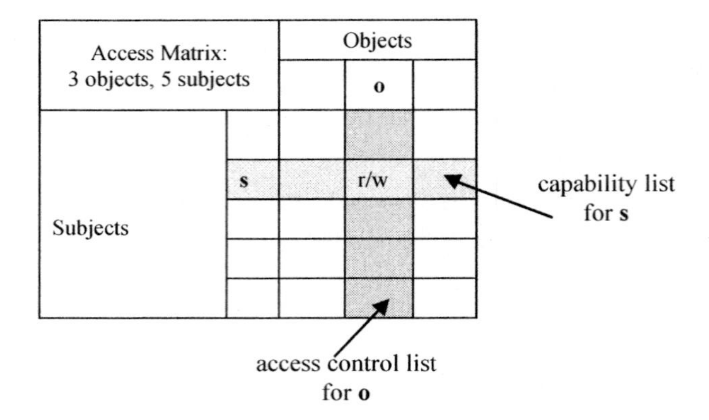

Table 10.3. Example role and access

Role	Access
Patient	all information for the patient
Doctor	all information
Voluntary caring agency	name, address, clinical data
Researcher	age, sex, clinical data
Organization staff	name and ID

Role hierarchies reflect the hierarchical structure of the enterprise (Ferraiolo, 2000). In the healthcare situation, a role called *specialist* could contain the roles of *surgeon* and *pediatrician*. This means that members of the role "surgeon" and "pediatrician" inherit the permissions for the role of "specialist" without the administrator having to explicitly assign the "surgeon" and "pediatrician" permissions (Griew & Currell, 2000).

RBAC deals well with confidentiality but less well with integrity. Integrity requires being clear about who can make what changes to which information and when. Getting the integrity specifications clear requires essentially scheduling the work of all staff on all information. This is an extension of role-based access control into *workflow management*.

Computer Mechanisms

Computer security mechanisms support computer security policies.

Cryptography

Cryptography encrypts and decrypts messages in secret code or cipher. Encryption converts data into a secret code for transmission over a network using an algorithm that allows only the intended receiver to decode it at the other end. The two main cryptographic methods are secret key and public key. In *secret key*, both sender and receiver must secretly share the information about how the message is encoded and decoded. *Public key* encryption involves both a private and a public key. The sender can use the receiver's public key to encrypt a message; the receiver uses his or her private key to decrypt it. Whereas the first method, secret key, requires first getting the key to the message recipient, in the second method owners never have to send private keys.

Encryption techniques mathematically transform a message into a *ciphertext*. Mathematical operations called *one-way functions* are particularly suited to this task. A one-way function is comparatively easy to do in one direction but much harder to do in reverse. For example, with a little concentration, many people can probably multiply 24 by 24 without using a pencil and paper. On the other hand, calculating the square root of the number 576 is much harder, even with a pencil and paper.

"Pig Latin" is a cryptographic technique that is good for children but not for serious work. The *pig Latin one-way function* is to take a word that begins with a consonant and move the consonant to the end of the word and append "ay." If the word begins with a vowel, simply append "ay." Thus the sentence:

"This is a cipher for simple messages."

Becomes in pig Latin:

"hisTay isay aay iphercay orfay implesay essagesmay."

To decrypt the encoded message one removes the "ay's" at the end of words and moves forward the last consonant. As soon as someone has the ciphertext and knows pig Latin, the person can decipher the message.

The RSA Algorithm is a one-way function and supports the possibility of public and private keys (Barrett, 1987). The RSA Algorithm has three steps:

1. **Key generation:** Two prime numbers, "p" and "q," are chosen and multiplied together to form "n." An encryption exponent "e" is chosen, and the decryption exponent "d" is calculated using "e," "p," and "q"
2. **Encryption:** The message M is raised to the power "e," and then reduced modulo "n" to form the ciphertext C
3. **Decryption:** The ciphertext C is raised to the power "d," and then reduced modulo "n" to re-recreate message M

When the RSA Algorithm is used in a public key system, the modulus "n" and the exponent "e" are published as the public key. The other exponent "d" is kept secret, as the private key. Each user holds his or her own private keys, and knows the public keys of the other user or users (see *Figure 10.6*). The factors of "n," "p," and "q" are not needed for encryption or decryption; they are only used in the key generation step. The difficulty of determining "p" and "q" from "n" and "e" is what protects the holder of "d" from someone computing "d" based on "n" and "e." An illustration of the public key method follows:

- Rosa knows her own public key (e_{rosa} and n_{rosa}), her own private key (d_{rosa}), and Ray's public key (e_{ray} and n_{ray})
- Ray knows the converse: his public key (e_{ray} and n_{ray}), his private key (d_{ray}) and Rosa's public key (e_{rosa} and n_{rosa})

Figure 10.6. Public-key encryption. The plaintext 'health information' goes through the public key encryption and becomes the ciphertext 'Xwa6fdl ;ka qrt ud'. The ciphertext is transmitted and is then decrypted with the private key.

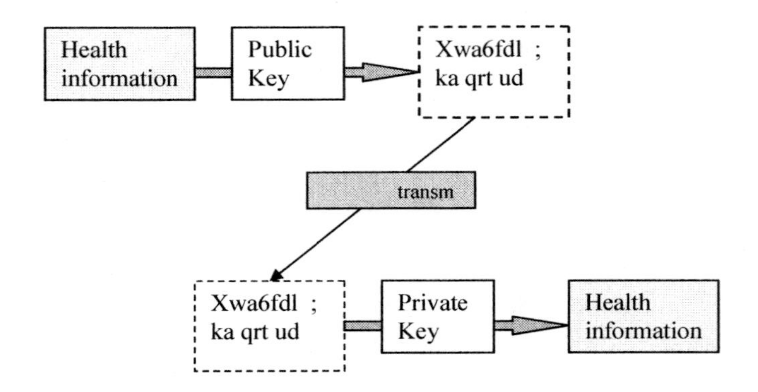

- For Rosa to send Ray a private message M that only Ray can read, she performs the following operation on the message M: $C_{M\ for\ ray}$ = (M raised to the power e_{ray}) modulo n_{ray}
- Ray, who is the only one to possess his private key (d_{ray}), performs the following to recover the message M: M = ($C_{M\ for\ ray}$ raised to the power d_{ray}) modulo n_{ray}
- To sign a message S, Rosa encrypts with her own private key: $C_{rosa\ signs\ S}$ = (S raised to the power d_{rosa}) modulo n_{rosa}
- Because only Rosa possesses d_{rosa}, only she can create this ciphertext $C_{rosa\ signs\ S}$. Anyone in possession of her public key (e_{rosa} and n_{rosa}) can verify the signature and obtain the deciphered message S by computing: S = ($C_{rosa\ signs\ S}$ raised to the e_{rosa}) modulo n_{rosa}

Thus to send a message to Rosa, Ray encodes it with Rosa's public key. Broadcasting a message to 20 people each with individual private keys would require 20 different encryptions.

Pretty Good Privacy (PGP) is a computer program that uses RSA. For example, PGP can encrypt "Rosa" so that it reads "457mRT%$354." The computer can decrypt this message into "Rosa" with PGP. *PGP* generates two keys that belong uniquely to the user. One PGP key is secret and stays with the user. The other key is public and is given by the user to his or her secret correspondents. The public key is simply a long string of characters (see *Figure 10.7*). Suppose the public key of *Figure 10.7* belongs to Rosa and that Rosa e-mails it to Ray. Ray can store Rosa's public key in his PGP program and use Rosa's public key to encrypt a message that only Rosa can read. One beauty of PGP is that Rosa can advertise Rosa's public key the same way that Rosa can give out Rosa's telephone number. If Ray has Rosa's telephone number, Ray can call Rosa's telephone; however, Ray cannot answer Rosa's telephone. Similarly, if Rosa has Ray's public key, Rosa can send Ray encrypted mail; however, Rosa cannot read Ray's encrypted mail.

PGP is easy to use. Windows versions allow users to encrypt and decrypt files and send or receive email messages with a *mouse click*. Versions are available for many operating systems. PGP is available to download from the Internet, and many PGP versions are *freeware* (meaning that they are free).

Public Key Infrastructure

Acquiring and using keys requires an infrastructure. Public key cryptography, on its own, is not enough to re-create the conditions for traditional paper-based commerce in an electronic world. Users also need an infrastructure of:

Figure 10.7. This string of characters is an example of a public key.

-----BEGIN PGP PUBLIC KEY BLOCK-----
Version: 5.0
mQCNAi44C30AAAEEAL1r6ByIvuSAvOKIk9ze9yCK+ZP
PbRZrpXIRFBbe+U8dGPMbXdJS4L/cy1fXr9R9j4EfFsK/rg
HV6i2rE83LjOrmsDPRPSaizz+EQTIZi4AN99iBomfLLZyU
zmHMoUoE4shrYgOnkc0u101ikhieAFje77j/F3596pT6nCx/
9/AAURtCRBbmRyZSBCYWNhcmQgPGFiYWNhcmRAd2
VsbC5zZi5jYS51cz6JAFUCBRAuOA6O7zYZz1mqos8BA
Xr9AgCxCu8CwGZRdpfSs65r6mb4MccXvvfxO4TmPi1DK
Qj2FYHYjwYONk8vzA7XnE5aJmk5J/dChdvfIU7NvVif=G
Qv9
-----END PGP PUBLIC KEY BLOCK-----

- Security policies to define the rules under which the cryptographic systems should operate
- Products to generate, store, and manage the keys
- Procedures to dictate how the keys should be generated, distributed, and used

This infrastructure is called, naturally enough, a *public key infrastructure* (PKI). PKI uses "digital certificates" which act like "electronic passports" and bind the user to his or her public key. Dealing with these certificates involves a:

- Security policy
- Certificate practice statement
- Certificate authority (CA)
- Registration authority (RA)
- Certificate distribution system
- PKI-enabled application

Details of these PKI attributes follow:

1. The security policy defines an organization's top-level direction on information security, as well as the processes and principles for the use of cryptography.

Typically, it will include statements on how the organization will handle keys and valuable information, and will set the level of control required to match the levels of risk.

2. A certificate practice statement gives the operational procedures on how the security policy will be enforced and supported in practice. It typically includes definitions on how the CAs are constructed and operated, how certificates are issued, accepted and revoked, and how keys are generated, registered and certified, where they will be stored, and how they will be made available to users.
3. CAs are the digital world's equivalent of passport offices. They issue digital certificates and validate the holder's identity and authority. Digital certificates are most trustworthy when they are vouched for by a trusted CA. CAs embed an individual's or an organization's public key along with other *identifying information* into each digital certificate and then cryptographically "sign" it as a tamper-proof seal, verifying the integrity of the data within it and validating its use.
4. A RA interfaces between the user and the CA. It captures and authenticates the identity of the users and submits the certificate request to the CA. The quality of this authentication process determines the level of trust that can be placed in the certificates.
5. The certificate distribution system distributes certificates in a number of ways depending on the structure of the PKI. For example, the users may distribute certificates themselves, or certificates may be distributed through a *directory service*. A directory service may already exist within an organization or one may be supplied as part of the PKI solution.
6. PKI-enabled applications are applications that support PKI as a secondary service. PKI-enabled applications exist for communications between Web servers and browsers, e-mail, electronic data interchange, and credit card transactions over the Internet. A PKI is a means to an end, providing the security framework by which PKI-enabled applications can be confidently deployed to achieve the end benefits.

Enterprises may create their own closed, private certificate infrastructure for internal use. However, public CAs, like those of VeriSign, are also available. All components of a PKI must interoperate, as it is unlikely that they will all be sourced from a single supplier. For example, the CA may have to interface with existing systems, such as directory servers already installed in the organization.

The CA should implement the organization's security policy. The *certificate management policy* must be accurately reflected in the roles of the CA and RA Operators and certificate users. For example, the CA Operator may decide to delegate the end-user certificate revocation to the RA Operators, while retaining revocation rights over RA Operator certificates.

The security of the CA and RA systems is critical for if compromised; then the whole PKI solution will be jeopardized. The PKI must ensure that the CA's private key is held in a tamper-resistant security module and provision made for disaster recovery purposes. Access to the CA and RA should be tightly controlled, for example, using smart cards to ensure strong user authentication. It should also be possible to configure the certificate management process such that more than one operator is required to authorize certification requests.

Healthcare PKI

Healthcare providers are a *mobile community* and are typically affiliated with multiple institutions. In the absence of an extensible infrastructure, the care provider could be faced with numerous identities, accounts, and technologies across these multiple environments making a complex environment for the end-user, and potentially impacting the time-sensitive nature of access efficiency. One of the primary goals of the security infrastructure, therefore, is to enable a single professional certificate to be used across all healthcare applications, institutions, and across multiple security technologies.

Several commercial entities exist today that provide CA services. However, these services are insufficient in the healthcare domain, as they do not certify the professional credentials of an individual. Healthcare applications must be able to ascertain not only the identity of an individual, but the individual's role, specialty, and the status of *professional credentials*. Furthermore, the certificate policies of the healthcare domain CAs must be consistent with the extensive validation processes that are currently conducted to establish trust and permissions that allow a clinician to practice medicine. Such policies must be consistent throughout the chain-of-trust relationships.

Many healthcare facilities are considering operating their own CA. While this option is sufficient for a self-contained operation, it is not scaleable for the level of *interoperability* required by healthcare. Healthcare transactions regularly involve unaffiliated entities. Under such a scenario, each organization must negotiate trust for the unaffiliated certificates. This negotiated trust must then be configured into each software product relying upon the certificates along with the appropriate access control. Most certificate-aware software does not currently support multiple "certificate mappings" and requires complex integration efforts for each CA recognized. Participating in a common CA model simplifies these relationships and configuration efforts. However, where a common CA does not exist, the use of automatic or semi-automatic certificate mappings is useful when the volume of traffic is high.

Several healthcare public key infrastructures (PKIs) have been developed. One such PKI, called *CHIME-Trust*, started in 1993 in Connecticut. CHIME-Trust well illustrates the technology and management issues germane to PKI. CHIME-Trust is managed by CHIME, an affiliate of the Connecticut Hospital Association. CHIME has established a trusted third-party service, which establishes a common chain-of-trust among healthcare organizations, enabling HIPAA compliant communications of patient care data (Lynch et al., 2000).

The statewide *healthcare domain, trusted, third-party services* architecture includes three primary components:

- Certificate authority (CA)
- Registration authority (RA)
- Lightweight directory access protocol (LDAP) directory server

All three of these components are extensible.

CHIME provides a number of services as a *trusted third party*. These core CA services include management of certificate revocation lists, certificate distribution, and time stamping. Some of these processes are unique to the healthcare professional certification environment, such as credential verification process. Other services, such as education, assist organizations in implementation and integration of the trusted third party infrastructure.

Small Provider Example

The size and organizational structure of the entities that are required to implement the Security Rule vary tremendously, and the appropriate approaches vary accordingly. The following example describes the manner in which a *small provider* might choose to implement the requirements.

For purposes of this example, a small provider is a one to four physician office, with two to five additional employees. The office uses a *PC-based* practice management system, which is used to communicate intermittently with a clearinghouse for submission of electronic claims. The number of providers is of less importance for this example than the relatively simple technology in use and the fact that there is insufficient volume or revenue to justify employment of a computer system administrator.

The office first assesses risks to its information assets. Then, to establish appropriate security, the office would develop policies and procedures to mitigate and manage those *risks*. These would include an overall framework outlining information security activities and responsibilities, and repercussions for failure to meet those responsibilities.

Next, this office might develop *contingency plans* to reduce or negate the damage resulting from processing anomalies. This office might establish a routine process for maintaining back-up media at a second location, obtain a PC maintenance contract, and arrange for use of a back-up PC should the need arise. The office would need to periodically review its plan to determine whether it still met the office's needs.

One person on staff might assume the role of "security officer" along with other roles. The office would need to create and document a personnel security policy and procedures to be followed. The *security officer* should be charged with seeing that the access authorization levels granted are documented and kept current. For example, records might be kept of everyone who is permitted to use the PC and what files they may access. Training in security must be provided to all personnel.

A small or rural provider may document compliance with many of the foregoing administrative security requirements by including them in an "office procedures" document that should be required reading by new employees and always available for reference. This *office procedures* document should include:

- Contingency plans
- Records processing procedures
- Information access controls (rules for granting access, actual establishment of access, and procedures for modifying such access)
- Security incident procedures (for example, who is to be notified if it appears that medical information has been accessed by an unauthorized party)
- Training

Periodic security reminders could include visual aids, such as posters or oral reminders in meetings.

The small or rural provider office would normally evaluate that the appropriate security is in place for its computer system and office procedures. This *evaluation* could be done by a knowledgeable person on the staff, by a consultant, or by the vendor of the practice management system as a service to its customers.

Large HMO Example

Kaiser Permanente (Kaiser) has a sophisticated security policy that was implemented a decade before the HIPAA Security Rule was formulated. What Kaiser was consistent with what the Security Rule subsequently mandated, and Kaiser has been a role model of other large organizations. Kaiser (www.kaiserpermanente.org) is a nonprofit, group-practice health maintenance organization with 8 million enrolled members, of whom 6 million live in California. Kaiser integrates health plan, hospitals, and medical groups.

History

Kaiser has been a leader in information systems use for decades. Kaiser made major extensions to its clinical data repository in 1994 and was then stimulated to also extend its security policy. The CEO asked that a security group be formed to develop policy. Physicians, nurses, and staff from medical records, clinical information systems, occupational health, legal, human resources, and internal audit were consulted. A 15-person *security group* was drawn from these constituencies and began meeting in 1995. Soon afterwards, the group contracted outside consultants; went through a self-education process; and then moved into the development of an over-arching set of policies to guide the organization's security implementation. From 1996 through 1997, the group developed its policies one-by-one and released them one-by-one throughout Kaiser via electronic mail (Hagland, 1997). The group also created a *training toolkit* to train people on these topics, and secured the cooperation of the local data processing staff to give everybody training. Portions of Kaiser's policies on roles of staff, local area networks, and e-mail and fax are presented next.

Roles of Staff

Kaiser has user, manager, and trustee roles. Kaiser (1999) has defined the security responsibilities of these roles. Through these definitions, Kaiser addresses the workflow of the organization.

Anyone accessing corporate data at any time for any reason is a user. A *User* must respect privacy, follow the rules, protect output, and report anyone else who violates the rules.

Managers lead an operational unit. *Managers* must determine user access privileges, follow the minimum necessary use guide, and update staff when any change in rules has occurred.

A Trustee leads activities related to one application from a user perspective. For information security, the *Trustee* is responsible for the policies regarding the application, including identifying the roles that may access what data inside the application. The Trustee also audits the use of the data and coordinates with managers corrective action against those who abuse the data.

Data Classification

Trustees classify Kaiser's data in their application according to its sensitivity. This supports access policies based on *data confidentiality*. Classification principles emphasize costs and damages. *Cost* refers to the amount of money required to replace the data. Damages are based on the impact on users or customers of misuse of the data. The classification affects the access controls to be placed upon the data.

Data is classified as public, internal, confidential, or registered confidential. An example of public data is a press release. An example of internal data is an internal phone directory. No auditing of access to public or internal data is performed. Patient treatment data is classified as confidential, and the trustee determines the situations in which its use is audited. Mental health treatment data is classified as *registered confidential* and any access is audited.

Local Area Network

The definition of roles is one approach to security, and a complementary approach defines how physical resources will be used. An example of a resource-based security policy is Kaiser's for local area networks (LANs).

Kaiser requires that LAN servers be in *physically secure areas* that are only used by LAN system administrators. Servers and workstations are configured to *prevent users* from modifying the software. LAN security administrators use access *control lists* to protect locally stored data. Users apply access controls to their personal business files.

Each user logs onto the LAN with a *unique user ID*. User IDs may not be shared. Passwords expire every month.

Fax and E-Mail

Fax machines must be inaccessible to the public. A recipient of a registered confidential fax must be contacted by phone before the fax is sent, and the recipient must agree to be waiting to receive the *fax*.

Kaiser encourages staff and patients to communicate via *e-mail* so long as both parties agree in advance and both adhere to Kaiser's policies. E-mail is not for urgent communications. If a message is not answered in a reasonable time, another channel of communication should be used. Parties must appreciate that messages might not be confidential because they could be intercepted by other. Staff must put in the medical record copies of clinically relevant e-mails that they send or receive.

The fax and e-mail policies highlight the importance of communicating in ways that are mutually agreeable and safeguard the confidentiality of the information communicated. Kaiser has a handful of other security policy documents, such as one on data retention and another on security training. Together these policy documents constitute an extensive and sophisticated approach to *security* in a large healthcare organization.

Conclusion

Naturally enough security has been important prior to HIPAA, but HIPAA's attempt to harmonize and regulate security nationally causes healthcare organizations to re-consider their approach to security. If security is seen primarily as a requirement to put a stronger *lock* on the door, then the investment in security will not show a profit to the implementing organization. If, instead, security is seen as precise, computer-supported workflow management, then investing in such security might be done in a profit-making way (Rada et al., 2002).

Maintenance costs for security compliance are high. In the case of privacy compliance, the costs for one year of maintenance are a small fraction of the costs of implementation. However, for security the maintenance costs in one year are higher than the implementation costs. The reason is that security takes time of every employee—procedures like security checks at doors—but for privacy most employees do nothing in maintenance mode.

The reaction to the Security Rule was much less than the reaction to the Privacy Rule in the years 2000 to 2005. For starters, the Privacy Rule compliance deadline was two years earlier than the Security Rule deadline. Then, the healthcare industry realized that enforcement of the Privacy Rule was largely supportive rather than punitive and expected the same for the Security Rule. Finally, while the Privacy Rule tends to require absolutes, such as every patient must see a notice of privacy practices, the Security Rule emphasizes addressable standards for which an entity can do whatever it can reasonably argue is appropriate. However, the Security Rule provides the framework.

Questions

Reading Questions

1. What is the relationship between workflow and security?
2. Compare and contrast gap analysis and risk analysis?
3. What is the meaning of "addressable" in the context of an addressable specification in the HIPAA Security Rule?
4. What is the relationship between cryptography and public key infrastructure?

Doing Questions

Imagine that you run a small medical clinic. The threats T to security of protected health information have been identified as:

- T1: cleaning crew that arrives during the night and might gain access to records left on desks.
- T2: cleaning crew that arrives during the night and might gain access to records stored on the computer.
- T3: claims that are transmitted unencrypted across the Internet from your office to a clearinghouse.

The possible remedial actions have been identified as:

- R1: locking any paper records in cabinets at the end of the day.
- R2: training cleaning crew about importance of not looking at records.
- R3: encrypting protected health information both on the hard drive and for Internet transmission.
- R4: increasing rate of changing passwords.

Provide a plausible expected loss and frequency for each threat and then a severity of threat based on the table "severity of threats." Then estimate:

- The cost of each remedial action (along with a one sentence explanation of why that cost)
- The percent reduction of a remedial action (or countermeasure) for each threat

Then complete an "analysis of countermeasures" table by entering the relevant preceding values into it and computing the:

- Total severity reduction
- Cost/benefit ratio

Finally, using a cutoff of 0.8, say what countermeasures should be implemented.

References

American Society for Testing and Materials. (1996). *Guide for electronic authentication of healthcare information: E1762*. West Conshohocken, PA: ASTM International.

Barkley, J., Beznosov, K., & Uppal, J. (1999). Supporting relationships in access control using role based access control. In *Fourth ACM Workshop on Role-Based Access Control* (pp. 55-65). Fairfax, VA: ACM Press.

Barrett, P. (1987). Implementing the Rivest Shamir and Adleman public key encryption algorithm on a standard digital signal processor. In *Advances in Cryptology—CRYPTO 86* (pp. 311-323). Santa Barbara, CA.

Dechow, J., Price, A., Kerber, J., Brancato, C., & Shaw, K. (2005). Readers' perspectives…The HIPPA security rule has contributed to better protection of patient information. Do you agree or disagree? *Health Data Management, 13*(12), 64.

Department of Health and Human Services. (2003). Health insurance reform: Security standards; Final Rule: 45 CFR Parts 160, 162, and 164; Department of Health and Human Services. *Federal Register, 68*(34), 8333-8381.

Ferraiolo, D. (2000). *Role-based access control.* National Institute for Standards and Technology. Retrieved May 2006, from http://hissa.ncsl.nist.gov/project/rbac.html

Government Accounting Office. (2000a). *Information security: Serious and widespread weaknesses persist at federal agencies: Report GAO/AIMD-00-295 to the House of Representatives*. Retrieved May 2006, from http://www.gao.gov/new.items/ai00295.pdf

Government Accounting Office. (2000b). *VA information systems: Computer security weaknesses persist at the Veterans Health Administration: Report GAO/AIMD-00-232 to the Acting Secretary of Veterans Affairs*. Retrieved May 2006, from http://www.gao.gov/new.items/ai00232.pdf

Griew, A., & Currell, R. (2000). Information, healthcare needs and security in the new NHS. *Health Informatics Journal, 6*, 61-66.

Group, H.C.T.W. (2005). *HIMSS CPRI Toolkit: Managing information privacy and security in healthcare*. Chicago: Health Information and Management Systems Society (HIMSS).

Hagland, M. (1997). Confidence and confidentiality. *Health Management Technology, 18*(12), 20-25.

Hagland, M. (1998). Six opinions on IT security. *Health Management Technology, 19*(12), 16-21.

Hellerstein, D. (1999). HIPAA's impact on healthcare. *Health Management Technology, 20*(3), 10-15.

Kaiser Permanente Medical Care Program. (1999). *Developing policies, procedures, and practices, section 4.3 sample security policies: Kaiser Permanente Northern California*. Retrieved May 2006, from http://www.health.ufl.edu/hipaa/full_toolkit.pdf

Lynch, J., Reed-Fouquet, L., Leung, W.-Y., Ruenhorst, P., & Martin, M. (2000). A healthcare public key infrastructure, The Connecticut experience. In *Annual Conference of Health Information and Managements Systems Society* (pp. 158-164). Dallas, TX: Health Information and Managements Systems Society. Retrieved from http://www.himss.org/content/files/proceedings/2000/sessions/ses116.pdf

Meissner, M., Kim, A., Collman, J., Hoffman, L., & Mun, S. (1997). *Case study: Project Phoenix - Risk analysis of a telemedicine system*. Retrieved May 2006, from http://www.health.ufl.edu/hipaa/full_toolkit.pdf

National Institute of Standards and Technology. (1996). *Generally accepted principles and practices for securing information technology systems: Special Publication 800-14*. Retrieved May 2006, from http://csrc.nist.gov/publications/nistpubs/

National Institute of Standards and Technology. (2001). *Underlying technical models for information technology security: Special Publication 800-33*. Retrieved from http://csrc.nist.gov/publications/nistpubs/

National Institute of Standards and Technology. (2002). *Risk management guide for information technology systems: Report NIST SP 800-30*. Rockville, MD.

National Research Council. (1991). *Computers at risk: Safe computing in the information age*. Washington, DC: National Academy Press.

National Research Council. (2002). *Cybersecurity today and tomorrow: Pay now or pay later*. Washington, DC: National Academies Press.

Rada, R., Haigh, P., Hebert, B., Klawans, C., & Newton, T. (2002). HIPAA best practices and tools. *HIMSS Annual Conference*. Chicago: Health Information and Management Systems Society. Retrieved from http://www.himss.org/content/files/proceedings/2002/sessions/ses133.pdf

Summers, R. (2000). *Secure computing: Threats and safeguards*. New York: McGraw-Hill.

Chapter XI

Personnel

Learning Objectives

- Observe patterns in healthcare personnel employment in the U.S. both in absolute number of employees and in relative number of employees in the allied healthcare sector
- Distinguish the hierarchical relations between administrators and some staff from the dotted-line relation from administrators to physicians
- Appreciate that while physicians have much independence, their cooperation with information systems development is crucial to the computer-based patient record
- Observe the role of nurses, as they are the most likely to routinely use computers in updating patient records
- Recognize the profession for medical records staff who have their own professional societies and certifications
- Formulate the responsibilities of the chief information officer and the structure of the organization that reports to this chief

Successful information systems depend more on people than on technology. What are the *roles* that are filled in a healthcare organization? Major roles are those of nurse and physician. Within the organizational hierarchy, the chief information officer is particularly important to information systems.

Patterns

The last one hundred years witnessed a dramatic growth in the number and types of *personnel* employed in the healthcare sector. The numbers rose from about 0.5 million in 1910 to about 7.5 million in 1990. This growth outstripped the American population growth and showed an increasing ratio of health personnel to the general population (see Table 11.1).

More extraordinary than the increased supply of health personnel has been the increasing number of categories of personnel. The U.S. Department of Labor recognizes *400 different job titles* in the health sector. Physicians constituted 30% of all health personnel in 1910 but 10% in 1990. Dentists and pharmacists fell in numbers from about 10% of the healthcare workforce in 1910 to about 2% of the healthcare workforce in 1990. Registered nurses rose in number from about 17% of the workforce in 1910 to 25% in 1990. What has been remarkable has been the growth in the categories of allied health technicians, technologists, aides, and assistants. They constituted 1 percent in 1910 and over half the health workforce in 1990. These figures should not mask the fact that all groups have increased in absolute number from year to year (Williams & Torrens, 2001).

The health services industry provided more than *11 million jobs* in 2000 (Bureau of Labor Statistics, 2006). Almost one-half of all salaried health services jobs were in hospitals. Another one-third of salaried jobs were in either nursing and personal care facilities or offices of physicians.

Workers in health services tend to be *older* than workers in other industries. They are also more likely to remain employed in the same occupation due, in part, to the high level of education and training required for many health occupations.

Health services firms employ large numbers of workers in *professional and service occupations*. Together, these two occupational groups cover 75% of the jobs in the industry. The next largest share of jobs is in office and administrative support. Management, business, and financial operations occupations account for only 5% of employment (Table 11.2).

Average earnings of non-supervisory workers in health services are slightly higher than the average for all private industry, with hospital workers earning considerably more than the average, and those in nursing and personal care facilities and home healthcare services earning less. Average earnings often are higher in hospitals because the percentage of jobs requiring higher levels of education and training is greater than in other segments. Segments of the industry with lower earnings employ large numbers of part-time service workers.

As in most industries, professionals and managers working in health services typically earn more than other workers do. Earnings in individual health services occupations vary as widely as their duties, level of education and training, and amount

Table 11.1. The ratio of health care employees to total population shows that for the years 1910, 1990, and 2000, one health care employee covers 186, 33, and 25 people, respectively.

People	1910	1990	2000
Employed in health sector	500,000	7,500,000	11,000,000
Total US population	93,000,000	250,000,000	280,000,000

Table 11.2. Employment statistics. Employment of wage and salary workers in health services by occupation in the year 2000. Will not add to totals due to omission of occupations with small employment. (Employment in thousands)

Occupation	Employment	
	Number	%
All occupations	11,065	100.0
Management, business, and financial	546	4.9
Professional and related occupations	4,975	45.0
Physicians and surgeons	459	4.1
Registered nurses	1,774	16.0
Dental hygienists	142	1.3
Radiology technologists and technicians	159	1.4
Health practitioner support technicians	210	1.9
Licensed nurses	552	5.0
Medical records and informatics	118	1.1
Service occupations	3,275	29.6
Dental assistants	237	2.1
Home health aides	261	2.4
Nursing aides and orderlies	1,053	9.5
Medical assistants	301	2.7
Maids and housekeeping cleaners	245	2.2
Personal and home care aides	160	1.4
Administrative support occupations	1,987	18.0
Administrative worker supervisor	147	1.3
Billing clerks and machine operators	166	1.5
Receptionists and information clerks	288	2.6
Office clerks, general	264	2.4
Medical secretaries	280	2.5

of responsibility (Table 11.3). *Earnings* vary not only by type of establishment and occupation, but also by size.

Unionization is more common in hospitals. In 2000, 14% of hospital workers and 10% of workers in nursing and personal care facilities were members of unions or covered by union contracts, compared with 14% of all workers in private industry.

Looking simply at *acute care hospitals* is enough to illustrate the complexity of the healthcare personnel situation. Hospitals are considered one of the most complex organizations in modern society. With the governing board holding legal authority and responsibility, and with the medical staff making decisions regarding patient care, administrators are delegated responsibility for day-to-day operation (see Figure 11.1). The organizational model suggests a hierarchical decomposition of responsibilities and authorities for the administration of the healthcare organization.

Physicians

The *physician* is traditionally the primary leader of the healthcare team. A physician is qualified by formal education and legal authority to practice medicine. Physicians earn high salaries and have traditionally enjoyed great independence.

An acute care organization, such as a hospital, has a medical staff that includes physicians and other qualified providers, such as dentists. The primary responsibility of the medical staff is the quality of the professional services given by members

Table 11.3. Hourly wages. Median hourly earnings of the largest occupations in health services in the year 2000.

Occupation	Hourly wage in $
Health services managers	27.12
Dental hygienists	24.70
Registered nurses	21.56
Radiology technicians	17.25
Licensed nurses	13.96
Dental assistants	12.47
Medical assistants	11.07
Receptionists and information clerks	10.15
Nursing aides and attendants	8.83
Home health aides	8.10

Figure 11.1. Organizational model. This community hospital organizational chart shows the president's relation to administrative vice-presidents, the medical staff, and the board (Mattingly, 1997). The five vice-presidents report to the president, and the units reporting to the vice president are listed after the vice president's title. The diagram omits much detail, and, for instance, does not show the Medical Records Department that might report to a vice-president or the chief of medical staff.

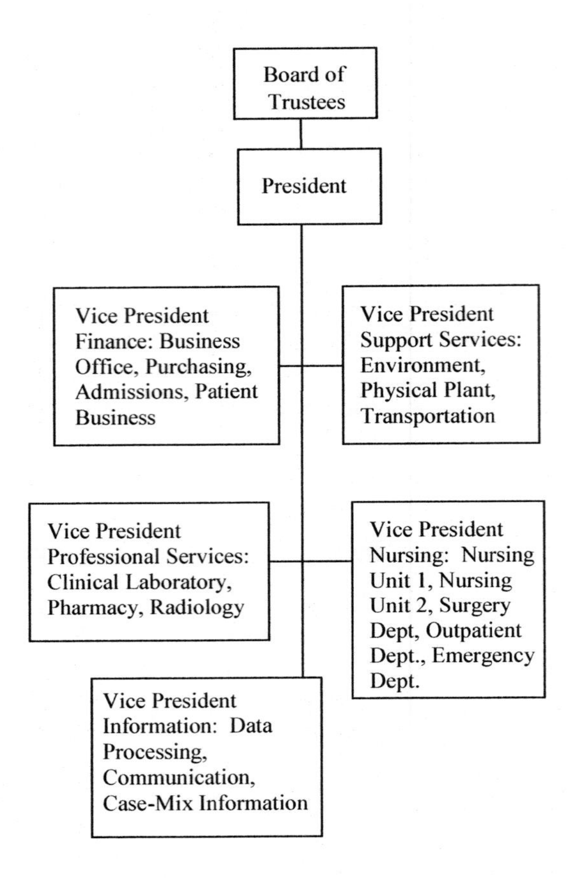

of the staff. *Medical staff* in an acute care organization is organized into officers, committees, and clinical services. Within the set of responsibilities that have to be discharged in the hospital, medical staff responsibilities include recommending staff appointments, delineating clinical privileges, continuing professional education, and maintaining a high quality of patient care. Members of the medical staff review the quality of most clinically significant functions, including, for instance, surgery, pediatrics, drug dosage, and blood usage.

Historically, physicians had little external review by non-physicians of their performance. Note in the hierarchy of the hospital that the chief of medical staff reports directly to the board of directors rather than to the president or CEO. The physicians have always preferred this relative autonomy.

While *peer-peer review* of physicians remains the predominant mode of quality control of doctors' services, the trend is toward having physicians measured by their outcomes in a quantitative way from data collected by the provider organization. The era of *profiling* hospitals arrived in the 1980s, when the Health Care Financing Administration began paying hospitals fixed case rates for Medicare patients. Hospitals, in turn, began to study the practice habits of physicians because their orders for services for Medicare inpatients determined whether or not the hospitals profited from the care they delivered.

Hospitals profile physicians' habits for economic credentialing. Hospitals may decide that certain clinicians do not warrant admitting privileges because their practice habits adversely affect the economic performance of the hospital.

When administrators at *Providence Medical Center* in Seattle presented profiling data to the medical staff, the medical staff first rebelled and said that the data was unreliable and unacceptable. Then the physicians became aware that they might lose a substantial proportion of their patients to other providers contracting with managed care plans if their outcomes were not as favorable as those of other providers. Medical staff then asked the hospital to initiate profiling. Every member of each clinical specialty department received his or her data compared to all other physicians in the same department. The range of variation discovered for most common diagnoses was much wider than members of staff had expected. After release of these findings, interest in development of practice guidelines appeared for the first time. After one year, a retrospective assessment of the program revealed a surprisingly large decline in average length of stay (from 5.3 days to 4.8 days). This accounted for a savings of 7,700 hospital bed days and made the hospital more attractive to health plans as a contract partner.

To correct for problems found in the profiles, *clinical practice guidelines* are appropriate. A clinical practice guideline codifies expectations for inputs, the features of treatment, and the outcomes. With guidelines and computerized information systems to identify inputs and outcomes, some surveillance of adherence to guidelines can be automated. Most healthcare institutions have simple clinical guidelines or protocols printed on paper for clinicians to memorize and to recall when they see a patient for whom the guideline applies.

Successful implementation of guidelines requires incentives, awareness, constant reminders, and systematic profiling of those who do and do not follow the guidelines. Achieving such conditions and trying gradually to get more and more information into digital forms that will facilitate semi-automation of *guideline adherence* is a big challenge. Yet meeting this challenge is critical to the long-term impact of health information systems. Until doctors use the information systems, the benefits of the systems will not increase much.

The realization of the importance of the physician to hospital information systems leads to the suggestion that the healthcare organization should have a clinician CIO who works in parallel with a technical CIO. The technical CIO would supervise and manage the organization that installs and maintains computer and communications technologies. The *clinical CIO* leads clinicians to successful data standardization, collection, and analysis for clinical quality improvement and outcomes management. The clinical CIO supervises a division of clinical informatics devoted to data collection to support profiling of physicians and clinical quality improvement exercises (Ruffin, 1999).

Nurses

Since Florence Nightingale founded modern nursing in the 19th century, *nurses* have been at the center of patient care. Nursing involves both simple tasks like administering medications and complex tasks like determining the response of a patient to treatment. The specific nurse's scope of practice varies with education, specialty, institutional policy, skill, and experience. Typically, a hospital pays a salary or an hourly wage to a nurse but pays doctors for the product of their labor. Thus, the nurse is more likely to have record-keeping tasks that are dutifully performed without fear that income will be reduced due to lack of time to produce more billable patient events.

Nursing consumes 40% of the typical hospital-operating budget. Nursing personnel systems track all human resource planning information necessary to manage the nursing workforce. *Personnel databases* can include information regarding every position (availability and specifications) and each individual (employment history, performance tracking, wage and salary history, professional registration, credentialing, and educational history). The staff scheduling system uses the database provided by the personnel management system and functions with the patient classification system to generate staff schedules based on specific patient care requirements (Mills, 1995).

When a health information system has come from multiple vendors, the nurse is likely to be the user most confronted with the dilemma of dealing with it. The nurse is often the *link* between the physician, the departments, and the patient. The nurse may need to have different passwords for different systems and to learn different computer commands and interface styles.

Nurses are responsible for collecting information from patients of the following sorts (Tranbarger, 1991):

- Vital signs, including temperature, pulse, blood pressure, and respirations
- Medications, including type of drug given, when, by what route, and dosage
- Intravenous fluids, including volume hung, amount infused, rate of flow, substances added, and location of access line
- Standard measures, including weight, height, intake and output, response to treatment, and laboratory values
- Other values monitored at bedsides, including arrhythmia patterns and blood pressure

Appropriate data elements are included in a nurse's *admission assessment* and updated at regular intervals. The information may have to be recorded in different parts of the patient record or in different online databases. This places a burden on the nurse who must identify what needs to be done, perform the function, and record the results. One function may cause the nurse to visit five different sites, look through several different forms, and then document the same information in multiple sites. Computerization can make this process easier or harder depending on how it is done. If all information has to be entered at computer terminals in a central location but most functions are performed at the bedside, then the difference between these two locations is a problem. Handheld data entry devices and bedside terminals might help the nurse perform the data entry functions.

Estimates of time spent by professional nurses on *documentation* vary from 40 to 75 percent. This is an enormous component of the hospital budget given the number of nurses and their hourly cost. Furthermore, nurses frequently do charting after their shifts end. When nurses work after their shift, they earn overtime pay, but also the opportunities for mistake through omission increase. Information systems should help the nurse effortlessly document workflow and patient results at the point of care.

Medical Record Staff

The *medical records department* includes several roles. For medical records, a director will primarily direct the work of a clinical data manager, a record processing manager, a transcription supervisor, and a coordinator of quality control and training (see Figure 11.2). These roles may themselves have sub-roles. For instance, the manager of clinical data supervises coder staff and data quality staff.

Medical records administrators receive special education and certification, as do physicians, nurses, and allied health professionals. The medical records administrator has these responsibilities:

Figure 11.2. Medical records roles. The role hierarchy for a Medical Records Department is depicted. Underneath each of the leaf nodes are multiple line staff, such as coding staff, processing staff, and transcription staff. Additionally, some roles are omitted for simplicity's sake, such as that of trainer.

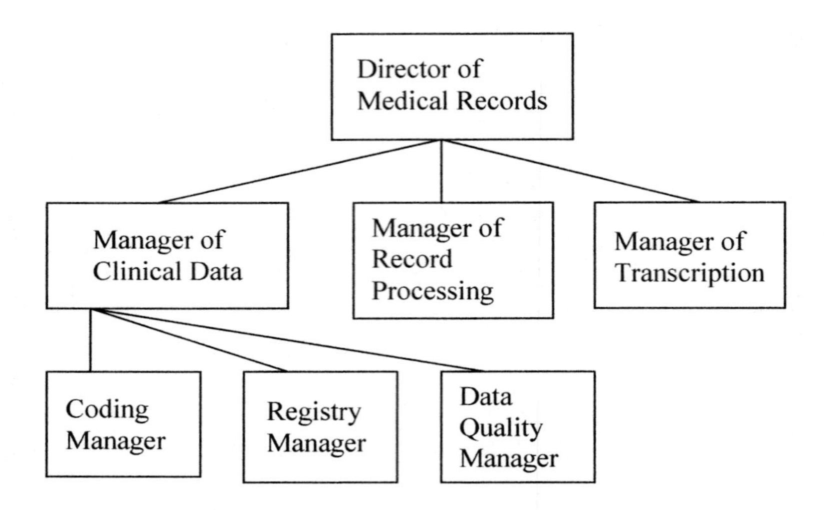

- Maintaining patient information systems consistent with legal, clinical, and accreditation requirements
- Processing, compiling, maintaining, and reporting patient data
- Abstracting and coding clinical data

In the United States the professional society most associated with medical records administrations is the *American Health Information Management Association* (www.ahima.org), which has 40,000 members. AHIMA issues credentials in health information management. Members earn credentials through a combination of education, experience, and performance on national certification exams. AHIMA two primary certificates are:

- Registered health information administrators (RHIAs) are skilled in the collection, interpretation, and analysis of patient data. Additionally, they receive the training necessary to assume managerial positions related to these functions. RHIAs interact with all levels of an organization—clinical, financial, and administrative—that employ patient data in decision-making and everyday operations. Historically, most RHIAs have held the title of director of the health information management department of an acute care facility. As patient records evolve toward computerization and as more entities such as third-party payers require health data, RHIAs benefit from a wider selection of roles in the industry. Information security and storage, data quality assurance, and advanced assistance to consumers with their health information are among the new domains.

- Registered health information technicians (RHITs) are health information technicians who ensure the quality of medical records by verifying their completeness, accuracy, and proper entry into computer systems. They may also use computer applications to assemble and analyze patient data for the purpose of improving patient care or controlling costs. RHITs often specialize in coding diagnoses and procedures in patient records for reimbursement and research. RHITs may serve as cancer registrars, compiling and maintaining data on cancer patients. The majority of RHITs are coders.

Historically, AHIMA members were basically coders. The Association encourages its members to assume aggressive professional careers and has evidence that that is happening. For instance, from 1999 to 2000 the number of AHIMA members who were compliance officers doubled; the number of information security officers has seen similar growth.

Each year, AHIMA collects professional data from its credentialed members as part of the annual membership cycle (Zender, 2003). The year 2001 survey includes responses from *31,000 credentialed members*. About 60% had RHIT and about 40% had RHIA certificates.

One-third of the respondents report *salaries* exceeding $40,000. Education is a key factor in determining salary levels and job opportunities. The data illustrate a dramatic progression in salary with higher educational levels: 7% of members with associate's degrees earned $50,000 to $74,999, while 22% of members with baccalaureate degrees earned $50,000 to $74,999, and 40% of members with master's degrees had income in this range. About half the members have earned a baccalaureate degree or higher.

Salaries are proportional to *managerial responsibility*:

- Director's average salary is about $50,000 per year
- Manager's average salary is about $42,000 per year
- Coder average salary is about $23,000 per year
- Consultant's average salary is about $50,000 per year

Working in a multi-hospital or diversified network is likely to mean a higher salary than in a single hospital, mental institution, or long-term care facility.

Earnings also increase with experience in the workplace. The biggest jump into salary brackets of $50,000 or more takes place after 10 years in the workplace. Salary gains stabilize after 20 years of experience.

IT Staff

Administrators approve *budgets* for information systems that amount in dollars to (Ruffin, 1999):

- Tens of thousands for small group practices
- Hundreds of thousands for group practices of 30 to 100 people
- Millions for single hospitals
- Tens of millions for multi-hospital systems

The healthcare organization may have various *structures* for dealing with information systems:

- In one extreme the entire information systems operation is outsourced and the only role in the healthcare organization itself for information systems is a liaison with the vendors, contractors, and consultants on hire to provide support.
- At the other extreme, the healthcare organization does everything itself, including developing its own unique software.

An IT department may be organized in various ways. An IT department may be organized by:

- Job function with, for instance, a communications unit to handle local and wide area networks and a data administration unit to handle databases
- Product lines with, for instance, a billing and administrative unit, a human and facility resource unit, and a clinical unit
- Organizational process with, for instance, a unit for patient revenue cycle and a unit for medical services
- Function and geography. This occurs for integrated delivery networks that have facilities in diverse geographical locations. The IT Department will have

some central units for core infrastructure, such as the wide-area network, but also some units for geographic regions

Of course, these four different approaches might occur in various combinations with one another and what is best for a given healthcare entity depends on a variety of factors not the least of which is the most natural fit with the organization of the parts of the healthcare entity outside the IT Department.

One factor that characterizes an IT Department is its degree of centralization or decentralization. Some functions may be *centralized*, such as database administration, and some decentralized, such as training and end-user support. The organization of the healthcare entity to which the IT Department belongs will also be critical. For instance, if the entity has several nearly autonomous hospitals, then one might expect the IT department to provide separate IT units for each of those hospitals.

As regards roles within a unit of an IT department, two examples are provided. The IT Department may have a unit for:

- Operations
- General user support

The *operations unit* is responsible for the ongoing operation of the data processing systems. Shifts of operators keep the systems operating 24 hours a day, 7 days a week. The unit may also be responsible for the communications system of the organization. The operation's unit might include these roles:

- Operations supervisor to schedule staff, maintain quality assurance, and establish directions
- Shift supervisor for the details of supervising a particular shift
- Senior and junior operators for daily work schedule implementation and troubleshooting
- Rounds technicians manage the user devices, such as terminals, printers, and telephones
- Data-entry staff for data like payroll data
- Document control clerk to supervise data-entry staff

A *general user support unit* is responsible for user coordination and support. Roles in that unit include:

- Support manager oversees allocation of staff to problems and set direction
- User support manager oversees the help desk and clinical operations
- Systems analyst evaluates application functionality required by user departments
- Programmers craft software programs based on specifications from the systems analysts
- Technical writers prepare documentation for internally developed applications
- Database managers create and maintain database software and data
- Help-line staff answer basic questions following help-line scripts
- Trainers develop and deliver training and maintain an information technology competency inventory of the staff in the healthcare organization

One or more individuals may fill a role based on the unit's size and available skill sets (Harmon et al., 2003).

CIO

The senior information systems role is the *CIO*. Responsibilities, qualifications, and career paths for CIOs are diverse.

Responsibilities

The CIO is responsible for:

- Information systems processing and development as the liaison between IS staff and senior management
- Telecommunications
- Systems maintenance and user support
- Liaising with medical records, admissions, patient accounting, and related information intensive departments of the health care organization
- Technology planning
- Vision and strategy with senior management

The CIO must develop an IS vision for the organization. This vision need not be obtainable in the mid-term but the organization should be able to work systematically toward it.

For a single hospital environment, the CIO may direct admissions, medical records, IS development, IS maintenance, IS operations, and IS user support (see Figure 11.3). The CIO would report to the *chief executive officer* and have a steering committee from throughout the hospital and an IS-specific administrative staff. In a multi-corporate environment, the CIO may be responsible for IS managers at each installation as well as for centralized systems planning, development, and maintenance.

As mentioned earlier in the section on physicians, a provider organization may want to have a medical CIO and a technical or administrative CIO. The *medical CIO* responsibilities broadly speaking are to:

- Support the development of clinical information systems that assist clinicians in the delivery of patient care
- Represent the needs and requirements of the physician community and serve as an advocate of management in promoting the use of information technology in the clinical setting

The responsibilities in further detail from one example are listed as (Sittig, 1999):

- Chairs clinical advisory groups to provide broad-based input into the design of the clinical information system
- Leads and facilitates clinician advisory groups in the design of clinical systems to support excellence in patient care and research
- Engages patient care providers with varying roles including physicians, nursing practitioners, nursing staff, ancillary department personnel, and medical records professionals to contribute to the development and use of the clinical information system
- Develops empathy and understanding of physician needs and builds relationships with physicians to gain support of IT initiatives
- Is highly responsive to users' needs, including training, to assure wide-spread acceptance and provider use of the clinical systems
- Reviews medical informatics trends, experiences and approaches, develops technical and application implementation strategies and assists in the development of strategic plans for clinical information systems
- Works in concert with information technology services to design and implement systems supporting patient care and research activities

Figure 11.3. CIO: Management structure for a CIO in a single hospital environment. CEO is synonymous with president.

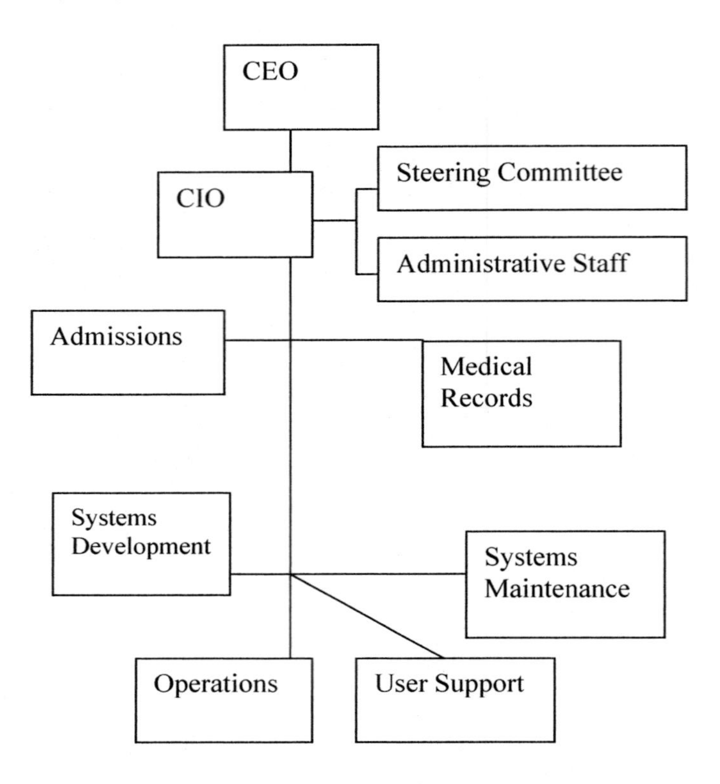

- Leads design of clinical pathway models with physician, nursing and administrative leadership, and will assist in modification of these models to gain maximum efficacy and support for patient care and research protocols
- Leads development of clinical "rules" supporting patient care and protocol research as well as the design of clinical system features supporting protocol management and the use of the system to leverage the clinicians' time and maximize communication with affiliates and referring physicians
- Designs and evaluates collection of data for clinical purposes, including tracking and interpretation of outcomes
- Participates in clinical activities: Provides patient care in appropriate clinical setting. Reviews patient assessments and management plans. Participates in applicable clinical research. Has active medical practice in area of specialty

The decision about who should be the *CIO* should be done with great care by a broad range of concerned individuals. By definition, the CIO will impact patient care, financial management, and administrative operations, and people from these units should all be consulted in the appointment of a CIO. The CIO should have a *background* in technical and managerial areas and should understand healthcare.

Career Paths

The CIO is responsible for managing information. This must be a collaborative effort involving both the policy setting and operational units of the organization. Three *biographical sketches* of CIOs are presented next and shed insight into the requirements for the position and the type of people who fill it.

Kay Carr is the CIO at St. Luke's Hospital in the Texas Medical Center in Houston, Texas (Schriner, 1998). She was educated in finance and became a *certified public accountant*. Her professional experiences demonstrated her managerial aptitude, and she rose through the ranks to become director of financial planning and controller. She was an outspoken critic of IT investments, and in 1995 when the hospital needed a new CIO, the CEO and CFO approached Kay. They wanted someone whose priority would be business decisions and not technical decisions. Carr brought her business experience, insider knowledge and the relationships she had developed with key stakeholders to her position. To assist her with the technical side, the hospital contracted for external technical support. Some IT staff did not want to see a CPA from the finance division become CIO and feared that IT would be overcome by finance concerns. While Carr utilizes her planning and management skill, she leaves the technical development to the technical experts. Carr says,

Sometimes I have to put my pride on the line and say, 'I don't know what that means.'

With internal expertise and external support, Carr rapidly deployed new IT projects, including new systems for payroll, human resources, pharmacology, radiology, medical records, and a new network.

Joan Hicks is the director of health system information services for the University of Alabama Health System. Hicks began her healthcare career as a *file clerk* in medical records at an acute care facility (Schriner, 1998). Fourteen years later, she was medical records director with responsibilities ranging from utilization and review to medical staff services and risk management. The CEO asked her to think about taking over the CIO position. Instead of accepting the offer, Hicks decided she needed more formal training. She took a position teaching medical records skills at the University of Alabama at Birmingham. While she was a faculty member, she also earned a master's of science in health informatics from the same university. After graduating, she spent two years in healthcare consulting in Atlanta before returning to Alabama to become director of medical information services for Children's Health System in Birmingham. Hicks feels that her technical knowledge is her weak suit, but she believes that technical expertise is not the most important skill for the top IT positions.

George Conklin started his career as a *research psychologist* and got progressively more involved in technology. He worked at New York State's Nathan Kline Institute for Psychiatric Research on database projects to help gauge and predict the behavior of mental health patients. His work led to a job managing the clinical information systems at Columbia Presbyterian Hospital in New York. Later Conklin joined the Sisters of Charity Healthcare System as the Houston organization's first VP of information management and CIO. Conklin's philosophy is to put trust in the business managers and win the respect of the people with whom you work. Conklin stays on top of ever-changing technology by reading IT journals and publications, meeting with vendors, and attending seminars. Conklin notes that in one job (McGee, 1998):

I was somewhat blinded by my successes and started to appreciate less the people who worked with me and helped me achieve them. This wasn't greeted well by others, and I've reaffirmed that I can't do it myself. The successes I've had in my career are the result of a lot of people.

In addition to winning the trust of business managers, CIOs must also win the respect of the other people with whom they work.

To summarize, the three CIOs did not start with formal training in IT nor initially worked in IT. CIOs are recruited from *diverse environments*. Technicians tend to put less emphasis on the financial aspects. The CEO, the CFO, and the board of directors are asking how much a project will cost and when it is delivered because "time is money."

Career opportunities for those already in CIO positions are multiple (Ummel, 2003). The healthcare industry is so pluralistic that different paths exist in different situations. CIOs with business and leadership strengths may achieve new accountabilities for enterprise-wide, information-related operations like registration and scheduling, central business offices, and medical records. In entities that are undergoing mergers, as many are, the CIO has further opportunities as the critical processes of internal integration and transformation rely partly on information systems.

CIOs may grow at times not through further line responsibility but through a shift in *reporting relationships*. Often the CIO reports to the CFO. However, a better situation for the CIO is to report directly to the CEO or the COO. Such a re-alignment is promising for a CIO.

Federal Workforce Surveys

A healthcare organization has many people involved directly in patient care. One category is doctors of dentistry, pharmacy, and optometry. Another category is "allied health professionals." More than *200 allied health occupations* exist, including medical technology, respiratory therapy, occupational therapy, and dietetics (Smith, 2000). These professionals may be involved in diagnosis, therapy, education, counseling, and management. As healthcare has become more complex, the allied health profession has grown. A health information system must be sensitive to the needs of this increasingly important population in the healthcare organization.

The *Bureau of Labor Statistics* projected that about 14 percent of all wage and salary jobs created between 1998 and 2008 would be in health services. The Health Resources and Services Administration collects workforce profiles. It does this for every state according to many categories. No specific category addresses information systems personnel. However, one gets a sense of the priorities in healthcare employment by reviewing this data. A snapshot is provided for an arbitrary state, in this case the state of Maryland (Health Resources and Services Administration, 2000). The proportions are similar for each state by population.

More than 204,000 people are employed in the health sector in *Maryland*, 9% of Maryland's total workforce. More Maryland health service workers were employed by hospitals (42%) than in any other healthcare setting. More than 16% of Maryland's health service workers were employed in nursing and personal care facilities. Further details are as follows:

- 13,000 active patient care physicians
- 48,700 licensed registered nurses and 10,000 licensed practical/vocational nurses
- 808 physician assistants practicing, 500 nurse practitioners, 174 certified nurse midwives, and 323 certified registered nurse anesthetists
- 2,891 dentists, 2,650 dental hygienists, and 4,050 dental assistants
- 3,320 pharmacists and 5,540 pharmacy technicians and aides
- 975 psychiatrists, 1,900 psychologists and 10,100 social workers
- 4,770 home health aides and 22,560 nursing aides and orderlies

The category that comes closest to intersecting with information technology staff is the category of technicians and technologists which for Maryland includes the following:

- 2,650 emergency medical technicians
- 6,760 medical and clinical laboratory technologists
- 1,340 medical records technicians
- 2,990 radiology technologists and 350 nuclear medicine technologists

There exists no generally recognized *license* for information systems specialists and particularly not within healthcare. Yet, healthcare is one of the most carefully licensed and controlled workforces in the U.S. The Health Information and Management Systems Society introduced a certification program effective 2002. Whether or not this program will gain acceptability and lead eventually to a category of health profession that is included in census taking remains to be seen.

Salaries

The *Health Information and Management Systems Society* (HIMSS) has members in hospitals, corporate healthcare systems, clinical practice groups, vendor organizations, healthcare consulting firms, and government settings in professional levels ranging from line staff to CEOs. The 1998 HIMSS Annual Compensation Survey represented 2,200 responding members of HIMSS. The typical respondent worked in information systems at a hospital. The average salary of respondents was $60,200, while the average IT salary across the U.S. was $71,000. For the HIMSS respondents:

- Average experience in the IT industry: 11.4 years
- Average weekly hours worked: 46.3

Number of employers in last three years:

- One: 53%
- Two: 37%
- Three: 10%

Highest level of education obtained:

- High school: 16%
- Associate's degree: 10%
- Bachelor's degree: 52%
- Master's degree: 21%

The following findings are an overview of each professional level surveyed in this study.

CEO/COO/CFO/Partner

- Earns $154,000 annually in total cash compensation
- Has been in current position for 10 to 14 years
- Directly supervises 6 to 10 people
- Works 54 hours per week

CIO

- Earns $125,000 annually in total cash compensation
- Has been in current position for 5 to 9 years
- Directly supervises 26 to 50 people
- Works 55 hours per week

Department Head

- Earns $81,000 annually in total cash compensation
- Received a 5% annual pay increase
- Has been in current position for 5 to 9 years
- Directly supervises 11 to 25 people
- Works 51 hours per week

Senior Staff

- Earns $70,000 annually in total cash compensation
- Has been in current position for 5 to 9 years

- Directly supervises 1 to 5 people
- Works 49 hours per week

Line Staff

- Earns $52,000 annually in total cash compensation
- Has been in current position for 2 to 4 years
- Has little, if any, supervisory responsibilities
- Works 45 hours per week

Clearly, the positions of higher managerial responsibility have higher salaries.

In the HIMSS survey, the average salary was $60,200 and this average ranged from $52,000 for a typical staff position to $116,000 for a senior management position. In the AHIMA survey described in the subsection about medical records staff, the salaries ranged from $23,000 for a coder to $50,000 for a director or consultant. Although a larger percentage of the HIMSS respondents had degrees than the AHIMA respondents (73% or the former and about 50% of the latter had Bachelors degrees or higher), this may not account for the large salary differences. AHIMA is an association that is mainly focused on medical records. HIMSS members are involved in healthcare applications of IT, and particularly innovative applications. IT staff in healthcare require higher salaries to attract and retain than medical records staff, since the IT staff have *options* of lucrative careers in other industries. Medical records professionals do not have the option of using their skills in a different industry in order to secure better salaries.

Retention

All industries *compete* for IT staff. The further one goes into the technical ranks, the less one needs healthcare knowledge. In the provider community, the move toward market-based compensation has been slow because these organizations are used to employees being captive to healthcare.

Retention strategies should be employed. Employees want progression paths and to understand how their career could grow. No one feels his or her career is enhanced through dedication to an organization utilizing "old" technology.

Mount Carmel Health System in Columbus, Ohio had 40% of its IT positions open, losing three to five people a month (Keener, 1999). They knew they had a problem, and the IT community did not hold the institution in high standing due to its high turnover. The central Ohio institution is across the street from Lucent Technologies, and their competitors also include banking, retail, insurance, and corporate headquarters. They seldom lose anyone to healthcare; it is other industries with which they are competing.

The goal of Mount Carmel's IT group is to have the "best IT department" in central Ohio, not the "best healthcare IT department." Mount Carmel competes against more than healthcare for human resources. The department did the usual things of looking at its hiring practices, but it went beyond that in restructuring its human resources approaches. Some of the more creative things included:

- The IT Department took on its own recruiter. Initially, Mount Carmel was losing people because salaries at Mount Carmel were lower than those at Lucent Technologies. The hospital made those salary adjustments.
- An employee survey revealed that people seldom left for the money, but for the opportunity for advancement. A system of career ladders was instituted, which are career paths or titles that define the levels and pay scale, based on skill levels.
- Every morning at 8:30 the IT area holds a coordination meeting for anyone who wants to attend. Lasting under 15 minutes, it addresses outstanding issues and problems, and personnel may ask for help or offer it. Over three years the department worked at retention strategies, compensation, quality of life, communications, training, recognition, a listening and open environment, and research into causes and needs.

Success has been measured in the high scores on employee surveys about the working environment, in the drop from forty to three open positions in the IT department, in the improved community comments about working at Mount Carmel, and in the movement of contractors under "contract with option to hire" agreements to employee status.

Healthcare, when forced to compete against other industries to retain IT employees, is often not successful because, historically, healthcare has been a relatively *low-paying industry*. Healthcare providers often use bonuses to try to compete more effectively with other industries for technical talent. Other industries often win a bidding war.

Questions

Reading Questions

1. How has the pattern of health personnel employment changed over the past one hundred years and what would it suggest for the patterns of the next one hundred years?
2. How is profiling affecting the physician?
3. How are the responsibilities of nurses significantly different from those for doctors?

Doing Questions

1. Consider the organizational hierarchies presented and discover information about some organization not presented, such as an ambulatory clinic, a pharmacy, or an insurance company, and indicate the personnel hierarchies that are used in that organization.
2. Physician billing is unlike lawyer billing in that lawyers charge for the hours they spend getting ready for a case, whereas doctors typically only charge for the time directly delivering care. What differences would you expect in physician involvement with healthcare information systems in these different situations and can you provide any evidence to support your expectations.
3. Nurses are the largest component of the healthcare workforce and also the portion most involved in the use of information systems. The University of Maryland at Baltimore Nursing School has one of the largest nursing informatics educational programs and many of its graduates proceed to high-level clinical information systems administrative functions in healthcare organizations. Some physicians think that physicians should be in the most senior position as regards directing clinical information systems. Explore what the current situation is (by interviewing people or studying Web sites) and discuss the changes that might occur over time.
4. Maintaining certification as a medical records administrator requires continuing education. Physicians and nurses must engage in continuing education to maintain certification. Find examples of continuing education to healthcare professionals that cover the topic of information systems and describe how you could develop a strategy for marketing such education online so as to take advantage of the need for re-certification.

5. The chief information officer has a relatively new but a vital role in the healthcare system. Find on the Web three descriptions of CIOs' positions in healthcare and summarize each briefly. You can find these from job advertisements on the Web, from magazine announcements about the accomplishments of some CIOs, or other places. For each position note the organization where the CIO is employed and your source of the information.
6. Provide a generic description of a CIO position specifically allowing you to identify by name, at least half a dozen of the roles described in this chapter. Provide this description in list format and highlight in red each reference to a role mentioned in the chapter.

References

Bureau of Labor Statistics. (2006). *Career guide to industries: Health care*. U.S. Department of Labor. Retrieved May 2006, from http://www.bls.gov/oco/cg/cgs035.htm

Harmon, B., Wah, R., & Inae, T. (2003). The military health system computer-based patient record. In *American Medical Informatics Association Annual Symposium* (p. 1068). Washington, DC: American Medical Informatics Association.

Health Resources and Services Administration. (2000). *State health workforce profiles: Maryland*. Retrieved May 2006, from ftp://ftp.hrsa.gov/bhpr/workforceprofiles/MD.pdf

Keener, R. (1999). Problems for everyone in IT staffing needs. *Health Management Technology*. Retrieved May 2006, from www.healthmgttech.com

McGee, M.K. (1998, September 28). What it takes to be a CIO. How did today's CIOs achieve their positions? Let us count the ways. *Information Week Online,* 1-4.

Mills, M.E. (1995). Computerization: Priorities for nursing administration. In M. Ball (Ed.), *Healthcare Information Management Systems: A Practical Guide* (pp. 247-258). New York: Springer Verlag.

Ruffin, M.d.G.J. (1999). *Digital doctors*. Tampa, FL: American College of Health Executives.

Schriner, M. (1998). Who's growing CIOs? *Healthcare Informatics*, (11), 77-89.

Sittig, D. (1999). *Chief medical information officer*. Association of Medical Directors of Information System. Retrieved May 2006, from http://www.informatics-review.com/jobdesc/sample3.htm

Tranbarger, R. (1991). Nurses and computers: At the point of care. In M. Ball (Ed.), *Healthcare information management systems: A practical guide* (pp. 95-102). New York: Springer Verlag.

Ummel, S. (2003). An interview with Stephen Ummel, Principal Cap Gemini Ernst & Young Health Consulting. *Journal of Healthcare Information Management, 17*(1), 27-30.

Williams, S.J., & Torrens, P. (Eds.). (2001). *Introduction to health services* (6th ed.). Albany, NY: Delmar Publishers.

Zender, A. (2003). AHIMA in the 21st century: Looking ahead. *Journal of American Health Information Management, 74*(10), 54-57.

Chapter XII

Vendors

Learning Objectives

- Identify the opportunity for consultants to provide insights from other institutions to help a healthcare organization with problems it has not routinely confronted
- Identify vendors that provide information system components for healthcare entities
- Develop a plan for large systems acquisition to begin on the provider's side with an evaluation of competing offerings and to follow with negotiations to maximize the mutual commitment to the project
- Develop a marketing plan for vendor of information systems to small clients that emphasizes a one-on-one relationship and simple, fast results
- Identify when outsourcing is appropriate

A *vendor* is any person or company that sells goods or services to someone else in the economic production chain. Parts manufacturers are vendors of parts to other manufacturers that assemble the parts into something sold to wholesalers or retailers. Retailers are vendors of products to consumers. In information technology, the term is applied to suppliers of goods and services to other companies. This chapter reviews attributes of IT vendors in healthcare. IT consultants who provide services to the healthcare industry are described and then the vendors of software and services.

IT Consultants

Cost-effective utilization of IT consultants is a skill essential to the healthcare chief information officer. In an interview of fifteen hospital administrators about consultants, the responses were varied but all said that they paid more than planned, the engagement took longer than expected, and accomplishments fell short of what was expected (Childs, 1997). Nonetheless, 11 of the 15 were relatively happy with their consultant's work, and all 15 indicated that they would be engaging another *consultant* within the year.

Services

Consulting is a *service industry* in the purest sense. A consulting firm's primary assets are its personnel. These assets produce revenue by providing services to clients. Individual consultants have specialized skills and proven experience, are established in their fields, and often have previously worked for a vendor, a hospital, or both.

The *services* that a typical healthcare information systems consultant offers are (Ball, 1991):

- Selection and evaluation of information systems
- Contract negotiations
- Implementation support
- Long-range information systems planning
- System testing
- Policy and procedure documentation
- Project management
- Quality assurance
- Reorganization
- Interface support

Healthcare institutions will request consultants for the following reasons:

- **Experience:** The consultant may have performed the task at other institutions or be familiar with the vendor whose solution is being installed in the institution. Thus the consultant can provide expertise that the healthcare institution is lacking.

- **Temporary solution:** A hospital may have need for a certain resource for a few months but no longer. In this situation of needing someone to perform a temporary job, a properly prepared consultant is more effective than a new employee who needs training but then is shortly no longer needed.
- **Objective:** Consultants are hired to review and evaluate organizational structures. The consultant brings objectivity and neutrality that the organization needs but may have difficulty obtaining internally.
- **Reference:** Consultants bring experience with systems and other hospitals that can help a hospital make a successful implementation of a new system.
- **Ownership:** Sometimes no one wants to finish some work that is required for some external reason. For instance, the Joint Commission on the Accreditation of Hospitals requires hospitals to have written policies. Typically staff does not want to write the policies in the form required for accreditation, so consultants may be hired to finish the job.
- **Risk:** Consultants may be hired when extra help is needed to complete a job or when the job seems in danger of failing. The hiring entity may want help and also a potential scapegoat in case the job is not finished successfully.

While these categories of experience, temporary solution, objective, reference, ownership, and risk are neither exhaustive nor mutually exclusive, they give a sense of what healthcare entities expect from consultants.

Consultant Perspective

From the *consultant perspective*, the attractiveness of the preceding roles could be as follows:

- **Experience:** The client needs something that I have done before, and I feel comfortable and confident to do it successfully. This is the best scenario for a consultant.
- **Temporary solution:** Not only might the job itself be temporary, but also the client may be inclined to treat the consultant in a lowly way in this "temporary solution" situation. Since the consultant might put such jobs on a low priority, the consultant might ironically ask for higher pay for such work.
- **Objective:** The client wants the consultant because the consultant is an outsider. The consultant can expect an active working environment, and people will pay attention to the views of the consultant rather than only expect the consultant to get the job done.

- **Reference:** This reference situation is also good for the consultant, as the client will be interested in the consultant's view.
- **Ownership:** The client has difficulty finding someone to take ownership, and that's why the consultant is there. The work may be less stressful given that no one else particularly cared to do the work, and the consultant might expect an easy job.
- **Risk:** The consultant is on the job because of the risk to fail. The consultant has an opportunity to show his capability but must be careful to not fail himself, even if the work may fail. Client staff may hesitate to help for fear of being associated with a likely failed effort. This is the worst situation for the consultant.

Of course, the preceding views of one consultant would not necessarily be the same as the views of another consultant. For the ownership situation, a different perspective is provided in the following scenario:

Suppose an organization hires you to write their policies and procedures. The medical staff told the administrators they are too busy to bother with this task. They want nothing to do with it, even when you ask them to review what you have written. You finish the task, without much input from the medical staff, and deliver the policy manual to the hospital administrator. Six months later, a suit is filed against the hospital because a doctor injured a patient. An investigation reveals that while the doctor performed the procedures in a similar manner to most of the doctors in that institution, he did not follow the written policy and procedures of the organization—a policy you wrote. The policy you wrote was based on what you thought the procedure should be rather than what was actually being done. You explain to the lawyers and hospital administrator that you asked the medical staff to review that particular policy, but they never did. What impact do you think this might have on your reputation as a consultant? Obviously, my point here is that the people who hired you may not care what result you get, unless something goes wrong. The darker, more troubling side of no one in the organization wanting to do a task is that they may be uninterested in or even resistant to your efforts. If you do not have adequate support for doing a task no one else wants to do, the risk of failure is significant.

Different People Will See a Job in Different Ways

The views of IT consultants on how to succeed in healthcare IT consulting are varied. The following quoted paragraphs are from Sam Wright who was a student in the author's class but also a practicing IT consultant to the healthcare industry.

His *view* is refreshingly direct:

Let me share my jaundiced view of the four rules of success for large healthcare consulting companies. This is information never put on the consulting company websites.

The first rule is charge very expensive rates. Healthcare consulting firms sell their services to hospitals and Health Maintenance Organizations (HMO) by saying that they are top healthcare experts and have experienced the problems experienced by the client, have resolved them, and will bring to the client invaluable experience. The firms charge clients anywhere from $85 per hour for a Staff Consultant to $300 per hour for a Vice President. Staff Consultants should be billable 90 to 100% of their employment time. Vice Presidents are billable 10 to 20% of the time. 80% of the Vice President's time is spent on marketing.

The second rule in consulting is selective hiring. Consulting firms hire workers that can open doors in the healthcare industry. If the consulting firm wants to compete in the private sector, they will pay employment agencies (head hunters) to search through existing hospitals and managed care organizations looking for IT directors, managers, and programmers who have skill sets needed for current or future projects. The firm offers the prospective candidates higher salaries and a chance (or requirement) to travel. The candidates bring knowledge and contacts into hospitals and HMO's. For the public sector, the consulting firms seek former congressmen or retired military officers. These people have connections into these markets, too. Next, to offset the high salaries being paid to the experienced executives, the consulting firms hire recent college graduates and pay them very little. Electronic Data Systems (EDS) uses this model. Basically, untrained college students are employed and sign a three-year financing commitment with EDS to pay for the programmer training given to them by EDS at the EDS Training facility in Dallas, Texas.

The third rule for the big consulting companies is to compete in guaranteed win situations. For example, all of the consulting firms provide Strategic Planning, System Selections, System Implementation (Management Consulting), and Facilities Management. Exploring Strategic Planning and Systems Selection in detail illustrates how a guaranteed win occurs:

Strategic planning has no risk. Basically, the consulting firm comes into a facility, reviews the existing software, hardware, and networking capabilities, and then creates a notebook or Power Point presentation recommending how the healthcare organization should plan for the future. This is no risk for the firm and is quick to accomplish. The firm will charge anywhere from 25,000 to 100,000 thousand dollars for this service depending on the size of the organization and number of consultants used.

System Selections are even more profitable. System Selections are when hospitals and HMO's desire to change their existing application for a new one. The hospital or HMO contracts a consulting firm to write the Request for Information (RFI) or Request for Proposal (RFP). Since these consulting firms have done RFI's and RFP's several times, the firm can supply the hospital or HMO with a standard set of questions that they can submit to software vendors. In other words, the hospital or HMO is paying the firm $25,000 dollars for an existing document.

The fourth and final rule for consulting success is fitting into the corporate image. Successful consulting firms require their consultants to dress in three-piece suits. CFO's of hospitals and HMO's want to see contracted labor that looks like it deserves the rates being paid.

In conclusion, consulting is a very profitable business. Firms that use the above rules make themselves very rich and very big.

While consulting can be a very profitable business, consultants also face hardships. A major challenge is to find the next contract. The parts of the job that are easy compared to a job as a regular employee of a firm are counterbalanced by the relative insecurity of the consulting job.

Companies

The healthcare entity will have a contract with the consultant. The entity will want precise *contract arrangements* that include precise deliverables at fixed times. There should be no learning curve to get immediate results from the consultants. The contract might stipulate precisely who will do the consulting work and not permit substitutes. If the consultants are local, then they might be required to work onsite.

A wide range of positions tends to be available for IT consultants in healthcare (see Figure 12.1). A national recruiter might be looking for experts in healthcare systems consulting, installation, development and sales. The companies doing the hiring would typically pay all fees.

There are many shapes and sizes of consulting company. According to the Gartner Group, the top three companies in the U.S. by *gross revenue* for health information

Figure 12.1. Sample IT consultant openings. This list of job availabilities comes from a recruiter of IT consultants in healthcare.

Data Dictionary Analyst: Near New York City, client looking for specialist to develop, test, implement and monitor data dictionaries. Wants understanding of ASTM, HL7, LOINC and or ANSI standards. ADT, billing, scheduling and clinical systems experience is a plus. Proficiency with current tools for multi-tiered database development tools.
Security Specialists: Requires knowledge of systems security, platforms, operating systems and networks. Moderate to high travel. HIPAA a plus. Location varies depending on experience.
Contracts Manager: East Coast location, consultant function. Responsible for the development and administration of IT/Telecommunications capital agreements. Aid provider clients with advice/direction on acquisition of major systems purchases.
Interim CIOs. High travel, usually involves temporary living arrangements. Ability to sell additional services a plus. High travel. Can be located anywhere.
Product Manager Benchmarking Systems: Low travel, great location on the East Coast.
Two Senior PACS Consultants: Preferably located on East Coast or willing to locate there. Responsibilities involve systems selection and strategic planning. Client wants one to be more marketing oriented.
Consulting Specialists Systems Selections: Help hospitals make critical decisions. Management-level position a possibility. Location depends on abilities. Moderate travel.
Senior Palm Developer needed in the **Northwest:** Small organization passing the breakeven point. Code Warrior required.
RN with oncology experience needed. Fairly high travel implementing new systems. Northwest, systems development opening.

systems consulting are (with their dollars earned in healthcare consulting in one year and their Web address):

- Cap Gemini Ernst & Young with $600 million (www.capgemini.com)
- SAIC with $435 million (www.saic.com)
- CSC Healthcare with $380 million (www.csc.com)

For these three, healthcare represents less than half of the company's total consulting revenue. However, numerous firms also do only healthcare consulting. For example, First Consulting Group (www.fcg.com) is a provider of information-based consulting, integration, and management services to healthcare.

Vendor Case Study

Cerner Corporation is one of the largest healthcare information systems companies. It will be described next to highlight features of a successful healthcare information systems vendor. In fact, Cerner is so successful that it is one of a few special companies that have been able to grow from zero dollars to one billion dollars in revenue in the past quarter century. Of the 7,454 U.S. companies that have issued initial public offerings since 1980 (and most companies do not get to that stage), only 5% have achieved one billion dollars in revenue, whereas 25% have gone bankrupt (Thomson, 2005). Cerner's keys to success are typical for companies that prosper (Murphy, 2006).

Background

Hospital clinical information systems tend to be purchased from a single vendor. Two-thirds of about 1,700 hospitals reported using a single vendor for their clinical information system (Gardner, 1989). However, only one-third of hospitals used the same vendor to both automate finance and clinical functions.

Single vendor systems tend to limit choice when more than one automated function is desired. Systems may have good order entry while offering only mediocre reporting functions. One way to get the best *components* is to purchase from different vendors and insist on the components being adequately connected on the computer network (Tranbarger, 1991).

Revenues for vendors of hospital information systems were $7 billion in 2003. Market participants range in size from small systems integrators to well-established firms with billions of dollars per year in revenues. Large enterprise software companies, including Oracle, SAP, and PeopleSoft, are in the healthcare market (Le, 2001). Manufacturers, such as General Electric and Siemens, also have significant healthcare information systems components. A handful of specialists in medical information management systems are also competing, such as Cerner and IDX Systems. No one company has more than a sliver of this highly fragmented business. Based on 2000 revenues, Siemens had the largest market share, with 4.9%, followed by McKesson with 4.8%, and Cerner with 2.1%. McKesson has the largest installed base, but the six biggest vendors together only have 16% of the market.

A few companies are *independent* and focused on healthcare IT. Cerner, IDX Systems Corporation, and Eclipsys Corporation have similar product lines, target audiences, client base, and corporate characteristics. Each company offers a suite of products that competes with the offerings of the other companies.

Cerner Founders

Cerner was founded by *three friends*: Neal Patterson, Clifford Illig, and Paul Gorup. They had been working for Arthur Anderson & Company in Kansas City when in 1979 they began to discuss a new venture. They would meet on Sunday afternoons in a Kansas City park and discuss their interest to create mission-critical software for an information intensive industry (Cerner, 2006). In 1979, they started a private company, called Patterson, Gorup, Illig & Associates (Cashill, 2005) and began entering into contracts to develop software. That company became Cerner Corporation.

Neal Patterson has been the chairman and chief executive officer of the company since the beginning. Illig has also been with the company non-stop and is the vice chairman. Gorup left the company for a 12-year sabbatical but returned and in 2006 held the position of vice president of knowledge and discovery. The biographical sketches of Patterson and Illig are presented next.

Patterson was raised on his family's farm near Manchester, Oklahoma. In 1972, he finished his bachelor's degree in finance and master's degree in business administration at Oklahoma State University. In 1973, Patterson joined Arthur Andersen & Company as an information system consultant.

Patterson articulates well in public forums and is committed to the *vision* that information technology creates value for health systems and their communities by reducing costs and improving quality. Additionally, Patterson is willing to take risks in the name of what he believes. In the 1990s, he bet the future of Cerner on its vision for a person-centric, information architecture, called Cerner Millennium, as Cerner invested all its assets in developing and marketing Millennium.

Illig graduated from the University of Kansas with a degree in accounting and business administration. Illig focuses on internal operations and finance, while Patterson focuses on vision and leadership. The partnership of Patterson and Illig is typical of what one finds in successful firms. A book about the keys to business success says (Thomson, 2005):

Dynamic duos are the stuff of corporate legend: Sears and Roebuck, Roy and Walt Disney, Hewlett and Packard, and the like.

Typically, in such partnerships, one person (Illig) concentrates on internal operations, while the other person (Patterson) represents the company for clients and investors.

Illig recognizes that the ability to share information within Cerner is as essential to Cerner, as it is to any of its clients. Under his leadership, Cerner emphasizes enterprise-wide technology for information sharing throughout the organization. Illig was also instrumental in the key *financial steps* of Cerner, including the company's initial public stock offering in 1986, secondary public offering in 1995,and its three, two-for-one stock splits.

Cerner History and Vision

Patterson, Gorup, Illig & Associates' first clients were not in healthcare but in other information intensive businesses, such as finance. However, when the company signed its first *healthcare client*, the founders decided that healthcare was the application industry on which to focus. The first healthcare client, St. John Medical Center in Tulsa, Oklahoma, purchased a pathology laboratory information system. The company called this product PathNet, and it was installed in 1982. About their "ah-ah experience" (see the description about Donald Lindberg in Chapter 1 for the meaning of "ah-ah experience"), the founders have said (Cerner, 2006):

In the early survival days, we discussed and even dabbled in a number of industries, but when we signed our first healthcare client, a laboratory, it was clear to all of us, we had found the industry that was everything we wanted and more. Healthcare was big. It was complex. It was propelled at its heart by information. Before long, we were hooked.

That healthcare was big was crucial because the new company intended to become a very large company. An information systems vendor that focuses its applications on one industry can not become large unless that industry has a massive information systems need, and healthcare meets that requirement.

In the course of building PathNet, the founders developed a vision for themselves as healthcare information systems vendors. They describe this vision thusly (Cerner, 2006):

Before we were done building PathNet, our first laboratory application, we had a vision for connecting the mission-critical information in healthcare on a common information platform. Our picnic-table concept of being mission-critical took on a crisp new meaning in our chosen healthcare industry: it meant being clinical—that is, being directly or indirectly involved in the diagnosis, treatment and monitoring of a person who needs medical care.

From the 1970s through the 1990s many healthcare information systems vendors built their products around the financial applications of their clients. Cerner was innovative in its focus on clinical issues. During that time, *clinically oriented systems* existed primarily in clinical support applications in laboratory, radiology, and pharmacy. In those support areas, Cerner focused in its initial products.

In its early days, Cerner took advantage of a government program to encourage small businesses. The *Small Business Investment Company* (SBIC) program is a public/private partnership that has provided approximately $50 billion in financing to approximately 100,000 small U.S. companies since the program's creation in 1958 (NASBIC, 1997). SBICs are private venture capital firms licensed by the U.S. Small Business Administration to make loans to small companies. In July 1986 a SBIC, called First Capital Corporation of Chicago, provided equity financing of $630,000 to Cerner. In 1986, Cerner employed 150 people and sold one product, PathNet. Cerner's prospectus for its first initial public offering in 1986 described its first-generation Health Network Architecture platform. The SBIC funding helped Cerner invest in the Health Network Architecture concept.

The Health Network Architecture was crucial to Cerner from 1986 to 1993. However, Cerner's vision evolved to a scalable architecture built around the person. In 1993 Cerner decided to rewrite all of its software (Cashill, 2005). The result was Cerner Millennium. *Cerner Millennium* can retrieve and disseminate clinical and financial information to and from every station in a given healthcare system. Millennium has been a success for Cerner. In 2006, Cerner employed 7,000 people.

Stock

Cerner went public in 1986, at a split-adjusted price of $1.00 per share. Cerner's *stock price* has increased an average of more than 20 percent annually since 1986. A benchmark is the composite index of the NASDAQ stock exchange that has increased an average of 10 percent annually for the same period. Ten thousand dollars invested in Cerner in 1986 was worth approximately half a million dollars in 2005.

The healthcare information systems vendor landscape rapidly changes. Mergers and acquisitions are one aspect of this changing landscape. Nevertheless, examining

Cerner's principal *competitors* at one spot in time might be educational. In Cerner's *2005 Annual Report* (Cerner, 2006) the following companies were listed as major competitors: Eclipsys Corporation, Epic Systems Corporation, GE Healthcare Technologies, iSoft Corporation, McKesson Provider Technologies, Medical Information Technology Incorporated, Misys Healthcare Systems, and Siemens Medical Solutions. Each of those eight companies offers a suite of software solutions and services that compete with Cerner's software solutions and services. Other competitors, such as Allscripts, focus on only a portion of the market that Cerner addresses and are not considered here. Of those eight competitors:

- Epic Systems and Medical Information Technology are privately owned and do not trade on the stock market
- Four entities are part of larger entities and do not trade shares separately from their parent: GE Healthcare (part of GE), McKesson Provider Technologies (part of McKesson), Misys Healthcare (part of Misys), and Siemens Medical (part of Siemens)

If one were to compare Cerner's stock performance to that of the stock performance of a company like GE or Siemens, then one would not be able to tell whether the stock performance of GE or Siemens was primarily related to its healthcare information systems products and services or something else.

Two of the eight companies are publicly held and focus on healthcare information systems: Eclipsys and iSoft. *Eclipsys Corporation* is headquartered in Boca Raton, Florida; began business in 1995; and was listed on the NASDAQ stock exchange in 1998. Its stock price opened in 1998 at approximately $18 per share, rose within a year to $40 per share, dropped by 2002 to $4 per share, and was in the teens in 2006. Between 1998 and 2006, the price of Cerner stock doubled.

iSoft PLC is headquartered in Manchester, England and its shares entered the London Stock Exchange in 2000 at a price of 180 pounds per share. The share price rose steadily till 2005 when it reached 450 pounds per share. Then in 2006 a serious accounting scandal surfaced (Bowers, 2006) and the share price dropped to 50 pounds.

As regards *government relations*, iSoft PLC has the following announcement on its corporate Web site (iSoft, 2006):

Following the merger with Torex plc in 2003, iSOFT no longer faces substantial competition from UK suppliers. In the UK, after the award of contracts under the National Health Service's National Programme for IT, current market share is 61%.

iSoft's relation with the National Health Service in the United Kingdom is a major part of the company's business.

Healthcare companies can be strongly affected by government legislation. For instance, the U.S. government implemented the *Balanced Budget Act* in 1997. The Balanced Budget Act reduced the payments that providers received from Medicare. With providers receiving less revenue, they were less prepared to pay vendors. Thus, Cerner's revenue declined shortly after the passage of the Balanced Budget Act. Between mid-1997 and mid-1999 Cerner's stock price dropped from approximately $15 per share to approximately $5 per share.

Considering the *market capitalization* of firms, one can see that the competitors that Cerner faces come in a wide range of sizes. Market capitalization is the total monetary value of all outstanding shares of a company. It is calculated by multiplying the number of shares outstanding by the current market price of one share. For instance, on October 3, 2006:

- ISoft Group had approximately 230 million shares outstanding
- The price per ISoft Group share was 0.57 British pounds
- Each British pound bought US$1.89

Thus, the market capitalization of ISoft Group was 248 million dollars. The market capitalization of the eight firms that Cerner listed as its competitors is shown in

Table 12.1. These companies (other than Cerner) were listed by Cerner in its 2006 Annual Report as its major competitors. The company name is in the leftmost column. Stock symbol in middle column may include between parentheses the stock exchange from which the data was collected (where exchange has been abbreviated as 'Exch'), if the stock is not traded on a U.S. exchange. The third column shows the market capitalization in units of one million U.S. dollars. Data from October 2006.

Company Name	Stock Symbol	Market Cap (US million dollars in)
iSoft	IOT (London Exch)	247
Eclipsys	ECLP	920
Misys	MSY (London Exch)	2,400
Cerner	CERN	3,500
McKesson	MCK	16,000
Siemens	SI (Frankfurt Exch)	77,000
General Electric	GE	370,000

Table 12.1. One sees that GE has a market capitalization that is 100 times larger than that of Cerner. The three largest companies by market capitalization, namely McKesson, Siemens, and GE, have another attribute worth noting. Those largest companies have products and services that are important to healthcare providers in addition to information systems. Both Siemens and GE are major producers of equipment, such as radiology equipment. Modern radiology equipment is extremely expensive and requires software to run. Furthermore, this same software must be connected with other information outside the radiology equipment in order to maximize the effectiveness and efficiency of the radiology equipment. Vendors such as Siemens and GE have a natural advantage in trying to sell a healthcare information system to a provider when that provider also needs other products from the vendor that will connect to the information system. McKesson is the largest pharmaceutical distributor in North America and can leverage its inside track with pharmacies into connections with the rest of the healthcare information systems of a healthcare provider. Cerner and iSoft do not have this "complementary product" attribute that McKesson, Siemens, and GE have.

Large Client

The relationship that a healthcare institution has with a IT vendor can significantly impact the implementation of applications. The probability of success is increased if those people involved assume the responsibility for creating a positive business relationship (Kock, 1991). Historically, business relationships have been formed between the vendor and the *purchasing department* or the information systems department, but this relationship must be broadened.

The purchase of a healthcare information system (HIS) is a complex undertaking. The first task is to obtain all the required, organizational approvals. The second task is to determine and manage a reasonable process timeline. The *timeline* will indicate five phases (Fox et al., 2001):

1. Window-shopping phase
2. Planning phase
3. Acquisition phase
4. Installation phase
5. Operations phase

Given that project personnel turnover is frequent and project expectations constantly change, the timeline must be flexible.

Evaluations

HIS *vendor evaluations* are most noticeable during the acquisition phase. However, evaluations should occur during each phase. The evaluations require top expertise and affect quality control. Unfortunately, the cost of the required expertise over time is rarely included in a healthcare organization's IT budget.

In general, a useful analogy for the management of a healthcare IT project, including the project's required evaluations of HIS vendors, is the management of an organization's *building projects*. Many healthcare organizations retain legal, architectural, construction, and maintenance firms throughout building projects to maximize the value from the projects' massive investments. IT investments are equally complex and massive, requiring comparable expertise throughout. HIS vendor evaluations should include a careful analysis of a limited number of pre-selected vendors. The analysis should be based on a series of "face-to-face" vendor meetings. These meetings should include follow-up documentation to be used as addenda to the contract; on-site, hands-on system demonstrations with scripts; off-site, telephone, and e-mail vendor reference checks; and, evidence of software "walk-throughs."

Contract Negotiations

After completion of the comprehensive vendor evaluation and selection of finalists, the organization is ready to proceed to the next phase, where the focus is on *contract negotiations*. Many companies make the mistake of advising a vendor that it has been selected as the winner of the "request for proposal" contest, and all that remains is to enter into a contract. By doing so, the purchaser has seriously undermined its bargaining position, since the vendor now knows that no one else is in the running. More effective is to select the top two vendors, then advise the preferred vendor that if negotiations break down or do not go as well as expected, the second choice is waiting in the wings.

Similarly, the healthcare entity need not disclose to the vendor the amount of money budgeted for the project. Often when this is done, the *contract price* will come in close to the budget price. Despite trying to negotiate low cost and high service, the healthcare entity must take care to maintain a positive relationship. Unlike other contract negotiations, when purchasing a complex and expensive healthcare information system, the purchaser and vendor will have to work together for an extended time. If the negotiations have been too mean-spirited, there may be, at least, two unpleasant outcomes: in the future, when the purchaser needs something from the vendor which is not covered by the contract, the vendor may impose a high charge in an attempt to make up for perceived losses at the outset. Or the purchaser has squeezed so much out of the initial pricing of the contract that the vendor's business ultimately fails.

The *definitions* section of the contract should cover terms like programs, software, system, hardware, third-party software, source code, installation, acceptance, documentation, and permitted users. How these terms are defined may well make the difference between a successful project and a failure. For instance, if the documentation does not include:

- Vendor's response to the RFP
- Listing of functional and performance specifications

then a warranty that "the system will operate in accordance with the documentation" will not be very helpful. Also, determining the correct type of license for the organization's particular use is essential. For example, there are:

- Site licenses, covering a specific geographical location
- Enterprise-wide licenses, encompassing an entire business or institution
- Licenses governing the right to use software on a subscription-type basis

Each of these and other types of licenses has its unique issues.

In reference to *payment terms*, objectively measurable performance milestones are best. These milestones should be coordinated with detailed acceptance testing criteria. For example:

- 10% of the contract price will be paid upon execution
- 20% upon delivery
- 30% upon completion of installation
- 40% upon final acceptance

The entire acceptance testing procedure should be detailed, including testing procedures and protocols, re-tests, and options if the tests are not successful.

Another significant contractual issue concerns access to the *source code*. Without it, the software cannot be adequately maintained. The issue may arise in the context of the vendor's bankruptcy, but is equally applicable if the vendor simply ceases to support the software. The purchaser wants access to the source code. This may be accomplished through a source code escrow arrangement or direct licensing of the code.

The inclusion of contract provisions for alternative dispute resolution may help avoid expensive litigation. An *escalation provision* defines the specific hierarchy of employees who are to be involved in resolving any problems that arise. If first level managers are unable to reach an agreement, the problem is escalated to the next level of management within a specified amount of time. If this informal process is unsuccessful, the contract may require binding arbitration, which offers advantages over a court battle.

WellSpan Health System

WellSpan Health System serves the healthcare needs of more than 500,000 people in Pennsylvania. WellSpan has developed specific guidelines for business analysis, RFP development, the vendor selection process, contract negotiations, and system implementation.

Wellspan and the vendor assume responsibilities as follows. WellSpan's responsibilities in the client-vendor partnership are to provide the designated resources to support the implementation plan, complete acceptance testing on schedule, notify the vendor in a timely manner of problems, serve as a positive reference if appropriate, attend executive and user conferences, provide constructive feedback and notify vendor of changes in WellSpan's business objectives. The vendor responsibilities in the partnership are to be a partner across the continuum of change, help WellSpan to achieve competitive advantage, deliver business results, and maintain strategic alliances with suppliers and competitors. An integral part of any client-vendor relationship is a sound *contract*.

Parkview Memorial Hospital

Parkview Memorial Hospital in Fort Wayne, Indiana has 600 beds. In 1986 the hospital decided to pursue the acquisition of an integrated hospital information system. A selection team was formed of the patient care system coordinator, the director of information systems, the vice president of finance, and a representative of nursing administration. Selection criteria were developed, and two vendors were identified as most suitable. Phone interviews and then site visits to other hospitals that had implemented the systems of the vendors were performed. During the product demonstrations and many meetings clarifying what the product would do, the business relationship continued to develop.

Following the selection of a system, the hospital and the vendor entered into a series of meetings to negotiate various terms of the contract. After a yearlong selection and negotiation process, Parkview Memorial purchased its total information system. The next step was implementation, and that step involved various hospital departments and the vendor over many *months*.

The *relationship* between vendors of health information systems and providers of healthcare is important to the successful implementation of a health information system. As healthcare systems become more complex and more dependent on information systems, the need for close fits between an organization's information system and every action taken within that organization increases. The differences in the actual functioning of the software provided by one vendor or another may be only one of many factors that enter into the determination of whether or not a vendor and a provider will work together successfully.

Small Client

When a vendor tries to sell a large product to a large healthcare entity, the stakes are high, the proposal tends to be detailed, and negotiations involve large teams from both the vendor and the provider. When a vendor tries to sell a small product to a *small healthcare entity*, the stakes are low, the proposal tends to be short, and negotiations involve a few one-on-one interactions. The client does not want to spend much time in the product review and wants clear results immediately demonstrated.

A successful vendor in this small client environment will promise to show *immediate results* and to take almost no time. A true story follows from a vendor representative:

It was interesting to market practice management to dentists. My approach was to walk into an office cold and talk to the receptionists. I would stay no longer than 5 minutes and just ask general questions to see if they were using computers and if so for what. Usually they were doing letters and other things in word processing. Some were doing general accounting in something like Peachtree (www.peachtree.com). This was in the late-1980s.

The next day I would send a letter to the receptionist thanking her for her time and asking if she thought the office manager would grant me a 15 minute appointment. The only question I wanted the office manager to answer for me was "If there was one problem you would like me to solve for you, then what would it be?"

I usually got the appointment. When I found out what their worst problem was I had my direction.

Then I would send another thank you letter to the office manager, which in dental offices was frequently the dentist's wife. In that letter I would indicate that perhaps I could help solve their problem and would they like for me to do a free analysis of their workflow to see if a computerized program would help solve the problem and save them money.

Again I seldom failed to get that meeting. But I would not grant that meeting unless the dentist signed-on at this point. The analysis was free, but I would not conduct it unless the dentist agreed that if I could show them how I could solve the problem for them and save them money, they would purchase the system from me.

At this point I got about a 50% positive. Sometimes when I did the analysis, I found it was management problems that were causing the problem and no computer was going to solve it. In that case I would terminate the analysis and report the problem as I saw it.

But of the ones for which I completed the analysis and made a recommendation, 90% ended in a sale.

We marketed a comprehensive modular system. The system saved the doctors money through EDI of claims and prompt payments. If the patient did not have dental insurance, then the dentist switched to presentation of the bill to the patient at the time of service and found that 80% of the patients paid during the visit. The cash flow improvements paid for the system.

We programmed the forms reports for each dental insurance company and the doctors paid us by the hour. We had one guy who had been a dentist, and he understood the workings in the dental office so he did the forms. That was lucrative "after-sales" money for our forms work.

The vendor representative has followed these steps:

- A 5-minute visit to learn the terrain
- A 15-minute appointment to identify a problem
- A free analysis for the solution to the problem

The free analysis is done under the condition that the dentist agrees to buy the vendor solution should the vendor representative convince the dentist of its cost-effectiveness. While 50% of the contacts are lost at this stage, the sales effort will not succeed until the decision-maker at the client (in the dentist office case the decision-maker is the dentist) supports the purchase. The term vendor representative is used rather than salesperson because this person has served not only the role of salesperson but also the role of business analyst.

In the role of *business analyst*, the vendor representative has been honest enough to note when a problem requires a solution that the software product does not support. For instance, the problem may be that the office intentionally does not respond to queries from the health insurance company for additional information on claims, and thus the insurance company does not pay the claims. The work process, as in responding to insurance queries, must be in the right direction before the software can help the work process be executed efficiently. The vendor finds that a good relationship with a customer can lead to further business.

Outsourcing

To *outsource* is to obtain goods or services from an outside supplier. Outsourcing IT means that an entity asks a third party to provide the IT staff and be responsible for the management of IT. Functions that healthcare entities outsource include software development, installation and integration, operations and management, employee support and training, applications and services, Web-related activities, and any combination of the preceding. Sometimes a healthcare entity will outsource its entire IT function. Outsourcing is a common way for healthcare entities to satisfy their IT needs. Hospitals outsource IT functions more than they outsource any other organizational task. According to survey results, healthcare managers remain typically satisfied with the overall results of outsourced IT tasks.

Entities outsource for two main reasons: cost minimization or strategic positioning. Rural hospitals and small hospitals are likely to outsource (Menachemi et al., 2004). This is, in part, because of the difficulty in recruiting qualified IT professionals to rural areas and the reduced availability of resources needed to produce IT functions in-house. The larger the hospital, the less likely it is to outsource its IT needs. Another important predictor of IT outsourcing behavior is the degree to which an organization places strategic importance on IT in its operations. In hospitals where the CIO believes that IT plays a major role in overall operations, outsourcing of IT is less common.

Questions

Reading Questions

1. List some of the largest companies by revenue from healthcare IT services.
2. What are differences between how a salesperson might approach a small client versus a large client?
3. List some key components of the contract negotiation process between a provider and a vendor.

Doing Questions

1. Explore what different vendors offer by way of clinical support department systems, such as radiology and pharmacy, and analyze the extent to which messages from one department to another are supported.
2. Draft a contract to be signed between a provider and an IT vendor.
3. Information systems consultants are needed by healthcare organizations for various reasons. Consider your own strengths and weaknesses as a potential consultant and describe what strengths you would emphasize in trying to successfully find a niche for yourself in the health information systems consulting business.
4. Identify a vendor of a healthcare information system and summarize the characteristics of the information system that the vendor provides. Distinguish the vendor's products that you describe relative to the other competing products on the market.
5. Compare and contrast what SAIC and CSC do for healthcare with IT.
6. Choose three companies in the healthcare IT arena. Go to the Web sites of the companies and search for the jobs available. Describe:
   - How easy or difficult was the work of finding relevant jobs on the Web
   - How many positions with the keyword "health" are available
   - What is the pattern of available positions in the "health" area in each company and across companies
   - What is the geographical distribution of positions
   - What are the fringe benefits of employment
   - Comment on the companies in terms of their market

The objective of this exercise is to learn about positions available in the industry and to use that also as a way to gain further insight about the employers.

References

Ball, E. (1991). Maximizing the benefits of using consultants. In M. Ball (Ed.), *HealthCare information management systems* (pp. 326-330). New York: Springer Verlag.

Bowers, S. (2006, August 9). ISoft suspends founder over accounts queries. *Guardian Newspaper*. Retrieved from www.guardian.co.uk

Cashill, J. (2005, July). *The drivers: Strong leadership key to consistent group for repeat winners of corporate report 100*. Ingram's: Kansas City Business Magazine. Retrieved October 2006, from http://www.ingramsonline.com/july_2005/cr100/cr-drivers.html

Cerner. (2006). *2005 Annual Report*. Cerner Corporation. Retrieved October 2006, from www.cerner.com

Childs, B. (1997). 9 keys to success. *Healthcare Informatics, 14*(5), 22-24.

Fox, S., Gillespie, W., & Kohn, D. (2001). *Vendor/product evaluations and contract negotiations under HIPAA*. Health Information and Management Systems Society 2001 Annual Conference. New Orleans, LA: Health Information and Management Systems Society.

Gardner, E. (1989). Finding a strategy that does the trick. *Modern Healthcare, 19*(27), 28-52.

iSoft. (2006). *Investor centre*. iSoft PLC. Retrieved October 4, 2006, from www.isoftplc.com/corporate/investor_centre/

Kock, L. (1991). Nursing's relationship with information system vendors. In M. Ball (Ed.), *HealthCare Information Management Systems* (pp. 125-131). New York: Springer Verlag.

Le, Y. (2001). The healthcare informatics 100. *Healthcare Informatics*, 35-76.

Menachemi, N., Burke, D.E., Diana, M., & Brooks, R. (2004). Characteristics of hospitals that outsource information system functions. *Journal of Healthcare Information Management, 19*(1), 63-69.

Murphy, R.M. (2006, April 28). *7 ways to join the billion-dollar club*. CNN. Retrieved October 2006, from money.cnn.com/2006/

NASBIC. (1997, February). *NASBIC success stories: Cerner Corporation*. National Association of Small Business. Retrieved October 2006, from www.nasbic.com/success/stories/cerner.cfm

Thomson, D.G. (2005). *Blueprint to a billion: 7 essentials to achieve exponential growth.* New York: Wiley.

Tranbarger, R. (1991). Nurses and computers: At the point of care. In M. Ball (Ed.), *HealthCare Information Management Systems* (pp. 95-102). New York: Springer Verlag.

Chapter XIII

Diffusion

Learning Objectives

- Apply the three phases of agricultural diffusion to healthcare information systems diffusion
- Develop a plan for encouraging diffusion of IT in a healthcare entity
- Identify four types of healthcare systems globally and provide examples of countries employing each type and relate this to information systems impact

To diffuse is to spread widely. Anthropologically, diffusion occurs when practices or innovations spread within a community or from one community to another. Diffusing a healthcare information system requires overcoming many barriers. Under what conditions is a healthinformation system successfully adopted by its intended target audience? In this chapter the theoretical issues for *diffusion* are presented. Then a detailed case of preparing to implement one large system shows some preparation needed to diffuse a system.

Theory

While many reports exist of successful health information systems implementations, the evidence suggests that the majority of implementations are failures (Heeks et al., 2000). These *failures* take many forms from:

- A complete collapse
- Working initially but failing later
- Working in the test site but not in the intended deployment site

The advice provided decades earlier by *Barnett* (1968) remains applicable today, namely, the system must be:

- Carefully attuned to the needs of its users
- Fit gracefully into the workflow of those who are expected to use it
- Show clear benefits to its usage

Students of history, sociology, and engineering note a number of *stages* that technical innovations go through before becoming accepted as traditional marketplace items or services. Frequently, the sequence is:

- Research
- Development
- Demonstration
- Commercial prototyping
- Production

Transitions between the stages occur at irregular intervals, and the cost of each phase is higher than the phase preceding it.

While many ideas and practices have moved rapidly through modern medicine, the spread of information systems has been irregular. For better or worse, the *rate of diffusion* of healthcare information systems (HIS) has been slow. Classical studies of diffusion of innovation have been made with respect to agricultural practices. The first bag of fertilizer applied to a farm essentially represents a commitment to testing, analysis, and correction of soil conditions ad infinitum. Lionberger (1960) constructed a taxonomy of *agricultural innovation* as follows:

- **Grade One:** Easily understood and demonstrated, use of pesticides for instance
- **Grade Two:** Somewhat more difficult to understand and demonstrable only over a minimum time of a crop cycle; use of improved fertilizers for instance

- **Grade Three:** More difficult to understand and demonstrable only over multiple years; for instance, improved genetic management of crops

Counterparts to these agricultural innovation examples can be found in the HIS field:

- **Grade One:** Automation of a current simple practice, such as patient accounting. This is easily understood, and the demonstration of feasibility and efficacy does not take long. This is especially true when a single package can be adopted to handle the entire patient accounting problem. More than 85% of all U.S. hospitals used computer systems in connection with their patient billing, collections, and third party reimbursements already by 1975.
- **Grade Two:** Automation of a current, more complex procedure such as analysis of electrocardiographic (EKG) signals. The general nature of the task is well understood—to interpret the EKG. The demonstration of successful operation of the automation is also rather easily shown over a matter of minutes. The automation of EKG interpretation has spread pervasively through the healthcare system.
- **Grade Three:** Automation of an entire system, such as a computerized medical record, is rather more difficult. The concept is not easily explained. It demands coordination of actions of many people. The execution must be timely. The beneficial results are indirect and relatively remote in time with respect to the actions of the system. Indeed, there may be no benefit unless all of the subsystem components perform their jobs properly. In these respects the concept of the computerized patient record is analogous to the concept of improved genetic practices in agriculture.

Nothing about the computer techniques in HIS makes them fundamentally different from such systems in non-medical fields. There are, however, two special *non-technical barriers*: medical knowledge and medical management.

Much of medicine remains an *art*. Mental health is a good example of an area in which the knowledge of the biological processes remains primitive. Unlike the monitoring of physiological parameters on a patient in the intensive care unit where alerts are readily generated for physiological signals gone askew, the monitoring of mental health patients is less precise. So what can be expected of a medical system for different patients with different conditions varies, and for some patients little scientific or algorithmically defined intervention seems relevant given the current understanding of disease.

The second barrier peculiar to healthcare is the management, social, or political environment. The healthcare system is composed of thousands of relatively *autonomous units*. Hospitals are themselves made of units that operate somewhat autonomously within the hospital. To the extent that healthcare institutions do not operate smoothly and sensibly with one another, the HIS cannot be shared or transplanted. To the extent that the institutions are Balkanized, so are their information systems.

Ruffin (1999) has gone so far as to say that the critical factor is *political,* as follows:

The successful selection, procurement, and implementation of information and communication systems are far more political than technical...Ignore the political issues and the technical issues will not matter, because implementation will fail and the potential benefits promised by the technology will not materialize. Attend to the politics, and deal with them, and which vendors your organization selects will not matter much, because, in a setting of consistent political interests, almost any vendor's product will perform well...Without excruciatingly exact formatting, data cannot flow from one computer to another. Without that excruciatingly exact formatting, data cannot flow from the laboratory system of a hospital to a communication network and into the computers in the offices of physicians.

To achieve this precise agreed formatting among units requires standardization, which in turn is essentially a political act.

Practice

IT will remain a cost center if it maintains the traditional practices. To overcome this, the IT plan must be fully integrated with the organization's *vision*. IT investments then are predicated on a return-on-investment (ROI) to both implement and sustain key business goals by automating newly redesigned processes. The following proactive measures can help transform an environment from one in which IT is an optional cost, to one in which IT is a critical enterprise investment (Ummel, 2003):

- The CEO assumes responsibility for the CIO.
- An IT Steering Committee is chaired by a senior executive other than the CIO and does knowledge gathering, planning, priority setting, and ROI-based investing. The members of the Committee are senior management, the CIO, some clinicians, and some departmental managers.
- A management incentive plan rewards achieving IT milestones.

- Operating managers and executives participate in vendor evaluation and selection.
- All IT projects are preceded by solid business cases, necessary and significant process redesign in applicable areas, and full accounting of the post-implementation results over the ensuing three years.
- Executives and managers are fully accountable for predetermined IT benefit realization in their annual performance review. Disciplinary actions are consistently enforced.

IT projects will be ineffectual until the people who control the business processes change their core processes as an adjunct to automation.

Information systems are critical to quality healthcare, but *clinician resistance* is a key barrier to diffusion. Paper records have the advantage of familiarity, portability, and *flexibility* for many users (Rada, 1991). While technologists contend that computer-generated "reminders" will improve care, clinicians fear that their professional autonomy is being limited (Dowling, 1987). Information systems may help identify *errors*, but when this information is used to punish doctors who make errors, they may be reluctant to use such systems.

The *education* of healthcare professionals may impact their view of information technology. Historically medical schools have de-emphasized education about the use of information systems or the functioning of healthcare enterprises in order to have enough time for the traditional topics, like anatomy, pharmacology, and pathology. Also, the increasing knowledge about the molecular basis of disease must fit into the curriculum, and time for information systems education is hard to find.

The National Library of Medicine has been active in funding physicians to study information systems but that impact has been small compared to the need for information systems *education for clinicians*. No ready solution to this education problem—namely the problem of reducing the gap between what clinicians might usefully know about information systems and what they have time to learn—is in sight.

Determining Strategy

The IT Department objectives must be aligned with those of the healthcare entity that it serves. Achieving this alignment of strategies is a complex process for which the CIO bears heavy responsibility. Strategy for an organization has two major components: formulation and implementation. *Formulation* involves determining the objectives that serve the mission of the entity. For instance, a high-level entity-wide objective might be to reduce the cost of care while preserving the quality of that care. *Implementation* involves making decisions about how the entity acquires skills, establishes capabilities, and alters processes to achieve its objectives. For instance, in implementation the entity may decide to outsource a major IT function.

In formulating and implementing IT strategy, the handling of IT assets and governing concepts is critical. The assets include IT applications, data, and staff. The *asset agenda* addresses issues such as the inventory of applications that needs to be maintained or newly developed, such as an application for an "enterprise master patient index." The *governing concepts* define how an entity views its IT. For example, the entity may want to be on the cutting edge of IT or to be conservative in that regard.

The *five forces* at work in helping determine how an entity handles its IT assets and its governing concepts are (Wager et al., 2005):

- **Entity-wide strategies:** For instance, the entity may intend to become the low-cost provider of care through disease management programs, and then the IT Department needs to focus on disease management program support.
- **Maintenance of core information management processes:** In this case the IT Department is continuously focused on improving core functions like ordering of tests and managing the revenue cycle.
- **New information technologies:** New technologies, such as wireless networks, may facilitate new work processes, such as nurses documenting the patient status while interacting with patients. The IT Department, in working with the entity, must decide whether or not striving to use these new technologies is consistent with the entity's objectives.
- **Assessment of trajectories of its existing strategies:** IT objectives invariably have a fixed time horizon and scope. For instance, computerized physician order entry may be expected to be implemented over a three-year period. A future role for genetic information in helping support decision-making about drug-drug interactions might be anticipated and thus factor into formulation of strategy.
- **Views about competition:** An entity must devise methods to counter competitive pressures. For instance, a hospital may be weakened if employers have significant power in determining whether or not their insured employees may use a particular hospital. The hospital may want to increase the relative bargaining power of patients over employers by supporting patient-oriented Web sites that rate hospitals.

An entity needs to employ these various forces in formulating and implementing its IT strategy.

Entities have *cultures* as regards how they strategize. Some entities have formal approaches that rely on multiple committees. Other entities have informal processes that rely on informal conversations. The approach to IT should be harmonious with the approach of the entity to other strategies.

Entity strategy is generally discussed in senior leadership meetings, and the CIO or a CIO liaison should be present at these meetings, at least whenever the meetings are scheduled to address IT. The IT Department should have a senior member of its staff function as a liaison with each major other department in the healthcare entity. Thus, in a hospital, the IT Department would have a liaison with the Finance, Nursing, Medical Staff, and Administrative Departments, at least. In the discussions that the liaisons have with members of other departments, insights about strategic imperatives may be obtained. The *liaisons* must convey these insights to the CIO who in turn digests and synthesizes them in recommendations to the senior executives of the entity.

IT can support the achievement of the entity's *objectives*. This occurs when the IT Department operates in ways consistent with those of other departments in the entity that they all serve. The path to formulating and implementing the IT objectives is a complex one involving formal and informal processes and must continually evolve.

As in other organizations, many of the aspects of strategic alignment in healthcare are *political* (Rada & Finley, 2004). The complex characteristics of healthcare with physician professionals, technicians, insurers, patients, government regulators, and so on complicate the pressures. While some factors speak to improvements in this situation in the future, the basic complexity remains and has led to this summarization (Wager et al., 2005): "The development of well-aligned IT strategies has been notoriously difficult for many years, and there appears to be no reason that crafting this alignment will become significantly easier over time."

Department of Defense

What are the detailed steps for implementing a major system to minimize user rejection of the system? An example from the military illustrates the necessary steps for implementation of an integrated health information system, in this case the *Composite Health Care System* (CHCS).

The *CHCS Program Office* is responsible for the diffusion of the CHCS. CHCS must be installed first in a treatment facility and pass an operational test and evaluation before worldwide implementation can begin. Implementation of the system requires commitment and teamwork at all levels from the Program Office to the sites.

The *Implementation Guide* describes the activities necessary for the successful implementation of the CHCS in medical treatment facilities (MTFs) worldwide. The Implementation Guide outlines roles and responsibilities, identifies points of contact, specifies business process changes, details key implementation and training activities, establishes timelines, and provides the framework for site level implementation planning and preparation.

The first step in planning for the CHCS implementation at a site is the acceptance of the CHCS *Site Agreement*. Experience with system implementation has shown that a clear understanding by all participants of the roles, responsibilities, and expectations is paramount to successful implementation, training, and testing activities. The Site Agreement was developed to ensure implementation participants understand the key success factors and to achieve consensual agreement to perform the required tasks. Only after signature by the CHCS program manager and the commanders of each of the participating facilities will implementation activities begin.

The CHCS Program Office (PO) interfaces with the personnel appointed by the MTF commanders. The MTF commander selects a military physician to serve as MTF *Project Officer*. This individual should be viewed as the commander's personal representative for this project, and should have sufficient rank, experience, and commitment to interact with higher headquarters staff, the CHCS PO staff, and to successfully orchestrate a myriad of tasks at the local level.

The CHCS Site Coordinator performs a *site survey* at each facility 7-9 months prior to scheduled installation. The purpose of the survey is to determine the requirements to prepare the MTF to receive CHCS. During the pre-implementation phase, site leaders ensure that CHCS site level data is contained in the *Health Data Dictionary* information model.

A set of core standardized templates is available to each MTF as part of CHCS. The *templates* include medical specialty specific templates as well as generic encounter templates. Documentation flexibility for providers is afforded through the use of encounter templates. Providers may use one of the templates in the core set or construct their own encounter templates by identifying the desired template components.

Training duration varies by user. Front desk and administrative personnel receive a 4-hour course. Support staff receive an 8-hour course. Medical providers, nurses, and nurse practitioners receive two days of CHCS training that includes guided exercises and hands on scenarios. Users receive their system identifiers and passwords after they have completed training.

International Health

Moving from the concerns of large global organizations, such as the American military to the concerns of countries, what does one see as the likelihood of diffusion of health information systems *internationally*? A person may travel from country to country and require healthcare wherever he or she may be. How will the health records of that individual be accessible to providers anywhere? Epidemics know no national boundaries. For example, AIDS originating in one country and spreading to another is of concern to both countries, and both countries want to know what is happening in the other to deal with this problem. The reasons for information systems to saddle national boundaries are many. However, the first problem to confront in this regard is that healthcare systems are different from country to country.

Expenditures

One dimension along which healthcare systems are measured is by the amount of money invested in them. The U.S. has the highest expenditure of any country on healthcare both nationally and per capita. In the year 2003, the U.S. spent 15.2% of its *gross domestic product* on healthcare or $5,700 per person (OECD, 2006). Other countries spent anywhere from 11% of their gross domestic product to 5% of it on healthcare. Likewise, per capita expenditure is much less in every country. By taking the local currency and converting the currency into U.S. dollars at official rates in 2003, one can normalize the per person expenditure. In 2003, Canada spent $3,000 per person on healthcare, United Kingdom spent $2,300, Japan spent $2,200, Korea spent $1,100, and Mexico spent $600 (see Table 13.1).

Life expectancy should be highest in the U.S., since the monetary investment in healthcare is highest in the U.S. However, this is not the case. The life expectancy in the U.S. in 2003 was 78 years. For the five countries aforementioned, the life expectancies are: Canada 80 years, United Kingdom 79 years, Japan 82 years, Korea 77 years, and Mexico 75 years. Of those five countries only Mexico has a lower life expectancy than the U.S., but Mexico's per capita investment in healthcare is approximately one-tenth that of the U.S.'s per capita investment. Figure 13.1 highlights the disparity between expenditures and life expectancy results across countries.

Policy

In all countries the *government* plays some role in health, but the extent of this role varies widely. In the United Kingdom the government essentially owns the healthcare system. In many countries the government owns some of the healthcare system and some is owned by other entities.

Table 13.1. Expenditures versus outcomes internationally: The first column shows arbitrarily selected countries with their names sorted alphabetically. The following three columns show data from the year 2003 that is acquired from the Organization for Economic Co-operation and Development. The column '%GDP' indicates the percent of the country's Gross Domestic Product spent on health. The column 'Per Capita' indicates in thousands of US dollar equivalents the amount a country spends per capita on health. The column 'LE' indicates the average Life Expectancy in decades for the population at birth.

Country	%GDP	Per Capita	LE
Australia	9.2	2.9	8.0
Austria	9.6	3.0	7.9
Canada	9.9	3.0	8.0
Czech Republic	7.5	1.3	7.5
France	10.4	3.0	7.9
Germany	10.8	3.0	7.9
Ireland	7.2	2.5	7.8
Italy	8.4	2.3	8.0
Japan	8.0	2.2	8.2
Korea	5.5	1.1	7.7
Mexico	6.3	0.6	7.5
Sweden	9.3	2.7	8.0
Turkey	7.6	0.5	7.1
United Kingdom	7.8	2.3	7.9
United States	15.2	5.7	7.8

In *countries* such as the United States, where private health insurance is widespread, the healthcare plans offered by insurers play a major role in setting the conditions for care. In countries with public or statutory healthcare insurance, there may be a single payer (usually a governmental unit, as in Canada). Alternatively, a plurality of insurers either quasi-public or private (as in Germany and France), may share these intermediary administrative tasks (Wessen, 1999).

Broadly speaking, healthcare systems nationally may be divided into 4 categories (Roemer, 1992):

Figure 13.1. Chart of expenditures versus outcomes. The legend for Table 13-1 applies to this figure. The dashed line with diamonds indicates percent of Gross Domestic Product spend on health; the dashed line with rectangles, the per capita health expenditure; and the line with triangles, the life expectancy per individual. The x-axis is countries and the y-axis is amounts. The chart makes clear that the highest costs are for the U.S. (which is to the far right of the x-axis), but the life expectancy for the U.S. is average. Data again comes from the Organization for Economic Co-operation and Development and is for the year 2003.

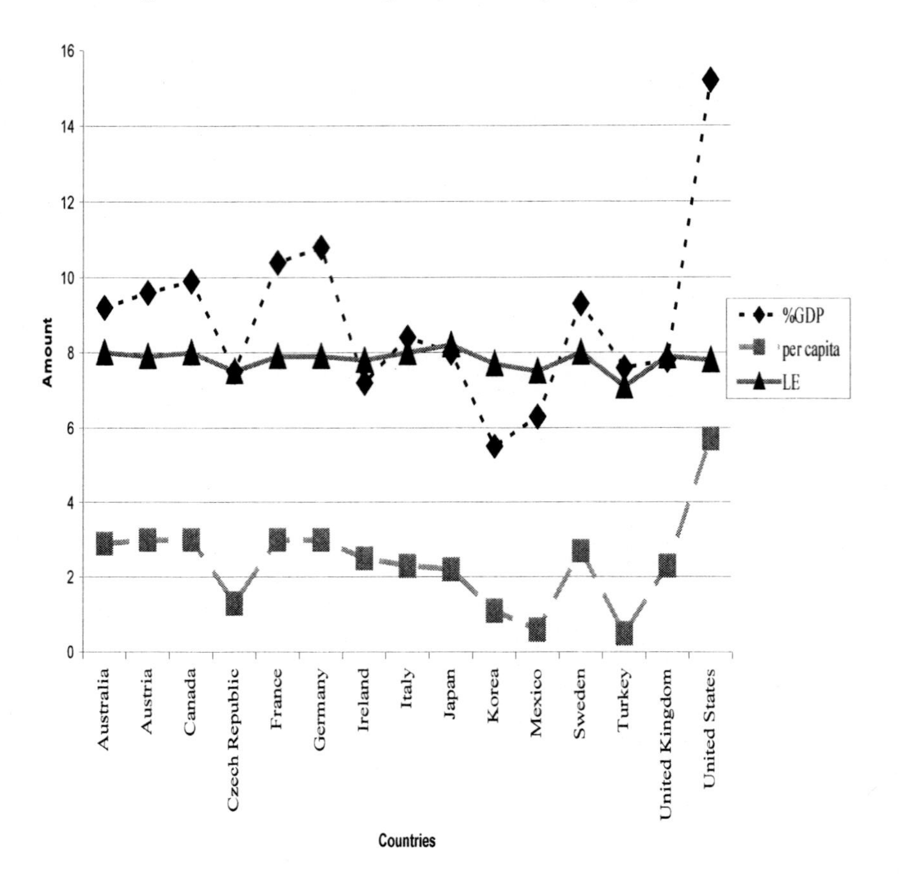

- Entrepreneurial
- Welfare-oriented
- Comprehensive
- Socialist

The only highly developed country with a basically entrepreneurial health system is the United States. Of middle-income, developing countries, the Philippines has an *entrepreneurial system* and of low-income, developing countries, Kenya provides an example of an entrepreneurial system.

Welfare-oriented systems are typical of Western Europe, Canada, Japan, and Australia. In 1883 Germany enacted legislation for mandatory health insurance. This insurance is now carried by hundreds of "sickness" funds financed by the government and regulated by the Ministry of Labor and Social Affairs at the federal level and in each "'lander" or province. The sickness funds enter into contracts with associations of physicians, which are paid periodic per capita amounts according to each fund's membership. Then the medical association reviews and pays the fees charged by the physicians. Government funds account for about 75% of the German health expenditure and about 25% comes from private funds. Peru and India are examples of low-income, developing countries with welfare-oriented healthcare systems.

The best-known *comprehensive health system* is that of Great Britain. From World War II until 1990, the British healthcare system could be characterized as one in which 100 percent of the population was entitled to complete healthcare, and the financial support was entirely from the government. Almost all health facilities were under the direct control of the government. The Scandinavian countries, Italy, and some other advanced countries have a similar comprehensive system. In a socialist health system the government controls all physical and human resources, and health services are available to everyone. Such is the case in Cuba, Russia, and China.

The debate about appropriate health system policies and strategies has been hampered by inadequate information about the extent to which systems contribute to a set of socially desirable goals. The World Health Report (WHO, 2000) proposed a framework for measuring the attainment of health systems in terms of socially desirable goals. The defining goal of health systems is to improve health. But people also expect them to be responsive to their legitimate non-health needs and to ensure that financial contributions to the system are distributed fairly across households. The goals of improving health and responsiveness contain two components—improving the average level and reducing inequalities. Accordingly, five indicators of goal attainment are the level of population health, inequalities in health outcomes, the level of responsiveness, inequalities in responsiveness, and the fairness of household financial contributions to health. The World Health Report measured the inputs used in achieving these goals—health system and non-health system inputs—and an index of the efficiency with which the goals were attained given these inputs. Major conceptual and methodological debates emerge. The major conceptual issues relate to the boundaries of the system, the concept of causality, the question of attribution of responsibility for outcomes, and whether goals are universal. Methodological debates focus on the measurement of healthy life expectancy, health inequalities, responsiveness, fairness of household financial contributions and efficiency. Information systems work is required to deal with the volume of data and the sophistication of analysis. Linking the measurement of outcomes and inputs with the analysis of the functions of health systems leads to the development of practical policy implications for ways to improve health system performance internationally (Murray & Frenk, 2000).

Technology

The *United Kingdom National Health Service* plan for information technology in healthcare is that local and national networks are integrated. In particular, integration of systems is encouraged so that any single data is collected only once. A network of shared administrative databases holding basic patient details has been replacing existing isolated databases.

The *Australian Institute of Health and Welfare* produced a National Health Information Model that provides a framework for the management of health information at the national level. It was developed using a "top-down" approach, allowing the model to reflect how health information should be structured rather than reflecting necessarily how health information is currently structured (Australian Institute of Health and Welfare, 1997). The model incorporates health information activities that meet agreed national priorities. These activities range from standard data charts of hospital accounts to health outcome measures. A key element of the model is a National Health Data Dictionary, which consists of a set of national standard definitions. The definitions extend beyond institutional healthcare and include the health labor force, outpatients, and mental health.

Fragmented health markets in the *European Union* hamper innovation and the spread of best practice. European Union governments spend, on average, 8% of their gross domestic product on health. Digital technologies can improve the productivity and scope of healthcare. This potential is not being fully exploited—only 1% of total health spending in Europe is used on information technology. The goals of the European Union are:

- Healthcare best practices in networking, health monitoring, surveillance of communicable diseases, and on links between hospitals, laboratories, pharmacies, doctors, primary care centers and homes are identified

- All European citizens have the possibility to have a health smart card to enable secure and confidential access to networked patient information
- All health professionals and managers are linked to a computerized health information infrastructure for prevention, diagnosis, and treatment

This does not mean controlling national healthcare at a European Union level. However, it does mean conducting health information systems research, agreeing health information standards, and building pan-European medical libraries.

The *United Nations* is involved in various global healthcare activities and information systems efforts. However, goals such as an international healthcare card for each citizen are only remote possibilities given the vast differences in health systems from country to country. The international activities in health information systems could benefit by further coordination at global levels, though this seems unlikely to happen anytime soon.

Questions

Reading Questions

1. Compare agricultural diffusion theory to healthcare information systems diffusion theory.
2. What kinds of healthcare systems do different countries have?

Doing Questions

1. The medical school curriculum has too much material to cover for the time available and under these conditions introducing new education about healthcare information systems is very difficult. How do you suggest that medical schools might introduce education about information systems into the curriculum? Please provide some evidence of your approach succeeding in some school(s).
2. Consider the three stages of diffusion as found in agriculture and health information systems. Find some examples of health information systems currently in use and categorize them according to where they would fit as to the type of diffusion that was necessary for them to succeed.

3. How might the wide diffusion of the World Wide Web have changed the conditions under which certain health information systems might be expected to diffuse? Provide arguments and examples.

References

Australian Institute of Health and Welfare. (1997). *The National Health Information Model*. Canberra, Australia: Institute of Health and Welfare.

Barnett, G.O. (1968). Computers and patient care. *New England Journal of Medicine, 279*, 1321-1327.

Dowling, A.F. (1987). Do hospital staff interfere with computer system implementation? In J.G. Anderson & S.J. Jay (Eds.), *Use and impact of computers in clinical medicine*. New York: Springer Verlag.

Heeks, R., Mundy, D., & Salazar, A. (2000). Understanding success and failure of health care information systems. In A. Armoni (Ed.), *Healthcare information systems: Challenges of the new millennium* (pp. 96-128). Hershey, PA: Idea Group Publishing.

Lionberger, H.F. (1960). *Adoption of new ideas and practices*. Ames: Iowa State University Press.

Murray, C.J.L., & Frenk, J. (2000). A framework for assessing the performance of health systems. *Bulletin of the World Health Organization, 78*(6), 717-731.

Organisation for Economic Co-operation and Development. (2006). *OECD health data 2006:Statistics and indicators for 30 countries*. Organisation for Economic Co-operation and Development. Retrieved November 4, 2006, from www.oedc.org

Rada, R. (1991). *Hypertext: From text to expertext*. London: McGraw-Hill.

Rada, R., & Finley, S. (2004). The aging of a clinical information system. *Biomedical Informatics, 37*(4), 319-324.

Roemer, M. (1992). National health systems throughout the world. In S. Jonas (Ed.), *An introduction to the U.S. health care system* (3rd ed.) (pp. 169-190). New York: Springer Verlag.

Ruffin, M.d.G.J. (1999). *Digital doctors*. Tampa, FL: American College of Health Executives.

Ummel, S. (2003). An interview with Stephen Ummel, Principal Cap Gemini Ernst & Young Health Consulting. *Journal of Healthcare Information Management, 17*(1), 27-30.

Wager, K., Lee, F., & Glaser, J. (2005). *Managing health care information systems: A practical approach for health care executives*. San Francisco: Jossey-Bass.

Wessen, A. (1999). The comparative study of health care reform. In F. Powell & A. Wessen (Eds.), *Health care systems in transition: An international perspective* (pp. 3-25). Thousand Oaks, CA: Sage Publications.

World Health Organization. (2000). *The world health report. Health systems: Improving performance*. Geneva, Switzerland: World Health Organization.

Chapter XIV

Conclusion

Learning Objectives

- Explain why healthcare information systems must fit into the workflow of people
- Relate trends in the healthcare industry to cost factors
- Synthesize a vision for healthcare information systems based on trends in information technology and economics

The study of health information systems is multi-disciplinary. In particular, the topic benefits from the fields of healthcare, management, and information systems. As distinct from a typical book in *management information systems*, this book looked exclusively at the experiences gained from healthcare.

Summary

Healthcare systems are so connected to the political and economic situation of a country that detailed, practical insights are hard to obtain that apply equally well across *countries*. The U.S. system has evolved over the past one hundred and fifty years from one that revolved around a solo private physician in a rural setting whose patients paid him directly for whatever services he rendered to a massive industry of insurance companies, multi-hospital networks, and mobile patients. This book focuses on healthcare information systems in the U.S.

Many of the insights of *pioneers* in health information systems from almost half a century ago remain equally valid today. Lindberg felt that information systems could make a big difference in the effectiveness and efficiency of healthcare. Barnett emphasized that the challenge is to fit into the workflow of those who are to use the system. Kissinger saw that the complexity of the environment continually increases and thus the challenge of fitting into the workflow also grows.

Many books have been written about health information systems with usually a distinct *audience* in mind each time. For instance, one can find books for:

- Physicians, with practical tips on how to use computers in the private office
- Chief information officers, on strategies for implementing enterprise-wide systems
- Nursing students, on support systems in the hospital that nurses use to help patient care
- Medical students, on computer-supported diagnosis

This book is for students of information systems and of healthcare administration and for professionals responsible for decisions about information systems in healthcare enterprises.

Challenges

Rising costs have been one of the greatest problems for the American healthcare system. The costs have risen more than costs of other services in the country. Some say this is due to the increase in costly treatments. However, in some other highly developed countries the portion of *gross national product* spent on healthcare is much less than in the U.S. and yet the quality of health for citizens on average in those countries is no less than that of citizens in the U.S.

Against the backdrop of high costs and sophisticated equipment, Americans are surprised at the large number of errors by healthcare providers. One hundred thousand people die each year in the U.S. from *medical errors* in hospitals. Information systems could reduce errors, if used properly.

To deal with high costs, the healthcare industry is moving towards less care in the hospital and more care in the *outpatient setting*. Information systems are likewise increasingly addressing the connections that are needed among the various parts of the healthcare enterprise, such as the hospital, the office, the insurer, and the consumer.

Most healthcare organizations spend less than five per cent of their budget on information systems. This is considerably less than one might expect for an *information intensive business*. The financial industry spends more than double that amount on information systems. However, the amount of investment in information systems in healthcare is increasing.

Design

The delivery of healthcare is a *professional business*. This contrasts with businesses that are either entrepreneurial or manufacturing in character. The professional business lends itself less to systematic use of information systems since the professionals prefer autonomy. The implication for design is that the design team has to work very closely with the users and carefully probe the nuances of the work environment. Whatever is proposed for implementation must very closely match the way the professionals are accustomed to work.

In addition to the close match to the work styles of the intended users, successful design projects in healthcare need to also pay close attention to the administrative situation. The support of all relevant levels of *administration* should be assured at the outset and carefully nurtured throughout the lifetime of the information systems project.

One approach to design of a hospital information system emphasizes the use of *pictures* to convey what happens in the healthcare entity. These pictures are produced by the designers in working closely with the end-users. The users give feedback based on the pictures, and refinements can proceed based on this iterative process of developing easy-to-interpret representations of the flow of information and work.

The kernel of a hospital information system provides the basic communication and processing capabilities. As such, it must make some assumptions about the control over the communication and decision-making in the hospital. This *kernel* thus must also be developed with great care in order to respect adequately the diverse political interests in the entity. A prototype should be constructed with which users can experiment so that they become comfortable with the basic assumptions.

Providers and Payers

The system components of a provider organization are reasonably well delineated. The initial component that patients typically face is the admissions or registration system. This system is connected to the *billing* and medical records system. The financial and resource management aspects of healthcare have been the first and most consistently computerized.

At the next stage of the patient experience is diagnosis and treatment. This stage remains dependent on subtle, imprecise factors that work against computerization. However, certain departments, such as the pathology laboratory, the radiology laboratory, and the pharmacy, have proven amenable to semi-automation, and computers are used in abundance in those departments. Connecting highly computerized facilities with manual facilities is difficult. Those components that revolve around the patient record and the collection of signs and symptoms from the patient are still often *paper-based.*

Some activities are readily digitized. Some departments proceed with their automation independently and move quickly. To achieve integration across departments is difficult. Departments must agree on *standard languages* for communicating parts of the patient record and other information. An example of a large military systems implementation reveals the extent of resource required to move even slowly forward in achieving integration across a healthcare system.

The basic *operations* of a health plan are to enroll members, contract with providers, accept claims from providers, adjudicate claims, make payments to providers, and audit the quality and efficiency of the healthcare delivery. The health plans are both part of the financial industry and part of the healthcare industry. The employees of a health plan are less autonomous than physicians and more readily cooperate with information systems staff in implementing systems that automate work. Health plans also place a greater fraction of their budget into information systems than do health providers.

The plans are involved with diverse entities. *Employers* often pay a large fraction of the premiums of an employee and this puts health plans and employers in intimate relationships. The U.S. government operates the U.S.'s largest health plan in the form of Medicare and Medicaid, but these are distinctly different from the private health plans due to the source of the money that the plan spends. Another entity that is important in the health plan scene is the clearinghouse. The clearinghouse is an intermediary between providers and health plans.

Health plans operate differently when serving individuals, small groups, and large organizations. They also face different laws and regulations at state and federal levels depending on the kind of customer they are serving. The laws and regulations represent a delicate balance between the government's intention to guarantee health for its citizens and at the same time to maintain a *capitalist health system.*

Regulations

Health care *regulations* cover access to, cost of, and quality of care. Complying with quality regulations incurs the most cost for the healthcare industry. Health insurance regulation, by contrast, tends to impose a cost on employers rather than on healthcare providers per se. Some associations help self-regulate the industry, such as the Joint Commission on Hospital Accreditation. When complying with a regulation, a healthcare entity must go through phases of awareness, training, implementation, and audit. This book has focused on regulation of provider-payer transactions, privacy, and security. One aspect of the provider-payer regulation is fraud control.

Fraud occurs when a claim is made that is not fair. The False Claims Act encourages citizens to "blow the whistle" on people or entities that defraud the government. Historically, insurance companies had little support legally for investigating or prosecuting fraud. Their easier approach was to raise rates if fraud ate into their profits. However, in the 1980s, the *National Healthcare Anti-Fraud Association* began to bring information from various insurers together and to focus on detecting and attacking fraud.

The government now uses semi-automated techniques to detect patterns of fraud. With the vast number of claims and with the many rules about how such claims should be made, computers are well suited to detect fraud. Much *software* exists both for generating claims that should avoid fraud and for detecting fraud in submitted claims.

E-Commerce and Transactions

A considerable portion of every healthcare dollar is spent on *provider-payer transactions*. HIPAA was passed in 1996 in part to reduce costs in healthcare by standardizing transactions between providers and payers. When the Congress realized that such standardization might also increase the accessibility of electronic health information to the wrong people, Congress added privacy and security requirements to HIPAA.

While not all aspects of a healthcare provider are touched by the provider-payer transactions, almost every healthcare entity is affected by this standardization. The standards apply to the envelope and format of the messages and to the codes used in the fields inside the messages. The major *codes* for diagnosis come from the "International Classification of Diseases" and the major codes for treatments come from "Current Procedure and Terminology."

Privacy and Security

The privacy component of HIPAA requires healthcare entities to treat *individually identifiable health information* with respect for privacy. Business associates cannot see the information without agreeing to certain contracts. Everyone in the healthcare entity should be careful to only use the information needed to do the job well.

The *Privacy Rule* gives patients new federal rights. Patients must be given copies of their medical records when the patients request it. The patient can request amendments to the medical record.

The *Security Rule* mandates common sense approaches to information security. Entities should have contingency plans, should ensure passwords are handled properly, should encrypt messages sent on the Internet, and so on.

Personnel and Vendors

People are the key to the success of any technology advance. The total number of people employed in the healthcare sector in the U.S. has grown from one million to eight million in the past hundred years. The patients and the front-line care providers, namely, the doctors, nurses, and allied health professionals, are the basis of the enterprise. The changes over the past one hundred years in the distribution of staff in the healthcare field are, however, particularly noteworthy. Originally, the system was served almost entirely by doctors working alone. Now over half of the workforce is allied health professionals. The next largest category is nurses, who number over three million in the U.S. Physicians number less than one million. This move to increasing reliance on diverse support staff makes sense in terms of the move to a cost-conscious, massive industry. The increasing reliance on support staff should also speak favorably to the likelihood of the industry increasing the use of computers because the support staff have proven more amenable to the use of information systems tools in their work.

Each large healthcare enterprise also has a staff of *information systems specialists*. The chief information officer is the senior members of this staff and is responsible for both vision and negotiating for resources with other components of the entity. The CIO's staff will both support users and engage in operations to continue the infrastructure activities of the entity.

Vendors of information systems play an important role in the health care industry. Hospital information systems would be difficult for the average hospital to build on its own. Some vendors are parts of massive information technology conglomerates with subsidiaries addressing the health sector. Other vendors focus exclusively on healthcare. In either case, a vendor with a large healthcare activity may offer a wide suite of systems to serve every part of the healthcare enterprise.

For diverse information systems problems, the healthcare entity may lack the staff with expertise to deal with the problems, and so the entity will hire consultants. *Consultants* assume roles not readily filled by anyone else, particularly when they have state-of-the-art technical knowledge and knowledge of best practices at comparable organizations. Consultants typically charge high prices, come from the environment in which they do consulting, and face the challenge of needing to continually find customers.

Knowledge and Diffusion

Knowledge-based systems can extend the value of information systems by adding intelligence to the processing of the information. For instance, a computer can look at a drug prescription, check a patient's record, check a knowledge base of adverse drug-drug interactions, and tell the care provider whether this new order is safe. Capturing the knowledge from people and encoding it into the computer is not easy. However, the greatest challenge is to get the knowledge-based systems to integrate with the workflow of the intended users.

Diffusion of technology has been studied in many disciplines. The basic conclusion is that the technology must fit easily into the workflow of the intended user and show immediate benefit. This is difficult to show with something like an integrated patient record system, whose gains may only be obvious after substantial effort to get information into the appropriate forms in the records. Analogies to agriculture are interesting. Pesticides can show immediate results, whereas genetic management of crops only reaps benefits over years. Automation of claims shows immediate results, whereas computerized patient records reap benefits after the entity's information systems are integrated.

A patient's or a society's health concerns go beyond a single hospital or city. *Countries* have healthcare systems that vary enormously from one to another. The European Union manifests some intriguing efforts to spread good practices across national boundaries.

Direction

The U.S. healthcare industry is highly fragmented (Cerner, 2000):

While science and medical technology continue to make significant progress in dealing with human disease and injury, the management and clinical processes of these complex delivery organizations have made little progress. ...This has resulted in an industry that is economically inefficient and produces significant variances in medical outcomes.

External forces have substantially directed administrative change in the health-care industry. Managed care organizations became intermediaries in the flow of funds. Other healthcare providers responded by consolidating and creating new, large delivery systems that were intended to realize economies of scale. For-profit business models were implemented in healthcare environments were they had not previously appeared. However, the attempts to create economies of scale and new profit models were largely *unsuccessful* in changing the economics of the American healthcare system.

All industries *evolve* in response to the marketplace, and the evolution of the healthcare information systems industry shows clear trends. In the early days (the 1960s), those systems focused on accounting—namely, generating bills and receiving payments. Later (the 1970s), clinical information systems began to appear but only in large hospitals and only in the clinical support areas, like laboratories. In those laboratories, the machines were being automated and the support staff accepted their changing roles relative to the machines. Also, the laboratories were cash cows for the hospitals.

During the 1980s, individual departments in large hospitals purchased their own systems tailored to their particular needs. This led to problems in connecting information systems within the larger entity. In the 1990s, the attention shifted to integrating systems across an entity. Clearly, *coordinating* across the enterprise requires agreement on a language for communicating among information systems. Such agreement can be achieved either when different vendors adhere to a common standard or when a healthcare entity purchases all its systems from one vendor that has integrated its products.

The first decade of the twenty-first century witnessed a focus on further levels of *connectivity* that exploited the Internet. Insurance companies, employers, providers, and patients are increasingly connected. Some patients can access their medical record at their healthcare providers' computer through the Internet. The extent to which patients will demand or take advantage of such opportunities remains to be seen.

Change is needed in healthcare information systems. The U.S. President's Commission said (*Quality First: Better Health Care for All Americans*, 1998):

Because of its decentralized nature, the health care industry arguably has a very complex business model consisting of a fragmented community of trading partners (i.e., hospitals, providers, group purchasers, pharmacies, clearinghouses, and others). Few other industries are decentralized to the same degree. ...The health care industry is so fundamentally decentralized and yet so critically in need of data-sharing that the use of common or cooperating information systems and databases becomes an operational imperative. ...Purchasers of health care services should insist that providers and plans be able to produce quantitative evidence of quality as a means of encouraging investment in information systems. ...The training of health care professionals should include the use of information technology in clinical settings.

That the Commission made specific recommendations on economics and on education is indicative of the importance of economics and education. *Economics and education* are the linchpins for the current healthcare system and thus are most in need of change in order that the system changes. While the problems of the healthcare industry could be reduced with the proper use of information systems, that use will only change after economics and education change.

While the vision and objectives of any given healthcare entity must be sensitive first to economics and education, they can ride the waves of change in information technology by following both healthcare trends and information systems trends. These *trends* call for increased support of the healthcare enterprise by information systems that will require enlightened participation of an increasingly large portion of those people who participate in the healthcare process.

This book has emphasized the information systems needs of the healthcare enterprise. However, the consumer trends that were described in an earlier chapter might become a dominating factor. The Web might allow for new socio-technical developments not previously anticipated. All of the developed countries have experienced powerful forces of demographic, cultural, and economic change that have shaped their healthcare systems. The industrial revolution and urbanization led to new health problems for the masses. The long-term result was the piecemeal development of state interventions into healthcare and the development of progressively more complex and specialized healthcare practices. This common heritage has led to patients demanding more and better care but society not satisfying these demands. One hope is that an enlightened citizenry through the advantages of global information systems might become better informed about health, more successfully treat itself, and turn the healthcare process into more of a *collaborative process* than it is now, thus leveraging the energy of the masses to help solve the health problems of the masses.

Questions

1. Which healthcare trends and information technology trends do you think are most significant for health information systems and why?
2. The vision calls for an integrated information system. One could imagine this achieved by having one vendor producing one masterful, comprehensive system or many vendors producing modules all of which communicated readily through standard interfaces with modules of all other vendors. Neither scenario

seems particularly likely. If you were to put your money on one approach or the other to win, which would it be and why?

References

Cerner. (2000). *1999 annual report*. Cerner Corporation. Retrieved October 2006, from www.cerner.com

Quality first: Better health care for all Americans. (1998). Washington, DC: President's Advisory Commission on Consumer Protection and Quality in the Health Care Industry.

About the Author

Roy Rada is a professor of information systems at the University of Maryland, Baltimore County. Previously, he was the Boeing distinguished professor of software engineering at Washington State University, the editor of *Index Medicus* at the National Library of Medicine, and professor of computer science at the University of Liverpool. Rada has worked as a consultant on computer-supported diagnosis in pathology and radiology, led a team developing medical informatics standards, developed online training material for doctors, and consulted with insurance companies and hospital networks about compliance with government regulations related to information systems. Rada's educational credentials include a PhD from the University of Illinois in computer science and a MD from Baylor College of Medicine. He has authored hundreds of scientific papers. His first journal article appeared in 1979 in the journal *Computers and Biomedical Research* and described a novel coding system for medical problem statements.

Index

Symbols

A

B

C

D

E

F

G

H

I

J

K

L

M

N

Q

R

S

T